INFANT, TODDLER, AND CHILD HEALTH

SOURCEBOOK

SECOND EDITION

Health Reference Series

INFANT, TODDLER, AND CHILD HEALTH SOURCEBOOK

SECOND EDITION

Basic Consumer Health Information on Infant, Toddler, and Child Health, including Newborn Care, Developmental Milestones, Birth Defects, Childhood Illnesses, and Safety Measures, Facts about Nutrition, Vaccination, Child Abuse, Early Intervention, and Injury Prevention, as well as Vital Insights into Promoting Health and Development from Infancy to Childhood

Along with Information about Home and Community Safety, a Glossary of Related Terms, and a Directory of Organizations for Additional Help and Information

OMNIGRAPHICS
An imprint of Infobase

Bibliographic Note

Because this page cannot legibly accommodate all the copyright notices, the Bibliographic Note portion of the Preface constitutes an extension of the copyright notice.

* * *

OMNIGRAPHICS
An imprint of Infobase
8 The Green
Suite #19225
Dover, DE 19901
www.infobase.com
James Chambers, *Editorial Director*

* * *

ISBN 978-0-7808-2136-1
E-ISBN 978-0-7808-2137-8

Library of Congress Cataloging-in-Publication Data

Names: Chambers, James, editor.

Title: Infant, toddler, and child health sourcebook / edited by James Chambers.

Description: Second edition. | Dover, DE: Omnigraphics, an imprint of Infobase, [2024] | Series: Health reference series | Preceded by: Infant, toddler and child health sourcebook / edited by Kevin Hayes. First edition. 2020. | Includes bibliographical references and index. | Summary: "Provides basic health information about the physical, mental, and developmental health of infants, toddlers, and children, including facts about the diseases and conditions that affect them and tips to bring them up in a healthy way. Includes an index, glossary of related terms, and other resources"-- Provided by publisher.

Identifiers: LCCN 2024010820 (print) | LCCN 2024010821 (ebook) | ISBN 9780780821361 (library binding) | ISBN 9780780821378 (eISBN)

Subjects: LCSH: Pediatrics--Popular works. | Child development--Popular works. | Children--Diseases--Popular works. | Children--Health and hygiene--Popular works.

Classification: LCC RJ61 .I623 2024 (print) | LCC RJ61 (ebook) | DDC 618.92--dc23/eng/20240404

LC record available at https://lccn.loc.gov/2024010820
LC ebook record available at https://lccn.loc.gov/2024010821

Printed in the United States

Table of Contents

Part 3. Birth Defects and Developmental Disabilities

Part 4. Childhood Illnesses and Conditions

Part 5. Healthy Infants and Toddlers (Ages 0–3)

Part 6. Healthy Children (Ages 4–11)

Part 7. Home and Community Safety

Part 8. Additional Help and Information

Preface

ABOUT THIS BOOK

The first years of life are a time of growth, discovery, and exploring potential. For parents and caregivers, navigating this period can be both exhilarating and overwhelming. From the newborn stage to the toddler years to childhood, each phase presents unique joys and challenges. While significant advancements have been made in prenatal, newborn, and child health care, ensuring optimal health for every child remains a critical challenge. In the United States, according to the Centers for Disease Control and Prevention (CDC), there were 3.66 million births in 2022, and the infant mortality rate (deaths within the first year of life) was approximately 5.6 deaths per 1,000 live births.

Infant, Toddler, and Child Health Sourcebook, Second Edition serves as a comprehensive resource, providing individuals with up-to-date information and practical guidance to navigate the complexities of caring for and nurturing young lives. Recognizing the importance of early intervention, this book explores developmental milestones and provides advice on addressing any concerns. It also addresses common childhood illnesses, birth defects, developmental disabilities, and the importance of nutrition and vaccination. Information on home and community safety, including childproofing, injury prevention, and mental health, is provided. Whether you are a new parent seeking insight or a seasoned caregiver looking for the latest information, this book offers a trusted and accessible resource to help you navigate the challenging and rewarding journey of raising healthy, happy children. The book concludes with a glossary of related terms and a resource list for further help and information.

HOW TO USE THIS BOOK

This book is divided into parts and chapters. Parts focus on broad areas of interest. Chapters are devoted to single topics within a part.

Part 1: Newborn Health Overview offers insights into the early stages of life, from assessing the vital signs of a newborn to understanding the Apgar score and key measurements. It includes crucial information on the importance of early breastfeeding initiation, caring for premature infants, common newborn and infant problems, and the dynamics of maternal, newborn, and child health.

Part 2: Child Development Milestones explores the essential milestones of child development, including speech and language development. It provides guidance for parents concerned about their child's development and emphasizes the importance of early intervention. The part also includes milestone checklists for infants, toddlers, and preschoolers, and addresses developmental milestones for puberty and adolescence.

Part 3: Birth Defects and Developmental Disabilities addresses various congenital issues such as neural tube defects, congenital heart defects, microcephaly, limb reduction defects, and cleft lip and palate. It also covers intellectual and developmental disabilities, including Down syndrome, cerebral palsy, autism spectrum disorder, sensory impairments, learning disorders, language and speech disorders, and Tourette syndrome.

Part 4: Childhood Illnesses and Conditions covers a range of common health issues in children, from respiratory illnesses and infections to growth-related issues and chronic conditions such as diabetes. It also addresses childhood mental health disorders, including attention deficit hyperactivity disorder (ADHD), obsessive-compulsive disorder (OCD), and posttraumatic stress disorder (PTSD). Additionally, it discusses pediatric injuries, antibiotic resistance, and childhood cancers.

Part 5: Healthy Infants and Toddlers (Ages 0–3) focuses on nurturing and caring for young children, including nutrition, vaccination, safe sleep practices, hygiene, oral health, childcare services, and physical activity during the preschool period. It provides guidelines on breastfeeding, weaning, and food safety, as well as information on the immunization schedule, cleaning and sanitizing infant feeding items, and dental care for baby teeth and gums.

Part 6: Healthy Children (Ages 4–11) talks about promoting health in older children, addressing diet and nutrition, hygiene, and managing food allergies and intolerances. It also focuses on positive parenting, the role of family structure, physical activity, and maintaining healthy habits.

Part 7: Home and Community Safety emphasizes the importance of creating safe environments for children. It covers topics such as preventing child abuse and neglect, safety measures against injuries, disaster preparedness, and internet safety. It also provides information about ensuring the safety of children with disabilities.

Part 8: Additional Help and Information includes a glossary of terms related to infant, toddler, and child health, along with a comprehensive resource list for further support and guidance.

BIBLIOGRAPHIC NOTE

This volume contains documents and excerpts from publications issued by the following U.S. government agencies: Agency for Healthcare Research and Quality (AHRQ); Centers for Disease Control and Prevention (CDC); Center for Parent Information and Resources (CPIR); ChildCare.gov; The Dru Sjodin National Sex Offender Public Website (NSOPW); Early Childhood Learning and Knowledge Center (ECLKC); *Eunice Kennedy Shriver* National Institute of Child Health and Human Development (NICHD); Federal Interagency Forum on Child and Family Statistics; Food and Nutrition Service (FNS); Foodsafety.gov; Health Resources and Services Administration (HRSA); MedlinePlus; National Cancer Institute (NCI); National Center for Injury Prevention and Control (NCIPC); National Center on Birth Defects and Developmental Disabilities (NCBDDD); National Heart, Lung, and Blood Institute (NHLBI); National Highway Traffic Safety Administration (NHTSA); National Institute of Arthritis and Musculoskeletal and Skin Diseases (NIAMS); National Institute on Deafness and Other Communication Disorders (NIDCD); National Institute of Dental and Craniofacial Research (NIDCR); National Institute of Diabetes and Digestive and Kidney Diseases (NIDDK); National Institute of Neurological Disorders and Stroke (NINDS); National Institutes of Health (NIH); National Youth Violence Prevention Resource Center; *NIH News in Health*; Office of Juvenile Justice and Delinquency Prevention (OJJDP); Office of Population Affairs (OPA); Office on Women's Health (OWH); StopBullying.gov; Substance Abuse and Mental Health Services Administration (SAMHSA); U.S. Consumer Product Safety Commission (CPSC); U.S. Department of Health and Human Services (HHS); U.S. Department of Homeland Security (DHS); U.S. Fire Administration (FA); and U.S. Food and Drug Administration (FDA).

It also contains original material produced by Infobase.

ABOUT THE *HEALTH REFERENCE SERIES*

The *Health Reference Series* is designed to provide basic medical information for patients, families, caregivers, and the general public. Each volume provides comprehensive coverage on a particular topic. This is especially important for people who may be dealing with a newly diagnosed disease or a chronic disorder in themselves or in a family member. People looking for preventive guidance, information about disease warning signs, medical statistics, and risk factors for health problems will also find answers to their questions in the *Health Reference Series*. The *Series*, however, is not intended to serve as a tool for diagnosing illness, in prescribing treatments, or as a substitute for the physician-patient relationship. All people concerned about medical symptoms or the possibility of disease are encouraged to seek professional care from an appropriate health-care provider.

A NOTE ABOUT SPELLING AND STYLE

Health Reference Series editors use *Stedman's Medical Dictionary* as an authority for questions related to the spelling of medical terms and *The Chicago Manual of Style* for questions related to grammatical structures, punctuation, and other editorial concerns. Consistent adherence is not always possible, however, because the individual volumes within the *Series* include many documents from a wide variety of different producers, and the editor's primary goal is to present material from each source as accurately as is possible. This sometimes means that information in different chapters or sections may follow other guidelines and alternate spelling authorities. For example, occasionally a copyright holder may require that eponymous terms be shown in possessive forms (Crohn's disease vs. Crohn disease) or that British spelling norms be retained (leukaemia vs. leukemia).

HEALTH REFERENCE SERIES UPDATE POLICY

The inaugural book in the *Health Reference Series* was the first edition of *Cancer Sourcebook* published in 1989. Since then, the *Series* has been enthusiastically received by librarians and in the medical community. In order to maintain the standard of providing high-quality health information for the layperson, the editorial staff felt it was necessary to implement a policy of updating volumes when warranted.

Medical researchers have been making tremendous strides, and it is the purpose of the *Health Reference Series* to stay current with the most recent advances. Each decision to update a volume is made on an individual basis. Some of the considerations include how much new information is available and the feedback we receive from people who use the books. If there is a topic you would like to see added to the update list, or an area of medical concern you feel has not been adequately addressed, please write to: custserv@infobaselearning.com.

Part 1 | **Newborn Health Overview**

Chapter 1 | Your Baby's First Hours of Life

After months of waiting, finally, your new baby has arrived! Mothers-to-be often spend so much time in anticipation of labor that they might not think about or even know what to expect during the first hours after delivery.

WHAT NEWBORNS LOOK LIKE

You might be surprised by how your newborn looks at birth. If you had a vaginal delivery, your baby entered this world through a narrow and bony passage. It is not uncommon for newborns to be born bluish, bruised, and with a misshapen head. An ear might be folded over. Your baby may have a complete head of hair or be bald. Your baby will also have a thick, pasty, whitish coating, which protected the skin in the womb. This will wash away during the first bath.

Once your baby is placed into your arms, your gaze will go right to their eyes. Most newborns open their eyes soon after birth. Their eyes will be brown or bluish-gray at first. Looking over your baby, you might notice that the face is a little puffy. You might notice small white bumps inside your baby's mouth or on his or her tongue. Your baby might be very wrinkly. Some babies, especially those born early, are covered in soft, fine hair, which will come off in a couple of weeks. Your baby's skin might have various colored marks, blotches, or rashes, and fingernails could be long. You might also notice that your baby's breasts and penis or vulva are a bit swollen.

Your baby's appearance will change from day to day, and many of the early marks of childbirth will go away with time. If you have any concerns about something you see, talk to your doctor. After a few weeks, your newborn will look more and more like the baby you pictured in your dreams.

BONDING WITH YOUR BABY

Spending time with your baby in those first hours of life is very special. Although you might be tired, your newborn could be quite alert after birth. Cuddle your baby skin-to-skin. Let your baby get to know your voice and study your face. Your baby can see up to about 2 feet away. You might notice that your baby throws his or her arms out if someone turns on a light or makes a sudden noise. This is called the "startle response." Babies are also born with grasp and sucking reflexes. Put your finger in your baby's palm and watch how he or she knows to squeeze it. Feed your baby when he or she shows signs of hunger.

MEDICAL CARE FOR YOUR NEWBORN

Right after birth, babies need many important tests and procedures to ensure their health. Some of these are even required by law. But as long as the baby is healthy, everything but the Apgar test (appearance, pulse, grimace, activity, and respiration) can wait for at least an hour. Delaying further medical care will preserve the precious first moments of life for you, your partner, and the baby. A baby who has not been poked and prodded may be more willing to nurse and cuddle. Therefore, before delivery, talk to your doctor or midwife about delaying shots, medicine, and tests. At the same time, please do not assume "everything is being taken care of." As a parent, it is your job to make sure your newborn gets all the necessary and appropriate vaccines and tests in a timely manner. The following tests and procedures are recommended or required in most hospitals in the United States.

Apgar Evaluation

The Apgar test is a quick way for doctors to figure out if the baby is healthy or needs extra medical care. Apgar tests are usually done twice: one minute after birth and again five minutes after birth.

Doctors and nurses measure five signs of the baby's condition. These are:

- heart rate
- breathing
- activity and muscle tone
- reflexes
- skin color

Apgar scores range from 0 to 10. A baby who scores seven or more is considered very healthy. But a lower score does not always mean there is something wrong. Perfectly healthy babies often have low Apgar scores in the first minute of life. In more than 98 percent of cases, the Apgar score reaches seven after five minutes of life. When it does not, the baby needs medical care and close monitoring.

Eye Care

Your baby may receive eye drops or ointment to prevent eye infections they can get during delivery. Sexually transmitted infections (STIs), including gonorrhea and chlamydia, are the main cause of newborn eye infections. These infections can cause blindness if not treated. Medicines used can sting and/or blur the baby's vision. Therefore, you may want to postpone this treatment for a little while.

Some parents question whether this treatment is really necessary. Many women at low risk for STIs do not want their newborns to receive eye medicine. But there is no evidence to suggest that this medicine harms the baby. It is important to note that even pregnant women who test negative for STIs may get an infection by the time of delivery. Plus, most women with gonorrhea and/or chlamydia do not know it because they have no symptoms.

Vitamin K Shot

The American Academy of Pediatrics (AAP) recommends that all newborns receive a shot of vitamin K in the upper leg. Newborns usually have low levels of vitamin K in their bodies. This vitamin is needed for the blood to clot. Low levels of vitamin K can cause a rare but serious bleeding problem. Research shows that vitamin K shots prevent dangerous bleeding in newborns. Newborns probably feel pain when the shot is given. But afterward, babies do not seem to have any discomfort. Since it may be uncomfortable for the baby, you may want to postpone this shot for a little while.

Newborn Metabolic Screening

Doctors or nurses prick your baby's heel to take a tiny sample of blood. They use this blood to test for many diseases. All babies should be tested because a few babies may look healthy but have a rare health problem. A blood test is the only way to find out about these problems. If found right away, serious problems such as developmental disabilities, organ damage, blindness, and even death might be prevented. All 50 states and U.S. territories screen newborns for phenylketonuria (PKU), hypothyroidism, galactosemia, and sickle cell disease (SCD). But many states routinely test for up to 30 different diseases. The March of Dimes recommends that all newborns be tested for at least 29 diseases. You can find out what tests are offered in your state by contacting your state's health department or newborn screening program. Or, you can contact the National Newborn Screening and Genetics Resource Center (NNSGRC).

Hearing Test

Most babies have a hearing screening soon after birth, usually before they leave the hospital. Tiny earphones or microphones are used to see how the baby reacts to sounds. All newborns need a hearing screening because hearing defects are not uncommon, and hearing loss can be hard to detect in babies and young children. When problems are found early, children can get the services they need at an early age. This might prevent delays in speech, language, and thinking. Ask your hospital or your baby's doctor about newborn hearing screening.

Hepatitis B Vaccine

All newborns should get a vaccine to protect against the hepatitis B virus (HBV) before leaving the hospital. Sadly, one in five babies at risk of HBV infection leaves the hospital without receiving the vaccine and treatment shown to protect newborns, even if exposed to HBV at birth. HBV can cause a lifelong infection, serious liver damage, and even death. The hepatitis B (HepB) vaccine is a series of three different shots. The AAP and the Centers for Disease Control Prevention (CDC) recommend that all newborns get the first HepB shot before leaving the hospital. If the mother has HBV, her baby should also get a hepatitis B immunoglobulin (HBIG) shot within 12 hours of birth. The second HepB shot should be given one to two months after birth. The third HepB shot should be given no earlier than 24 weeks of age but before 18 months of age.

Complete Checkup

Soon after delivery, most doctors or nurses also:

- measure the newborn's weight, length, and head
- take the baby's temperature
- measure the baby's breathing and heart rate
- give the baby a bath and clean the umbilical cord stump[1]

[1] Office on Women's Health (OWH), "Your Baby's First Hours of Life," U.S. Department of Health and Human Services (HHS), February 22, 2021. Available online. URL: www.womenshealth.gov/pregnancy/childbirth-and-beyond/your-babys-first-hours-life. Accessed March 4, 2024.

Chapter 2 | **Assessing Newborn Health**

Chapter Contents

Section 2.1 | **Key Measurements for Newborns**

When a child is born, health-care professionals perform several vital measurements to assess the newborn's health status and development. These include their birth weight, length, head circumference, gestational age, and Apgar score. These measurements are crucial in monitoring the newborn's growth and development in the early stages of life, so it is important for parents and caregivers to understand them.

WEIGHT

The weight of a newborn, one of the first measurements recorded after birth, is an essential indicator of the baby's health. Birth weight can vary significantly and is influenced by factors such as genetics, maternal nutrition, and gestational age. A healthy newborn typically weighs between 5.5 and 8.8 pounds. Low birth weight, defined as less than 5.5 pounds, may indicate a premature birth or intrauterine growth restriction (IUGR). In comparison, a high birth weight, defined as exceeding 8.8 pounds, can sometimes signal gestational diabetes or other maternal health conditions. Monitoring the baby's weight gain in the weeks and months following birth is crucial for assessing growth and nutritional status. Health-care providers typically recommend weight checks during regular visits and checkups. Adequate weight gain is a positive sign of healthy growth and development, while poor weight gain may warrant further evaluation and intervention to address any underlying issues.

LENGTH

Another key measurement taken at birth is the length of the newborn, also known as "crown-heel length." The average newborn typically measures 18–22 inches long, although variations in length are normal. Length measurement provides valuable information about the baby's overall growth and development, indicating future height potential. Although genetics significantly influences height, monitoring growth over time can help identify potential abnormalities or developmental issues that may require intervention.

HEAD CIRCUMFERENCE

Measuring the circumference of the baby's head helps assess brain growth and development. The average head circumference for a newborn ranges from 13 to 14 inches, with variations depending on factors such as gestational age and birth weight. Head circumference increases rapidly during the first few months as the brain grows and develops. Regular head circumference measurements are needed to identify abnormalities that may require further evaluation. Rapid or slowed growth in head circumference may indicate underlying conditions such as hydrocephalus (excessive fluid in the brain) or microcephaly (abnormally small head size). Early detection of these conditions is essential for timely intervention and to manage the baby's long-term outcomes. Health-care providers closely monitor head circumference during routine visits to ensure the baby's brain development is progressing normally.

GESTATIONAL AGE

The baby's gestational age at birth is used to assess developmental milestones and potential health risks. Gestational age refers to the length of time the baby has spent in the womb. It is typically measured in weeks from the first day of the mother's last menstrual period (LMP) to the date of birth. In some cases, ultrasound measurements taken during pregnancy may determine gestational age more accurately. Preterm babies (between 37 weeks, 0 days and 38 weeks, 6 days) and post-term babies (after 42 weeks) may have different needs and potential health concerns compared to full-term babies (between 39 weeks, 0 days and 40 weeks, 6 days). Preterm birth can increase the risk of complications such as respiratory distress syndrome (RDS), while post-term birth may be associated with meconium aspiration (when the baby inhales their first feces into the lungs) or macrosomia (excessive birth weight). Health-care providers will adjust care and monitoring based on the baby's gestational age.

APGAR SCORE

Health-care providers utilize the Apgar score to quickly assess a newborn's overall health and well-being at one minute and five minutes after birth. The Apgar score evaluates five key indicators, namely the appearance, pulse, grimace, activity, and respiration. Apgar scores provide valuable information about the baby's adaptation to life outside the womb and can help health-care providers identify any immediate concerns that require intervention. While most babies receive an overall score of seven or above, lower scores may indicate the need for additional support or medical attention. Apgar scores are used in conjunction with other assessments to provide immediate care. Monitoring key measurements for newborns is essential for assessing their health, growth, and development in the early stages of life. From birth weight to Apgar scores, each measurement provides valuable insights into the baby's well-being and helps guide health-care decisions.

References

"Assessments for Newborn Babies," Stanford Medicine Children's Health, November 17, 2016. Available online. URL: www.stanfordchildrens.org/en/topic/default?id=assessments-for-newborn-babies-90-P02336. Accessed April 3, 2024.

Belleza, Marianne. "The Newborn and Normal Developmental Milestones," NursesLabs, July 22, 2023. Available online. URL: https://nurseslabs.com/the-newborn. Accessed April 3, 2024.

Jamshed, Saira, et al. "Frequency of Normal Birth Length and Its Determinants: A Cross-Sectional Study in Newborns," *Cereus*, 12, no. 9 (2020): e10556. https://doi.org/10.7759/cureus.10556.

Knisley, Kimberly. "How Early Can You Safely Give Birth?" Healthline, February 28, 2020. Available online. URL: www.healthline.com/health/pregnancy/how-many-weeks-is-it-safe-to-give-birth. Accessed April 3, 2024.

"Newborn Measurements," Stanford Medicine, July 31, 2018. Available online. URL: www.stanfordchildrens.org/en/

topic/default?id=newborn-measurements-90-P02673. Accessed April 3, 2024.
"Newborn Measurements," UC San Diego Health, March 1, 2022. Available online. URL: https://myhealth.ucsd.edu/Library/DiseasesConditions/Pediatric/NormalNewborn/90,P02673. Accessed April 3, 2024.

Section 2.2 | **Understanding the Apgar Score**

The Apgar is a noninvasive test for newborns at one minute and five minutes after birth. It was developed by Dr. Virginia Apgar in 1952 to assess newborns experiencing breathing difficulties and other issues upon delivery. The test helps doctors and nurses determine the kind of medical attention or emergency action a newborn may need shortly after birth based on five categories, each assigned a score between zero and two. The nurse or midwife scores the newborn based on each category at one minute to assess their endurance during the birthing process and again at five minutes to determine their overall health. The scoring system measures the following:

- **Appearance**. The nurse assesses the baby's blood oxygenation through skin color. A healthy pink color indicates good oxygen levels, scoring two points; a pink body but blue extremities indicate poor oxygen circulation to the hands and feet, scoring one point; bluish or pale tones might suggest breathing difficulties, scoring zero points. Observing a baby's lip and tongue color is more precise in determining their health. Color assessment can be subjective by observer and is not always an effective measure for dark-skinned babies.
- **Pulse**. A healthy heart rate for a newborn typically ranges between 100 and 160 beats per minute (bpm).

Slower or faster rates warrant further evaluation. The scoring involves two points for heart rates above 100 bpm, one point for rates below 100 bpm, and zero points for no pulse.

- **Grimace**. The nurse checks the baby's involuntary response to mild irritation by touching the soles of their feet. A strong response to stimulation such as crying, sneezing, or coughing indicates good muscle tone and nervous system function, scoring two points, while a grimace or weak cry scores one, and no response scores zero.
- **Activity**. The nurse evaluates the baby's muscle tone. Active body movements score two points, flexing of arms and legs alone scores one point, and no movement scores zero points.
- **Respiration**. The nurse assesses the baby's breathing rate and effort. A healthy newborn typically breathes 30–60 times per minute with minimal effort. The scoring involves two points for strong and normal breathing, one for irregular or slow breathing, and zero for no breathing. An overall score of 7–10 indicates that the baby is in good health, 4–6 is considered moderately abnormal and suggests that some resuscitation measures may be required, and a score of 4 or under suggests that the newborn needs immediate medical attention.

A low score at one minute often becomes normal at the five-minute mark. Newborns with low blood oxygen levels or a low heart rate may score between four and six at the one-minute mark. If the newborn does not breathe independently, oxygen is given to help stabilize the oxygen supply to the lungs. Medications are administered through the umbilical cord to normalize the newborn's heartbeat. If the score remains below seven points, even after 5 minutes, the test is repeated at 5-minute intervals for at least 20 minutes.

FACTORS INFLUENCING LOW APGAR SCORES

Newborns may score low on the Apgar test due to these additional reasons:

- difficult labor experience: prolonged labor, traumatic birth, or other complications
- emergency cesarean birth
- premature birth
- maternal medical condition
- umbilical cord issues

LIMITATIONS OF APGAR SCORES

The Apgar score is limited to assessing a newborn's physiological condition in the early minutes of their life. The score alone is not recommended to predict adverse health issues in newborns. For instance, a premature newborn with no indication of asphyxia may score low on the Apgar test due to immaturity.

The newborn's score can also be influenced by the mother's sedation during labor or a cesarean section, the newborn's congenital malformations, gestational age, and other factors. Assessing certain categories, such as skin color, can also be subjective. In recent years, there have been some reconsiderations to modify the terms used in the scoring system. For instance, characterizing healthy skin as "pink" may not be accurate for assessing newborns with darker skin.

References

"The Apgar Score," The American College of Obstetricians and Gynecologists, October 15, 2015. Available online. URL: www.acog.org/clinical/clinical-guidance/committee-opinion/articles/2015/10/the-apgar-score. Accessed March 28, 2024.

Dalili, Hosein, et al. "Comparison of the Combined versus Conventional Apgar Scores in Predicting Adverse Neonatal Outcomes," *PLoS ONE*, 11, no. 2 (2016). https://doi.org/10.1371/journal.pone.0149464.

Nall, Rachel. "Apgar Score: What You Should Know," Healthline, October 18, 2023. Available online. URL: www.healthline.com/health/apgar-score#Limitations-of-Apgar-score. Accessed March 28, 2024.
Repine, Kelsey; and Chatterjee, Debnath. "Apgar Score," OpenAnesthesia, December 13, 2022. Available online. URL: www.openanesthesia.org/keywords/apgar-score. Accessed March 28, 2024.
Schwartz, Charles I. "Apgar Score," Medline Plus, October 22, 2022. Available online. URL: https://medlineplus.gov/ency/article/003402.htm. Accessed March 28, 2024.

Chapter 3 | **Early Initiation of Breastfeeding**

BREASTFEEDING

Breast milk is a great source of nutrition for your baby. The *U.S. Dietary Guidelines for Americans* recommend that infants be exclusively breastfed for about the first six months and then continuing breastfeeding while introducing appropriate complementary foods until your child is 12 months old or older. The American Academy of Pediatrics (AAP) and the World Health Organization (WHO) also recommend exclusive breastfeeding for the first six months, with continued breastfeeding and appropriate complementary foods for up to two years or longer.

Vitamins and Minerals

Breastfed babies need additional vitamin D and may need additional iron. Although breast milk is an excellent source of the nutrition your baby needs, he or she will need to get extra vitamin D (beginning at birth) and possibly iron from supplements.

BENEFITS OF BREASTFEEDING

Breastfeeding is good for both you and your baby. Breast milk is the best source of nutrition for most babies. As your baby grows, your breast milk will change to meet his or her nutritional needs. Breastfeeding can also help protect you and your baby against some short- and long-term illnesses and diseases.

Benefits to the Baby

Babies who are breastfed have a lower risk of:

- asthma
- obesity
- type 1 diabetes
- severe lower respiratory disease
- acute otitis media (AOM; ear infections)
- sudden infant death syndrome (SIDS)
- gastrointestinal infections (diarrhea/vomiting)

YOUR FIRST BREAST MILK OR COLOSTRUM

At birth, your breasts will produce a thick, yellowish substance called "colostrum." Colostrum is packed with nutrients and other important substances that help your baby build his or her immune system. There will not be a lot of this liquid at first, but the amount will gradually increase over the first couple of days. Most babies will get all the nutrition they need through colostrum during the first few days of life. As you begin breastfeeding, your baby's sucking will tell your body to start making milk. For most mothers, this thinner, whiter form of milk comes in about three days after birth, but may take longer for first-time moms. You may notice your breasts feeling full, hard, and warm as this happens. Your baby may want to breastfeed more frequently around this time. If you are concerned about your milk coming in, talk to a lactation consultant or your doctor or nurse.

AS YOUR BABY GETS OLDER

Teething/Biting

You can continue to breastfeed once your baby starts to get teeth. Babies use their tongues, not their teeth, to breastfeed. If your baby is latched well and sucking, you should not feel the teeth while your baby is feeding. Once in a while, babies might bite the nipple or breast, especially when they are teething. Talk to a lactation consultant for tips on how to teach your baby not to bite.

Refusing to Breastfeed

Sometimes babies will suddenly stop wanting to breastfeed. Many times it is hard to know why this happens. Refusing to breastfeed is usually temporary, and your baby will start breastfeeding again within a few days. Some reasons your baby may refuse breastfeeding include teething, illness, stress, a change in environment, such as a new childcare situation, or a major change in routine. This usually does not mean your baby is ready to wean. Take the following steps to help your baby return to breastfeeding:

- Keep offering your baby the breast or breast milk from a bottle if bottle feeding.
- Spend extra time cuddling and holding your baby.
- Offer the breast in quiet spaces and when your baby is sleepy or relaxed.
- Pump or express milk frequently to keep your breast milk supply up until your baby starts breastfeeding again.

Distracted Breastfeeding

Your baby is starting to notice all the things going on around him or her. This can mean that your baby might get distracted while breastfeeding. Help your baby focus by turning off the TV, dimming the lights, or feeding in a quiet place.

Weaning

Although breastfeeding is recommended until your baby is at least 12 months old, weaning may happen before then.

ARE YOU BREASTFEEDING CORRECTLY?

Breastfeeding is a learning process. Each baby and mother's experience with breastfeeding is different. It is important that your baby has a good latch. This helps your baby get enough breast milk. The following are signs of a good or bad latch.

Signs of a Good Latch

- Your baby's mouth is open wide over the areola (the darker area around your nipple), with lips turned out.
- Your baby's chin is resting against the breast, baby's chest and stomach are against your body, and baby's head is straight and not turned to the side.
- You can see and hear your baby swallowing while breastfeeding.
- Your baby is swallowing regularly.

Signs of a Bad Latch

- Your baby is only suckling on the nipple.
- Your baby's lips are curled inward.
- Breastfeeding hurts.
- Your nipples are cracked or bleeding.
- Your nipples look flat or misshapen after breastfeeding.
- Your baby keeps coming off the breast while breastfeeding.

How Do You Build a Full Milk Supply?

- Make sure your baby has a good latch.
- Breastfeed often in the first few weeks. Your baby may want to eat as often as every one to three hours, including during the night.
- If you are not breastfeeding at the breast, express or pump your breast milk as often as your baby normally eats.
- Breastfeeding, or expressing or pumping breast milk, sends a signal to your breasts to keep making milk.

HOW MUCH AND HOW OFTEN TO BREASTFEED

Every baby is different. How much and how often your baby feeds will depend on your baby's needs. Here are a few things to expect about breastfeeding during the baby's first days, weeks, and months of life.

First Days

- **Your newborn baby's belly is tiny**. He or she does not need a lot of milk with each feeding to be full.
- **Your baby may want to eat as often as every one to three hours**. Frequent feeding helps increase your milk supply and gives your baby practice at sucking and swallowing.
- **Hear your baby**. You may be able to hear your baby sucking and swallowing the breast milk.
- **Most babies who are getting breast milk should not be fed infant formula in the first few days**. If you are concerned about meeting your baby's needs, talk to a lactation consultant, or your baby's nurse or doctor, right away. They can help you address any breastfeeding problems and determine the best way to meet your baby's needs.

First Weeks and Months

- **As babies grow, their bellies also grow**. Your baby will gradually be able to drink more breast milk at each feeding.
- **Over the first few weeks and months, the time between feedings will start to get longer**. On average, most exclusively babies will feed about every two to four hours. Some babies may feed as often as every hour at times, often called "cluster feeding." Or, they may have a longer sleep interval of four to five hours.
- **How often your baby feeds might change depending on the time of day**. Some feeding sessions may be long, and others, short. Babies will generally take what they need at each feeding and stop eating when they are full. They should seem content and drowsy after feeding when they have had enough milk.
- **Breastfeeding frequency**. Your baby will breastfeed about 8–12 times in 24 hours.

6–12 Months

- How long and how often babies breastfeed will change as they grow and start eating more solid foods.
- Continue to follow your baby's cues and breastfeed when you notice signs of hunger. This is sometimes called "breastfeeding on demand."
- If your baby seems less interested in breastfeeding after you introduce solid foods, try breastfeeding before you offer other foods.
- Your breast milk is the most important source of nutrition, even after you start feeding your baby solid foods.

12–24 Months

- The number of times a day a toddler breastfeeds varies. Some want to breastfeed only before bed or in the morning. Others continue to drink breast milk as a bigger portion of their daily diet. Continue to follow your child's cues to decide when he or she is hungry and wants to breastfeed.

PUMPING BREAST MILK

There are many reasons you might want to pump, hand express breast milk, or feed your baby pumped breast milk. Having expressed breast milk can allow your baby to drink your breast milk from a bottle.

When to Start Pumping

If you are planning to return to work or school or will be away from your baby for other reasons, you may want to start pumping a few weeks beforehand. This will give you the chance to practice pumping and will give your baby time to get used to feeding from a bottle.

How Often to Pump

When away from your baby or if you exclusively pump your milk, try to pump as often as your baby is drinking breast milk. This will help remind your body to keep making the amount of milk your baby needs.

How Much to Pump

Pumping as often as your baby normally drinks breast milk should help your body make about the amount of milk your baby needs. This amount may differ from baby to baby and can change as babies grow. If you find that you are not able to pump as much milk as your baby wants to eat while you are away, you may want to consider adding another pumping session to increase your milk supply.

How to Keep Your Pump Clean

Keeping the parts of your pump clean is very important. For information on how to keep your pump parts clean before and after use, visit How to Keep Your Breast Pump Kit Clean: The Essentials (www.cdc.gov/hygiene/childcare/breast-pump.html).

How to Make Pumping Work for You

There are many different types of breast pumps on the market and factors to consider when choosing the best pump for your situation. Talk with a lactation support provider for tips on how to help make pumping work for you.[1]

ARE THERE ANY SPECIAL CONDITIONS OR SITUATIONS IN WHICH YOU SHOULD NOT BREASTFEED?

In special cases, women may be advised not to breastfeed. These instances include when a woman is taking certain medications or drugs, when she has been diagnosed with a specific illness, or when other specific conditions apply.

[1] "Breastfeeding," Centers for Disease Control and Prevention (CDC), March 7, 2023. Available online. URL: www.cdc.gov/nutrition/InfantandToddlerNutrition/breastfeeding/index.html. Accessed March 5, 2024.

Medications/Other Drugs and Breastfeeding

Certain medications are known to be dangerous to infants and can be passed to your infant in your breast milk. Women taking the following medicines should speak with their health-care providers before considering breastfeeding:

- antiretroviral medications (for human immunodeficiency virus (HIV) and acquired immunodeficiency syndrome (AIDS) treatment)
- birth-control medications containing estrogen, until breastfeeding has been well established
- cancer chemotherapy agents
- illegal drugs
- certain medications prescribed to treat migraines, such as ergot alkaloids
- mood stabilizers, such as lithium and lamotrigine
- sleep-aid medicines

In addition, women who are undergoing radiation therapy should not breastfeed, although some therapies may require only a brief interruption of breastfeeding. The abovementioned list of medications and other drugs is only a guideline. Before breastfeeding, you should speak with your health-care provider about all medications that you are taking. These include prescribed medications, over-the-counter (OTC) medicines, vitamins, and herbal therapies. Medications that are safe during pregnancy may also be safe for you to continue while you are breastfeeding, although you should check with your health-care provider to make sure they are safe before you breastfeed. Contact your infant's health-care provider if you see any signs of a reaction to your breast milk in your infant, such as diarrhea, excessive crying, or sleepiness.

Health Conditions and Breastfeeding

Women with certain illnesses and infections may be advised not to breastfeed because of the danger of passing the illness or infection to the breastfed infant. If you have any of the following conditions, breastfeeding your infant is not advised:

- infection with HIV
- infection with human T-cell lymphotropic virus (HTLV) type I or type II
- untreated, active tuberculosis

If you are sick with the flu, including the H1N1 flu (also called the "swine flu"), you should not stop feeding your infant expressed milk. You should avoid being near your infant, however, so that you do not infect him or her. To avoid infecting your infant, someone who is not sick should give your infant your expressed milk.

If you have Zika virus or live in areas where Zika virus is found, the Centers for Disease Control and Prevention (CDC) recommends you continue to breastfeed your infant. Although Zika virus has been detected in breast milk, there are no reports of transmission of the virus through breastfeeding, and the benefits of breastfeeding are thought to outweigh the risks. If possible, breast milk will be collected from the mothers.

Domestic and International Guidelines on HIV/AIDS and Breastfeeding

In the United States, the AAP and the CDC recommend against breastfeeding if you are HIV positive; the same advice applies in other developed countries. Without any specific interventions to reduce transmission, infants breastfed by HIV-positive mothers have an increased chance of acquiring HIV through the breast milk. This rate increases if infants are breastfed longer and for mothers with newly acquired HIV.

Only HIV-positive mothers living in developing countries should consider breastfeeding their babies, especially if a safe and reliable source of infant formula is unavailable. This is because breast milk may protect against malnutrition and diarrhea, which are major causes of infant mortality in some areas of the developing world. If an HIV-positive woman decides to breastfeed her baby, research indicates that the risk of transmitting HIV to her baby is reduced if she exclusively breastfeeds (does not use a combination of formula and breast milk) and if she and her infant take antiretroviral drugs.

Other Considerations for Breastfeeding

In some additional situations, or if women or infants have certain health conditions, women may be advised not to breastfeed or may have difficulty breastfeeding.

- **Women with certain chronic illnesses may be advised not to breastfeed or will be advised to take steps to ensure their own health while breastfeeding.** For example, women who have diabetes should monitor their blood sugar levels regularly, may need to reduce their insulin, and may need a snack containing carbohydrates before or during breastfeeding. Also, women who are underweight, including those with thyroid conditions or certain bowel diseases, may need to increase their calories to maintain their own health during breastfeeding.
- **Breastfeeding challenges.** Women who have had breast surgery in the past may face some difficulties with breastfeeding.
- **Breastfeeding caution for substance use.** Women who actively use drugs or do not control their alcohol intake, or who have a history of these situations, also may be advised not to breastfeed.
- **Infants who have galactosemia—a rare metabolic disorder in which the body cannot digest the sugar galactose—should not be breastfed.** Galactosemia is detected by newborn screening (NBS), allowing proper treatment and diet to begin immediately. If not detected, the galactose builds up and becomes toxic for the infant, leading to liver problems, intellectual and developmental disabilities, and shock.[2]

[2] "Are There Any Special Conditions or Situations in Which I Should Not Breastfeed?" *Eunice Kennedy Shriver* National Institute of Child Health and Human Development (NICHD), January 31, 2017. Available online. URL: www.nichd.nih.gov/health/topics/breastfeeding/conditioninfo/special-conditions. Accessed March 5, 2024.

Chapter 4 | **Premature Infant Care**

Chapter Contents

Section 4.1 | **Understanding Preterm Births**

In general, a normal human pregnancy is about 40 weeks long (9.2 months). Health–care providers now define "full-term" birth as birth that occurs between 39 and 40 weeks and six days of pregnancy. Infants born during this time are considered full-term infants. Infants born in the 37th and 38th weeks of pregnancy—previously called term but now referred to as "early term"—face more health risks than do those born at 39 or 40 weeks. Deliveries before 37 weeks of pregnancy are considered "preterm" or "premature":

- **Preterm or premature labor**. Labor that begins before 37 weeks of pregnancy.
- **Preterm or premature birth**. A birth that occurs before 37 weeks of pregnancy.
- **Preterm or premature infant**. An infant born before 37 weeks in the womb. (These infants are commonly called "preemies" as a reference to being born prematurely.)

"Late preterm" refers to 34 through 36 weeks of pregnancy. Infants born during this time are considered late-preterm infants, but they face many of the same health challenges as preterm infants. More than 70 percent of preterm infants are born during the late-preterm time frame. Preterm birth is the most common cause of infant death and is the leading cause of long-term disability in children. Many organs, including the brain, lungs, and liver, are still developing in the final weeks of pregnancy. The earlier the delivery, the higher the risk of serious disability or death.

Infants born prematurely are at risk for cerebral palsy (CP; a group of nervous system disorders that affect control of movement and posture and limit activity), developmental delays, and vision and hearing problems. Late-preterm infants typically have better health outcomes than those born earlier, but they are still three times more likely to die in the first year of life than full-term infants. Preterm births can also take a heavy emotional and economic toll on families.

WHAT CAUSES PRETERM BIRTH?

The causes of premature birth are numerous, complex, and only partly understood. Medical, psychosocial, and biological factors may all play a role in preterm birth. There are three main situations in which premature birth may occur:

- **Spontaneous preterm birth.** This term refers to unintentional, unplanned delivery before the 37th week of pregnancy. This type of preterm birth can result from a number of causes, such as infection or inflammation, although the cause of spontaneous preterm birth and delivery is usually not known. A history of delivering preterm is one of the strongest predictors for subsequent preterm births.
- **Medically indicated preterm birth.** If a serious medical condition—such as preeclampsia—exists, the health-care provider might recommend a preterm delivery. In these cases, health-care providers often take steps to keep the baby in the womb as long as possible to allow for additional growth and development while also monitoring the mother and fetus for health issues. Providers also use additional interventions, such as steroids, to help improve outcomes for the baby.
- **Nonmedically indicated (elective) preterm delivery.** Some late-preterm births result from inducing labor or having a cesarean delivery even though there is not a medical reason to do so, even though this practice is not recommended. Research indicates that even babies born at 37 or 38 weeks of pregnancy are at higher risk for poor health outcomes than babies born at 39 weeks of pregnancy or later. Therefore, unless there are medical problems, health-care providers should wait until at least 39 weeks of pregnancy to induce labor or perform a cesarean delivery to prevent possible health problems.

The National Child and Maternal Health Education Program (NCMHEP), led by the *Eunice Kennedy Shriver* National Institute of Child Health and Human Development (NICHD) in collaboration with 33 other agencies, organizations, and groups focused on maternal and child health, offers videos and other information about why it is best to wait until at least 39 weeks of pregnancy to deliver unless there is a medical reason.

WHAT ARE THE SYMPTOMS OF PRETERM BIRTH?

Preterm birth is any birth that occurs from 20 through 36 weeks of pregnancy. Here are the symptoms:

- contractions (tightening of stomach muscles or birth pains) every 10 minutes or more often
- change in vaginal discharge (leaking fluid or bleeding from the vagina)
- feeling of pressure in the pelvis (hip) area
- low, dull backache
- cramps that feel like menstrual cramps
- abdominal cramps with or without diarrhea

It is normal for pregnant women to have some uterine contractions throughout the day. It is not normal to have frequent uterine contractions, such as six or more in one hour. Frequent uterine contractions, or tightenings, may cause the cervix to begin to open. If a woman thinks that she might be having a preterm birth, she should call her doctor or go to the hospital to be evaluated.

WHAT ARE THE RISK FACTORS FOR PRETERM BIRTH?

There are several risk factors for preterm birth, including ones that researchers have not yet identified. Some of these risk factors are "modifiable," meaning they can be changed to help reduce the risk. Other factors cannot be changed. Health-care providers consider the following factors to put women at high risk for preterm birth:

- Women who have delivered preterm before, or who have experienced preterm labor before, are considered to be at high risk for preterm birth.
- Being pregnant with twins, triplets, or more (called "multiple gestations") or the use of assisted

reproductive technology is associated with a higher risk of preterm birth. One study showed that more than 50 percent of twin births occurred preterm, compared with only 10 percent of births of single infants.
- Women with certain anomalies of the reproductive organs are at greater risk for preterm birth than women who do not have these anomalies. For instance, women who have a short cervix (the lower part of the uterus) or whose cervix shortens in the second trimester (fourth through sixth months) of pregnancy instead of the third trimester are at high risk for preterm delivery.

Certain medical conditions, including some that occur only during pregnancy, also place a woman at higher risk for preterm delivery. Some of these conditions include:

- urinary tract infections (UTIs)
- sexually transmitted infections (STIs)
- certain vaginal infections, such as bacterial vaginosis and trichomoniasis
- high blood pressure (HBP)
- bleeding from the vagina
- certain developmental anomalies in the fetus
- pregnancy resulting from in vitro fertilization (IVF)
- being underweight or obese before pregnancy
- short time period between pregnancies (less than six months between a birth and the beginning of the next pregnancy)
- placenta previa, a condition in which the placenta grows in the lowest part of the uterus and covers all or part of the opening to the cervix
- being at risk for rupture of the uterus (when the wall of the uterus rips open; rupture of the uterus is more likely if you have had a prior cesarean delivery or have had a uterine fibroid removed)
- diabetes (high blood sugar) and gestational diabetes (which occurs only during pregnancy)
- blood clotting problems

Other factors that may increase the risk for preterm birth include the following:

- Ethnicity:
    - Preterm birth occurs more often among certain racial and ethnic groups. For example, infants of African-American mothers are more likely to be born preterm than infants of white mothers.
    - American-Indian/Alaska Native mothers are also more likely to give birth preterm than are white mothers.
- Age of the mother:
    - Women younger than age 18 are more likely to have a preterm delivery.
    - Women older than age 35 are also at risk of having preterm infants because they are more likely to have other conditions (such as high blood pressure and diabetes) that can cause complications requiring preterm delivery.
- Certain lifestyle and environmental factors:
    - late or no health care during pregnancy
    - smoking
    - drinking alcohol
    - using illegal drugs
    - domestic violence, including physical, sexual, or emotional abuse
    - lack of social support
    - stress
    - long working hours with long periods of standing
    - exposure to certain environmental pollutants

CAN WE PREDICT WHO IS MORE LIKELY TO EXPERIENCE PRETERM BIRTH?

There is no definitive way to predict preterm birth. Many research studies are focusing on this important issue. By identifying which women are at increased risk, health-care providers may be able to provide early interventions, treatments, and close monitoring of these pregnancies to prevent preterm delivery or to improve health outcomes. However, in some situations, health-care providers know that a preterm delivery is very likely. Some of these situations are described in the following sections.

Shortened Cervix

As a preparation for birth, the cervix (the lower part of the uterus) naturally shortens late in pregnancy. However, in some women, the cervix shortens prematurely, around the fourth or fifth month of pregnancy, increasing the risk for preterm delivery. In some cases, a health-care provider may recommend measuring a pregnant woman's cervical length, especially if she previously had a preterm birth. Ultrasound scans may be used to measure cervical length and identify women with a shortened cervix.

Incompetent Cervix

The cervix normally remains closed during pregnancy. In some cases, the cervix starts to open early, before a fetus is ready to be born. Health-care providers may refer to a cervix that begins to open as an "incompetent" cervix. The process of cervical opening is painless and unnoticeable, without labor contractions or cramping. To try to prevent preterm birth, a doctor may place a stitch around the cervix to keep it closed. This procedure is called "cervical cerclage." The NICHD-supported research has found that, in women with a prior preterm birth who have a short cervix, cerclage may improve the likelihood of a full-term delivery.

HOW DO HEALTH-CARE PROVIDERS DIAGNOSE PRETERM LABOR?

If a woman is concerned that she could be showing signs of preterm labor, she should call her health-care provider or go to the hospital to be evaluated. In particular, a woman should call if she has more than six contractions in an hour or if fluid or blood is leaking from the vagina.

Physical Exam

If a woman is experiencing signs of labor, the health-care provider may perform a pelvic exam to see if:

- the membranes have ruptured

- the cervix is beginning to get thinner (efface)
- the cervix is beginning to open (dilate)

Any of these situations could mean the woman is in preterm labor. Providers may also do an ultrasound exam and use a monitor to electronically record contractions and the fetal heart rate.

Fetal Fibronectin Test

This test is used to detect whether the protein fetal fibronectin (fFN) is being produced. fFN is like a biological "glue" between the uterine lining and the membrane that surrounds the fetus. Normally fFN is detectable in the pregnant woman's secretions from the vagina and cervix early in the pregnancy (up to 22 weeks, or about five months) and again toward the end of the pregnancy (one to three weeks before labor begins). It is usually not present between 24 and 34 weeks of pregnancy (5½–8½ months). If fFN is detected during this time, it may be a sign that the woman may be at risk of preterm labor and birth. In most cases, the fFN test is performed on women who are showing signs of preterm labor. Testing for fFN can help predict which pregnant women showing signs of preterm labor will have a preterm delivery. It is typically used for its negative predictive value, meaning that if it is negative, it is unlikely that a woman will deliver within the next seven days.

WHAT TREATMENTS ARE USED TO PREVENT PRETERM BIRTH?

Currently, treatment options for preventing preterm birth are somewhat limited, in part because the cause of preterm birth is often unknown. But there are a few options, described in the following sections.

- **Hormone treatment**. Progesterone, a hormone produced by the body during pregnancy, was thought to prevent preterm birth in certain groups at high risk of preterm birth, such as those with prior preterm birth. The NICHD Maternal-Fetal Medicine Units (MFMU) Network found that progesterone given to women at risk of preterm birth due to a prior preterm birth reduces the chances of a subsequent preterm birth by one-third, when started at 16 weeks of gestation and continued to 37 weeks of gestation. Because subsequent research did not show the same effect, the use of progesterone to prevent preterm birth is now under review by the U.S. Food and Drug Administration (FDA).

- **Cerclage**. A surgical procedure called "cervical cerclage" is sometimes used to try to prevent early labor in women who have an incompetent (weak) cervix and have experienced early pregnancy loss accompanied by a painless opening (dilation) of the cervix (the bottom part of the uterus). In the cerclage procedure, a doctor stitches the cervix closed. The stitch is then removed closer to the woman's due date.
- **Bed rest**. Contrary to expectations, confining the mother to bed rest does not help prevent preterm birth. In fact, bed rest can make preterm birth even more likely among some women. Women should discuss all of their treatment options—including the risks and benefits—with their health-care providers. If possible, these discussions should occur during regular prenatal care visits, before there is any urgency, to allow for a complete discussion of all the issues.[1]

Section 4.2 | **Managing Respiratory Challenges in Preemies**

Almost 1 of every 10 infants born in the United States are premature, or preemies. A premature birth is when a baby is born before 37 completed weeks of pregnancy. A full-term pregnancy is 40 weeks. Important growth and development happen throughout pregnancy, especially in the final months and weeks. Because they are born too early, preemies weigh much less than full-term babies.

[1] "About Preterm Labor and Birth," *Eunice Kennedy Shriver* National Institute of Child Health and Human Development (NICHD), May 9, 2023. Available online. URL: www.nichd.nih.gov/health/topics/preterm. Accessed March 5, 2024.

They may have health problems because their organs did not have enough time to develop. Problems that a baby born too early may have include the following:

- breathing problems
- feeding difficulties
- cerebral palsy (CP)
- developmental delay
- vision problems
- hearing problems

Preemies need special medical care in a neonatal intensive care unit (NICU). They stay there until their organ systems can work on their own.[2]

WHAT IS RESPIRATORY DISTRESS SYNDROME?

Respiratory distress syndrome (RDS) is a common breathing disorder that affects newborns. RDS occurs most often in babies born before their due date, usually before 28 weeks of pregnancy. Less often, RDS can affect full-term newborns. Most newborns who have RDS survive. However, these babies may need extra medical care after going home. Some babies have complications from RDS or its treatment, including the development of another lung condition called "bronchopulmonary dysplasia" (BPD).

WHAT ARE THE SYMPTOMS OF RESPIRATORY DISTRESS SYNDROME?

Symptoms of RDS include:

- fast and shallow breathing
- grunting
- flaring of the nostrils with each breath
- bluish tone to a baby's skin and lips
- pulling inward of the muscles between the ribs when breathing

[2] MedlinePlus, "Premature Babies," National Institutes of Health (NIH), November 27, 2015. Available online. URL: https://medlineplus.gov/prematurebabies.html. Accessed March 5, 2024.

HOW WILL A DOCTOR FIND OUT WHETHER A NEWBORN HAS RESPIRATORY DISTRESS SYNDROME?

Respiratory distress syndrome is common in premature newborns, but doctors may need to run tests to rule out other types of newborn breathing conditions. After doing a physical examination to look at a newborn's symptoms, your provider may order one or more of the tests listed subsequently.

- **Lung imaging tests.** Tests such as chest x-rays show how well the lungs and heart are working. X-rays are used to diagnose most types of newborn breathing conditions.
- **Heart tests.** Tests such as an echocardiogram can check for a possible congenital heart defect (CHD).
- **Blood tests.** These tests look for an infection.

WHAT CAUSES RESPIRATORY DISTRESS SYNDROME?

Respiratory distress syndrome is caused by a lack of surfactant in the lungs. The lungs of a fetus start making surfactant during the third trimester, which starts after the 26th week of pregnancy. Surfactant is a foamy substance that keeps the lungs fully expanded so that newborns can breathe in air once they are born. Without it, the lungs collapse, and the newborn must work hard to breathe. This can cause the baby's organs to be without necessary levels of oxygen. If a full-term baby develops RDS, it may be because they have faulty genes that affect how their bodies make surfactant.

HOW IS RESPIRATORY DISTRESS SYNDROME TREATED?

The earlier a baby is born, the more likely they are to have RDS that cannot be prevented. Nearly all babies born before 28 weeks of pregnancy will have RDS. With treatment, many newborns that are diagnosed with RDS will recover. Some common treatments include:

- **Nasal continuous positive airway pressure (nCPAP).** This device provides breathing support by gently pushing air into the baby's lungs through prongs placed in the nose.

- **Surfactant replacement therapy**. This can be used if a newborn struggles to breathe despite the use of nCPAP. Sometimes, giving an infant surfactant requires the use of a breathing tube. If so, because of the possible complications, your baby's provider will help you consider the risks and benefits of the procedure.
- **Mechanical ventilation**. This is used only in very serious cases of RDS. A ventilator is a machine that takes over the work of breathing and is a form of life support. The machine connects to a breathing tube that runs through a newborn's mouth or nose and into the windpipe. Babies that require ventilation are more likely to develop BPD. They may also develop health problems from the breathing tube or ventilator, such as an airway or lung injury.
- **Fluids and nutrients**. These may be given to help prevent malnutrition and promote growth. Nutrition is critical to the growth and development of the lungs.

If a baby born with RDS still requires breathing support by the time they reach their original due date, they are diagnosed with a condition called "BPD." Depending on how serious their RDS is, they may also develop other medical conditions, including:

- bleeding in the brain, which can delay cognitive development or cause intellectual disabilities or CP
- lung complications, such as air leaking from the lung into the chest cavity, called "pneumothorax," or bleeding in the lungs
- impaired vision
- infections that can cause sepsis[3]

[3] "Neonatal Respiratory Distress Syndrome," National Heart, Lung, and Blood Institute (NHLBI), March 24, 2022. Available online. URL: www.nhlbi.nih.gov/health/respiratory-distress-syndrome. Accessed March 5, 2024.

Section 4.3 | Neonatal Intensive Care Transition Planning

When infants are born before their due date or with health problems, families often need help managing their baby's health care after leaving the hospital. Since they spend the first part of their lives in the hospital, the babies and their families may find it helpful to have extra support. A health coach will work with your family to teach you to care for your infant, connect with the right doctors and specialists for treatment, and find resources in your area. The role of the health coach is as an educator, not as a caregiver.

Planning must start before hospital discharge and continue through follow-up with the primary care provider. After discharge from the hospital, your infant's care must be well coordinated and clearly communicated to avoid medical errors that could harm the baby. After your infant is discharged, your health coach should follow up with you by phone within a few days to make sure the transition is going well. Your health coach will want to know how your baby is doing, whether you have any questions or concerns, if your infant has been to the scheduled appointments, and so on.

GETTING CARE

Tips for Finding a Pediatrician

- Your family will need to visit a pediatrician within the first week after leaving the hospital.
- Plan ahead to avoid the pressure and frustration of finding a pediatrician right before your baby is discharged from the hospital.
- Ask your health coach or social worker if you need help finding a doctor for your baby.
- Decide whether the pediatrician's office needs to be close to your home, job, or daycare.
- Call the pediatrician's office to ask if they accept your current health insurance and if they are accepting new patients.
- Ask the pediatrician's office what your copayment and responsibilities are.

- Ask the pediatrician's office which doctor your baby will see at every visit.
- Ask the pediatrician's office if a doctor is on call 24 hours a day for emergencies.

Tips about Health Insurance

- Your baby will need to visit the doctor regularly after birth.
- You have only 30 days to add your newborn to your insurance plan. Call your current insurance company as soon as possible to add your newborn.
- Ask your social worker if you qualify for Medicaid, and apply while your baby is still in the hospital.
- Ask about Children's Medicaid—Children's Health Insurance Program (CHIP), Project Medical Home, and other low-cost care benefits if you do not qualify for Medicaid.

UNDERSTANDING SIGNS AND SYMPTOMS OF ILLNESS

Call the doctor if your baby:

- has a fever of more than 100 °F (37.78 °C)
- has diarrhea for more than one day
- is throwing up forcefully
- is not eating well
- has not had at least six to eight wet diapers per day
- has a very yellow eye color or skin color
- is hard to wake up
- has fast or difficult breathing
- makes jerking movements
- is not looking well or acting well

CRYING

Common Causes

- hunger
- pain

- sleepy
- clothes too tight
- soiled diaper
- too hot or too cold

Call your doctor if:

- your baby looks or acts sick (is throwing up, appears to be in pain)
- you are exhausted from the crying and fear you might hurt your baby

COLIC

What Is Colic?

- unexplained crying for three or more hours a day
- excessive crying
- usually begins suddenly and for no clear reason
- difficult to comfort
- usually goes away as your baby gets older than three months of age

Remember that colic is normal in a lot of babies and is simply part of their personality. It has nothing to do with your parenting or any illness. It is important to remain calm and never shake your baby.

MEDICINES AND IMMUNIZATIONS

Medication Safety

- Keep a list of your baby's medications with you at all times.
- Speak to your baby's health-care professional, and ask specific questions about your baby's medicines.
- When picking up refills, check the label carefully for the correct medicine, strength, and dose.
- Read over-the-counter (OTC) labels to make sure the product is appropriate for your child's age.
- Use medicines only as directed.

- Use the measuring devices that come with the products, and use these devices as instructed.
- Keep medicine bottles away from other small children.
- Never allow a child to drink directly from a medicine bottle.

GIVING YOUR BABY ORAL MEDICINES

Know the name of the medicine and what it is for.

- Carefully read the label of each medicine before giving it to your baby.
- Know why your baby needs to take this medicine.

Know the dose.

- It is best to use an oral syringe to give liquid medicine to a baby.
- Avoid using teaspoons because they are not precise.
- Ask the pharmacist to mark the syringe at the dose you need to give.
- Keep the syringe with the corresponding bottle and color code them.
- Know how often to give the medicine.

Ask your baby's doctor or pharmacist what to do in case you miss a dose.

Know possible side effects.

- Always observe your baby for any bad reactions to the medicine.
- Call your baby's doctor in case of a bad reaction.

PREVENTING INFECTION

Everyone must wash their hands or use hand sanitizer before and after they touch your baby.

- Avoid large crowds.
- Avoid sick people.
- Have people cover their mouth and nose with a tissue when they cough or sneeze.
- Do not allow anyone to smoke around the baby.

PREMATURE BABY IMMUNIZATION SCHEDULE

What Is an Immunization?

Immunizations protect us from contracting serious diseases. They are often given by shot, but sometimes by mouth or nose.

Premature Babies

Immunizations are given to premature babies at the same age as full-term infants.

At Birth

- Hepatitis B (HepB) vaccine
    - the first dose is usually given at birth before leaving the hospital
    - should complete the doses by 6–18 months of age

Six to Eight Weeks Old

- diphtheria, tetanus, and pertussis (DTaP) vaccine
- *Haemophilus influenzae* type b (Hib) vaccine
- pneumococcal vaccine
- poliovirus (IPV) vaccine

Benefits of Vaccines

- Vaccines prepare your baby's body to fight illness.
- Vaccines protect you and others around you.
- It costs less to prevent a disease than to treat it.

How Can You Manage Your Child's Breathing Problems at Home?

- Visit the neonatal intensive care unit (NICU) often, and help care for your baby as much as possible in the hospital.
- Learn how to use equipment: pulse oximeter, oxygen tank, and nasal cannula.
- Know the signs of difficulty breathing.
- Learn cardiopulmonary resuscitation (CPR).
- Learn how to give your child's medicines.

- Plan ahead for extra help at home.
- Schedule routine follow-up doctor visits.
- Wash your hands frequently.
- Avoid crowds.
- Have your child immunized.

CRIB SAFETY

What Is Sudden Infant Death Syndrome?

- "SIDS" stands for sudden infant death syndrome.
- It refers to the sudden, unexplained death of an infant less than one year old.

What Should You Know about Sudden Infant Death Syndrome?

- Babies sleep safer on their backs.
- Babies should be placed on a firm sleep surface.

What Can You Do to Lower Your Baby's Risk of Sudden Infant Death Syndrome?

- Babies should be put on their backs to sleep for naps and at night.
- Keep toys, objects, and loose bedding out of your baby's sleep area.
- Do not allow smoking around your baby.
- Do not allow your baby to overheat while sleeping.

What about "Tummy Time"?

- Daily tummy time is necessary for normal development.
- Make sure your baby spends several hours on their tummy when they are awake, and someone is watching.

BRONCHOPULMONARY DYSPLASIA

What Is Bronchopulmonary Dysplasia?

- type of chronic lung disease
- common in babies born early

- damaged lung tissue causes breathing and health problems
- lungs trap air, fill with fluid, and produce extra mucus

What Causes Bronchopulmonary Dysplasia?

- being born early
- having a virus called "respiratory syncytial virus" (RSV)
- having a heart condition
- being on a ventilator
- lack of nourishment
- fluid in the lungs

What Are the Symptoms of Bronchopulmonary Dysplasia?

- grunting
- breathing heavily
- flaring nostrils
- sucking in air
- tiring easily
- pale or grey skin

How Is Bronchopulmonary Dysplasia Diagnosed?

- if your baby still needs oxygen at 36 weeks old
- if your baby has been on a ventilator

How Is Bronchopulmonary Dysplasia Treated?

- Bronchopulmonary dysplasia (BPD) is treated with oxygen to support breathing, diuretics to control fluid in the body, and medicine to relax the airway.
- Treatment does not cure BPD.
- Treatment helps your baby breathe better.
- Lungs will eventually heal.
- Your baby needs nutrients for healthy growth.

RESPIRATORY SYNCYTIAL VIRUS

What Is Respiratory Syncytial Virus?

- a common virus that affects babies and infants
- leading cause of two lung infections: pneumonia and bronchitis

Symptoms of Respiratory Syncytial Virus

- starts out like a cold with a fever or runny nose
- can also include:
  - coughing
  - problems breathing
  - fast breathing
  - not eating well

How Is Respiratory Syncytial Virus Spread?

- contact with someone who is coughing or sneezing
- enters the body through the eyes, nose, or mouth

How to Prevent the Spread of Respiratory Syncytial Virus

- Wash your hands before and after handling a baby.
- Avoid exposing your baby to others with cold symptoms.
- Cover coughs/sneezes and throw away used tissues.
- Keep your baby away from crowded areas.
- If your baby is at high risk for RSV, talk to your doctor about a monthly shot that can help lower the risk of a baby getting severe RSV.
- Your baby may be eligible for palivizumab (brand name: Synagis®), a treatment given to prevent and reduce RSV.
- The shot, given monthly during RSV season, reduces the chance of your baby getting pneumonia and bronchitis.
- Babies may still get RSV but will be less sick.

FEEDING

Bottle Feeding

- Feed your baby only infant formula and breast milk for their first four to six months.
- Feed your baby at least every three hours, day and night.
- Before each feeding, warm the breast milk or formula to room temperature by placing the bottle in warm water; do not leave cold bottles on the counter to warm up.
- Never heat breast milk or formula in a microwave oven.
- Throw away any remaining breast milk or formula after each feeding.
- When traveling, keep the breast milk or formula cold in a cooler.

Formula Preparation

Infant formulas are available in the following three ways.

READY TO FEED

Do not add water.

LIQUID CONCENTRATE

Add sterile water.

POWDER

Add sterile water.

To Make Sterile Water

- Boil water for two minutes.
- Cover the pot.
- Let water cool to room temperature.

Formula Storage and Use

- Store the prepared formula in a refrigerator.
- Use the formula in 24–48 hours.

BOTTLE CLEANING

- Clean bottles and nipples by washing them with hot, soapy water or on the top rack of the dishwasher.
- Allow bottles and nipples to air dry.

BREASTFEEDING YOUR BABY

Breastfed babies have:

- fewer ear infections
- lower chance of asthma, food allergies, and dental cavities
- protection against diarrhea, stomach, and lung infections
- better nervous system development and higher intelligence quotient (IQ) levels
- lower risk of some childhood cancers
- lower chance of becoming overweight

GASTROSTOMY TUBE (G TUBE OR BUTTON)

The following are the steps for giving medicines and feeding if your baby has a gastrostomy tube:

- Clear the G tube or button as your health-care provider showed you.
- Check for placement of the G tube or button.
- Slowly push in liquid medicine or feed with a syringe.
- If the pharmacist says it is ok, pills and capsules may be dissolved in 10–20 cc of warm tap water.
- All medicines and feedings should be flushed in with 5–10 cc of warm tap water.
- Ask your baby's doctor, nurse, or pharmacist how to measure the tap water.

It is important to use the specific tube adapter made by the manufacturer of your button.

- In fluid-restricted babies, flush medicines with only 1–5 cc of warm tap water.
- Vent the tube after feeding to remove excess air or fluid and reduce leaking.

Protecting the G Tube or Button

- Snap T-shirts and onesies work best to prevent babies from pulling on the tube or button.
- You may also use a sticky wrap or stretchy dressing.[4]

[4] Agency for Healthcare Research and Quality (AHRQ), "Transitioning Newborns from NICU to Home," U.S. Department of Health and Human Services (HHS), December 2013. Available online. URL: www.ahrq.gov/sites/default/files/wysiwyg/patient-safety/settings/hospitals/nicupacket.pdf. Accessed March 5, 2024.

Chapter 5 | **Common Newborn and Infant Problems**

Some physical conditions and issues are very common during the first couple of weeks after birth. Many are normal, and the infant's caregivers can deal with them if they occur. Mostly, it is a matter of the caregivers learning about what is normal for their infant and getting comfortable with the new routine in the household. New parents and caregivers often have questions about several aspects of their infant's health and well-being.

BOWEL MOVEMENTS

Infants' bowel movements go through many changes in color and consistency, even within the first few days after birth. It is import ant to keep track of your infant's bowel movements. Some things to look for include:

- **Color**. A newborn's first bowel movements usually consist of a thick, black, or dark green substance called "meconium." After the meconium is passed, the stools (poop) will turn yellow-green. The stools of breastfed infants look mustard-yellow with seed-like particles.
- **Consistency**. Until the infant starts to eat solid foods, the consistency of the stool can range from very soft to loose and runny. Formula-fed infants usually have stools that are tan or yellow in color and firmer than those of breastfed infants. Whether your baby is breastfed

or bottle-fed, hard or very dry stools may be a sign of dehydration.

- **Frequency**. Infants who are eating solid foods can become constipated if they eat too many constipating foods, such as cereal or cow's milk, before their system can handle them. The U.S. Food and Drug Administration (FDA) and the American Academy of Pediatrics (AAP) do not recommend cow's milk for babies under 12 months.

Also, because an infant's stools are normally soft and a little runny, it is not always easy to tell when a young infant has mild diarrhea. The main signs are a sudden increase in the number of bowel movements (more than one per feeding) and watery stools. Diarrhea can be a sign of intestinal infection, or it may be caused by a change in diet. If the infant is breastfeeding, diarrhea can result from a change in the mother's diet. The main concern with diarrhea is the possibility of dehydration. If fever is also present and your infant is less than two months old, you should call your health-care provider. If the infant is over two months old and the fever lasts more than a day, check the infant's urine output and rectal temperature and consult a health-care provider. Make sure the infant continues to feed often.

Starting around the age of three to six weeks, some breastfed babies have only one bowel movement a week. This is normal because breast milk leaves very little solid waste to pass through the digestive system. Formula-fed infants should have at least one bowel movement a day. If a formula-fed infant has fewer bowel movements than this and appears to be straining because of hard stools, constipation may be the cause. Check with your health-care provider if there are any changes or problems with your infant's bowel movements.

CARE OF THE UMBILICUS

The umbilical cord delivers oxygen and nutrients to the fetus while it is in the womb. After delivery, the umbilical cord is cut. The remaining part of the cord dries and falls off in about 10 days, forming the belly button (navel). Follow your health-care provider's recommendations about how to care for the umbilicus. This care might include:

- keeping the area clean and dry
- folding down the top of the diaper to expose the umbilicus to the air
- cleaning the umbilicus gently with a baby wipe or with a cotton swab dipped in rubbing alcohol

Contact your health-care provider if there is pus or redness.

COLIC

Many infants are fussy in the evenings, but if the crying does not stop and gets worse throughout the day or night, it may be caused by colic. According to the AAP, about one-fifth of all infants develop colic, usually starting between two and four weeks of age. They may cry inconsolably or scream, extend or pull up their legs, and pass gas. Their stomachs may be enlarged. The crying spells can occur anytime, although they often get worse in the early evening. The colic will likely improve or disappear by the age of three or four months. There is no definite explanation for why some infants get colic. Sometimes, in breastfeeding babies, colic is a sign of sensitivity to a food in the mother's diet. Rarely, colic is caused by sensitivity to milk protein in formula. Colic could be a sign of a medical problem, such as a hernia or some type of illness. If your infant shows signs of colic, the first step is to consult with your health-care provider. Sometimes, changing the diet of a breastfeeding mother or changing the formula for bottle-fed infants can help. Some infants seem to be soothed by being held, rocked, or wrapped snugly in a blanket. Some like a pacifier.

DIAPER RASH

A rash on the skin covered by a diaper is quite common. It is usually caused by irritation of the skin from being in contact with stool and urine. It can get worse during bouts of diarrhea. Diaper rash usually can be prevented by frequent diaper changes.

Your health-care provider can recommend care for diaper rash, which may include:

- rinsing the skin with warm water, using soap only after bowel movements. Because baby wipes may leave a film of bacteria on the skin, their use is often not recommended
- exposing the rash to air as much as possible by loosely attaching the diaper at the waist or removing the diaper entirely during naps
- laying the infant on a towel to absorb urine

Caregivers should contact a health-care provider if the rash is not better in three days or if the child becomes worse.

SPITTING UP/VOMITING

Spitting up is a common occurrence for newborns and is usually not a sign of a more serious problem. After feeding, try to keep the infant calm and in an upright position for a little while. Keep a burp towel handy, just in case. Contact your health-care provider immediately if your infant:

- is not gaining weight
- is spitting up so forcefully that stomach contents shoot out of the infant's mouth
- spits up green or yellow liquid, blood, or a substance that looks like coffee grounds
- has blood in the stool
- shows other signs of illness, such as fever, diarrhea, or difficulty with breathing

Some parents worry that their infant will spit up and choke if they are put to sleep on their backs, but this is not the case. Healthy infants naturally swallow or cough up fluids—it is a reflex all people have. Where the opening to the windpipe is located in the body makes it unlikely for fluids to cause choking. Babies may actually clear such fluids better when on their backs.

The Safe to Sleep® Campaign (formerly the Back to Sleep campaign) by the *Eunice Kennedy Shriver* National Institute of Child

Health and Human Development (NICHD) recommends placing infants to sleep on their backs to reduce the risk for sudden infant death syndrome (SIDS). Since the recommendation for back sleeping began in 1992, the number of fatal choking deaths has not increased. In fact, in most of the few reported cases of fatal choking, an infant was sleeping on his or her stomach.

TEETHING

Although newborns usually have no visible teeth, baby teeth begin to appear generally about six months after birth. During the first few years, all 20 baby teeth will push through the gums, and most children will have their full set of these teeth in place by age three. An infant's front four teeth usually appear first, at about six months of age, although some children do not get their first tooth until 12 or 14 months. As their teeth break through the gums, some infants become fussy, sleepless, and irritable; lose their appetite; or drool more than usual. If an infant has a fever or diarrhea while teething or continues to be cranky and uncomfortable, contact your baby's health-care provider. The FDA does not recommend gum-numbing medications with an ingredient called "benzocaine" because they can cause a potentially fatal condition in young children. Talk to your health-care provider for advice on using these products for your teething infant. Other potential forms of relief for your infant include a chilled teething ring or gently rubbing the child's gums with a clean finger.

URINATION

Infants urinate as often as every one to three hours or as infrequently as every four to six hours. In case of sickness or if the weather is very hot, urine output might drop by half and still be normal. Urination should never be painful. If you notice any signs of distress while your infant is urinating, notify your child's health-care provider because this could be a sign of infection or some other problem in the urinary tract. In a healthy child, urine is light to dark yellow in color (The darker the color, the more concentrated the urine; the urine is more concentrated when the child is not drinking much liquid.). The presence of blood in the urine or a bloody spot on the diaper is not normal and should prompt a call to the health-care provider. If this bleeding occurs with other symptoms, such as abdominal pain or bleeding in other areas, immediate medical attention is needed.

JAUNDICE

Jaundice can cause an infant's skin, eyes, and mouth to turn a yellowish color. The yellow color is caused by a buildup of bilirubin, a substance that is produced in the body during the normal process of breaking down old red blood cells and forming new ones. Normally the liver removes bilirubin from the body. But, for many infants, in the first few days after birth, the liver is not yet working at its full power. As a result, the level of bilirubin in the blood gets too high, causing the infant's color to become slightly yellow—this is jaundice. Although jaundice is common and usually not serious, in some cases, high levels of bilirubin could cause brain injury. All infants with jaundice need to be seen by a health-care provider. Many infants need no treatment. Their livers start to catch up quickly and begin to remove bilirubin normally, usually within a few days after birth. For some infants, health-care providers prescribe phototherapy—a treatment using a special lamp—to help break down the bilirubin in their bodies.

If your infant has jaundice, ask your health-care provider how long the child's jaundice should last after leaving the hospital, and schedule a follow-up appointment as directed. If the jaundice lasts longer than expected, or an infant who did not have jaundice starts to turn yellowish after going home, a health-care provider should be consulted right away. If you intend to get discharged early, particularly within 48 hours of birth, your infant's jaundice may peak later in the first week. It is almost impossible to say how severe the jaundice level is by just looking at the baby's skin, especially for infants of color. Therefore, make every effort to keep follow-up appointments so the health-care provider can check the level of jaundice with a simple blood test.[1]

---

[1] "What Are Some of the Basics of Infant Health?" *Eunice Kennedy Shriver* National Institute of Child Health and Human Development (NICHD), September 7, 2021. Available online. URL: www.nichd.nih.gov/health/topics/infantcare/conditioninfo/basics. Accessed March 8, 2024.

Chapter 6 | Maternal, Newborn, and Child Health

Chapter Contents

Section 6.1 | Benefits of Prepregnancy Care and Counseling

There are things you can do before and between pregnancies to increase the chances of having a healthy pregnancy. Getting your body ready for pregnancy may look different for different people.

Your health before pregnancy is very important and can affect the health of your future baby. By making a plan before getting pregnant, you can take steps toward a healthier you and baby-to-be.

PLANNING FOR PREGNANCY

Talk to Your Health-Care Provider

Before getting pregnant, talk to your health-care provider about your health history and any medical conditions you currently have.

Take a list of talking points so you do not forget anything. Be sure to talk to your doctor about:

- any current medical conditions you have
- all medicines you take, including prescriptions, over-the-counter (OTC) medicines, supplements, and vitamins
- vaccinations
- lifestyle and behavior

Get 400 Micrograms of Folic Acid Every Day

Folic acid is a B vitamin. Having enough folic acid in your body at least one month before and during pregnancy can help prevent major birth defects of the developing baby's brain and spine (neural tube defects (NTD)).

Stop Drinking Alcohol, Smoking, and Using Certain Drugs

Smoking, drinking alcohol, and using certain drugs can cause many problems during pregnancy, such as premature birth, birth defects, and infant death. If you are trying to get pregnant and cannot stop drinking, smoking, or using drugs, contact your health-care provider, local Alcoholics Anonymous, or local alcohol treatment center.

Avoid Toxic Substances and Environmental Contaminants

Avoid harmful chemicals, environmental contaminants, and other toxic substances such as synthetic chemicals, some metals, fertilizer, bug spray, and cat or rodent feces around the home and in the workplace. These substances can hurt the reproductive systems of men and women.

Reach and Maintain a Healthy Weight

People who are overweight or obese have a higher risk for many serious conditions, including complications during pregnancy. People who are underweight are also at risk for serious health problems.

Learn Your Family History

Collecting your family's health history can help you identify factors that might affect your baby or your ability to become pregnant. Based on your family health history, your doctor might refer you for genetic counseling. Other reasons for genetic counseling include having had several miscarriages, infant deaths, trouble getting pregnant (infertility), or having a genetic condition or birth defect that occurred during a previous pregnancy.

Get Mentally Healthy

Mental health is how we think, feel, and act as we cope with life. To be at your best, you need to feel good about your life and value yourself. Everyone feels worried, anxious, sad, or stressed sometimes. However, if these feelings do not go away and interfere with your daily life, get help. Talk with your health-care provider about your feelings and treatment options.

Health-care professionals can also help with counseling and other support services if you are in a stressful or abusive environment.[1]

[1] "About Planning for Pregnancy," Centers for Disease Control and Prevention (CDC), May 15, 2024. Available online. URL: www.cdc.gov/pregnancy/about/index.html. Accessed June 26, 2024.

Having a healthy pregnancy is one of the best ways to promote a healthy birth. Getting early and regular prenatal care improves the chances of a healthy pregnancy. This care can begin even before pregnancy with a prepregnancy care visit to a health-care provider.

PREPREGNANCY CARE

A prepregnancy care visit can help women take steps toward a healthy pregnancy before they even get pregnant.[2]

Section 6.2 | Role of Prenatal Care in Child Health

What happens during prenatal visits varies depending on how far along you are in your pregnancy. Schedule your first prenatal visit as soon as you think you are pregnant, even if you have confirmed your pregnancy with a home pregnancy test. Early and regular prenatal visits help your health-care provider monitor your health and the growth of the fetus.

THE FIRST VISIT

Your first prenatal visit will probably be scheduled sometime after your eighth week of pregnancy. Most health-care providers will not schedule a visit any earlier unless you have a medical condition, have had problems with a pregnancy in the past, or have symptoms such as spotting or bleeding, stomach pain, or severe nausea and vomiting.

You have probably heard pregnancy discussed in terms of months and trimesters (units of about three months). Your health-care provider and health information might use weeks instead. Here is a chart that can help you understand pregnancy stages (see Table 6.1) in terms of trimesters, months, and weeks.

---

[2] "What Is Prenatal Care and Why Is It Important?" *Eunice Kennedy Shriver* National Institute of Child Health and Human Development (NICHD), January 31, 2017. Available online. URL: www.nichd.nih.gov/health/topics/pregnancy/conditioninfo/prenatal-care. Accessed March 8, 2024.

Table 6.1. Pregnancy Stages

Trimester	Months	Weeks
1	0–3	0–17
2	4–6	18–30
3	7–9	31–42

Because your first visit will be one of your longest, allow plenty of time. During the visit, you can expect your health-care provider to do the following:

- Answer your questions. This is a great time to ask questions and share any concerns you may have. Keep a running list for your visit.
- Check your urine sample for infection and to confirm your pregnancy.
- Check your blood pressure, weight, and height.
- Calculate your due date based on your last menstrual cycle and ultrasound exam.
- Ask about your health, including previous conditions, surgeries, or pregnancies.
- Ask about your family health and genetic history.
- Ask about your lifestyle, including whether you smoke, drink, or take drugs, and whether you exercise regularly.
- Ask about your stress level.
- Perform prenatal blood tests to do the following:
    - Determine your blood type and Rhesus (Rh) factor. Rh factor refers to a protein found in red blood cells. If the mother is Rh-negative (lacks the protein) and the father is Rh-positive (has the protein), the pregnancy requires a special level of care.
    - Do a blood count (e.g., hemoglobin, hematocrit).
    - Test for hepatitis B (HepB), human immunodeficiency virus (HIV), rubella, and syphilis.
    - Do a complete physical exam, including a pelvic exam, and cultures for gonorrhea and chlamydia.

- Do a Pap test or test for human papillomavirus (HPV) or both to screen for cervical cancer and infection with HPV, which can increase the risk for cervical cancer. The timing of these tests depends on the schedule recommended by your health-care provider.
- Do an ultrasound test, depending on the week of pregnancy.
- Offer genetic testing: screening for Down syndrome and other chromosomal problems, cystic fibrosis (CF), and other specialized testing depending on history.

PRENATAL VISIT SCHEDULE

If your pregnancy is healthy, your health-care provider will set up a regular schedule for visits that will probably look like this:

- **Before 28 weeks**. Monthly.
- **Weeks 28–36**. Every two weeks.
- **Week 36 to birth**. Weekly.

LATER PRENATAL VISITS

As your pregnancy progresses, your prenatal visits will vary greatly. During most visits, you can expect your health-care provider to do the following:

- Check your blood pressure.
- Measure your weight gain.
- Measure your abdomen to check your developing infant's growth—"fundal height" (once you begin to "show").
- Check the fetal heart rate.
- Check your hands and feet for swelling.
- Feel your abdomen to find the fetus' position (later in pregnancy).
- Do tests such as blood tests or an ultrasound exam.

Talk to your health-care provider about your questions or concerns. It is a good idea to write down your questions and bring them with you. Several of these visits will include special tests to check for gestational diabetes (usually between 24 and 28 weeks) and other conditions, depending on your age and family history.[3]

[3] "What Happens during Prenatal Visits?" *Eunice Kennedy Shriver* National Institute of Child Health and Human Development (NICHD), January 31, 2017. Available online. URL: www.nichd.nih.gov/health/topics/preconception-care/conditioninfo/prenatal-visits. Accessed March 8, 2024.

Part 2 | **Child Development Milestones**

Chapter 7 | **Child Developmental Monitoring and Screening**

HEALTHY DEVELOPMENT

The early years of a child's life are very important for their health and development. Healthy development means that children of all abilities, including those with special health-care needs, are able to grow up where their social, emotional, and educational needs are met. Having a safe and loving home and spending time with family—playing, singing, reading, and talking—are very important. Proper nutrition, exercise, and sleep can also make a big difference.

Effective Parenting Practices

Parenting takes many different forms. However, some positive parenting practices work well across diverse families and settings when providing the care that children need to be happy, healthy, and to grow and develop well. A comprehensive report looked at the evidence in scientific publications for what works and found the following key ways that parents can support their child's healthy development:

- responding to children in a predictable way
- showing warmth and sensitivity
- having routines and household rules
- sharing books and talking with children
- supporting health and safety
- using appropriate discipline without harshness

Parents who use these practices can help their children stay healthy, be safe, and be successful in many areas—emotional, behavioral, cognitive, and social.

DEVELOPMENTAL MILESTONES

Skills such as taking a first step, smiling for the first time, and waving "bye-bye" are called "developmental milestones." Children reach milestones in how they play, learn, speak, behave, and move (e.g., crawling and walking).

Children develop at their own pace, so it is impossible to tell exactly when a child will learn a given skill. However, the developmental milestones give a general idea of the changes to expect as a child gets older.

As a parent, you know your child best. If your child is not meeting the milestones for their age or if you think there could be a problem with your child's development, talk with your child's doctor and share your concerns. Do not wait.[1]

DEVELOPMENTAL MONITORING

Developmental monitoring observes how your child grows and changes over time and whether your child meets the typical developmental milestones in playing, learning, speaking, behaving, and moving. Parents, grandparents, early childhood providers, and other caregivers can participate in developmental monitoring. If you notice that your child is not meeting milestones, talk with your doctor or nurse about your concerns.

When you take your child to a well-child visit, your doctor or nurse will also do developmental monitoring. The doctor or nurse might ask you questions about your child's development or will talk and play with your child to see if he or she is developing and meeting milestones. A missed milestone could be a sign of

[1] National Center on Birth Defects and Developmental Disabilities (NCBDDD), "Child Development Basics," Centers for Disease Control and Prevention (CDC), February 23, 2023. Available online. URL: www.cdc.gov/ncbddd/childdevelopment/facts.html. Accessed February 23, 2024.

a problem, so the doctor or another specialist will take a closer look by using a more thorough test or exam. Your childcare provider can also be a valuable source of information on how your child develops.

Facts about Developmental Monitoring

- **Who**. Parents, grandparents, or other caregivers.
- **What**. Look for developmental milestones.
- **When**. From birth to five years of age.
- **Why**. To help you:
  - celebrate your child's development
  - talk about your child's progress with doctors and childcare providers
  - learn what to expect next
  - identify any concerns early
- **How**. With easy, free checklists available at www.cdc.gov/milestones.

DEVELOPMENTAL SCREENING

Developmental screening takes a closer look at how your child is developing. Your child will get a brief test, or you will complete a questionnaire about your child. The tools used for developmental and behavioral screening are formal questionnaires or checklists based on research that ask questions about a child's development, including language, movement, thinking, behavior, and emotions.

Developmental screening can be done by a doctor or nurse but also by other professionals in health care, early childhood education, community, or school settings.

Developmental screening is more formal than developmental monitoring and normally done less often than developmental monitoring. Your child should be screened if you or your doctor have a concern. However, developmental screening is a regular part of some of the well-child visits for all children even if there is no known concern.

The American Academy of Pediatrics (AAP) recommends developmental and behavioral screening for all children during regular well-child visits at the following ages:

- 9 months
- 18 months
- 30 months

In addition, the AAP recommends that all children be screened specifically for autism spectrum disorder (ASD) during regular well-child visits at the following ages:

- 18 months
- 24 months

If your child is at higher risk for developmental concerns due to preterm birth, low birth weight, environmental risks such as lead exposure, or other factors, your health-care provider may also discuss additional screening. If a child has an existing long-lasting health concern or a diagnosed condition, the child should have developmental monitoring and screening in all areas of development, just like those without special health-care needs.

If your child's health-care provider does not periodically check your child with a developmental screening test, you can ask that it be done.

Facts about Developmental Screening

- **Who**. Health-care provider, early childhood teacher, or other trained provider.
- **What**. Look for developmental milestones.
- **When**:
  - developmental screening at 9, 18, and 30 months of age
  - autism screening at 18 and 24 months of age
- **Why**. To find out:
  - if your child needs more help with development because it is not always obvious to doctors, childcare providers, or parents
  - if more developmental evaluations are recommended

- **How**. With a formal, validated screening tool available at www.acf.hhs.gov/archive/ecd/child-health-development/watch-me-thrive.

DEVELOPMENTAL EVALUATION

A brief test using a screening tool does not provide a diagnosis, but it indicates if a child is on the right development track or if a specialist should take a closer look. If the screening tool identifies an area of concern, a formal developmental evaluation may be needed. This formal evaluation is a more in-depth look at a child's development, usually done by a trained specialist, such as a developmental pediatrician, child psychologist, speech-language pathologist, occupational therapist, physical therapist, or other specialist. The specialist may observe the child, give the child a structured test, ask the parents or caregivers questions, or ask them to fill out questionnaires. The results of this formal evaluation determine whether a child needs special treatments or early intervention services or both.

Facts about Developmental Evaluation

- **Who**. Developmental pediatrician, child psychologist, or other trained provider.
- **What**. Identify and diagnose developmental delays and conditions.
- **When**. Whenever there is a concern.
- **Why**. To find out:
    - if your child needs specific treatment
    - if your child qualifies for early intervention
- **How**. With a detailed examination, formal assessment tools, observation, and surveys from parents and other caregivers, often in combination, depending on the area of concern.

WHY DEVELOPMENTAL MONITORING, SCREENING, AND EVALUATION ARE IMPORTANT

Many children with developmental delays or behavior concerns are not identified as early as possible. As a result, these children must wait to get the help they need to do well in social and educational settings (e.g., in school, at home, and in the community).

In the United States, about one in six children aged 3–17 has one or more developmental or behavioral disabilities, such as autism, a learning disorder, or attention deficit hyperactivity disorder (ADHD). In addition, many children have delays in language or other areas that can affect how well they do in school. However, many children with developmental disabilities are not identified until they are in school, by which time significant delays might have occurred and opportunities for treatment might have been missed.

SERVICES FOR CHILDREN WITH DEVELOPMENTAL DISABILITIES

Research shows that early intervention treatment services can improve a child's development. Early intervention services can help children from birth through three years of age (36 months) learn important skills.

For children aged three and older with an identified developmental delay or disability, special education services may be provided.

Services can include a variety of options, depending on the child's need, such as therapy to help the child talk, move and walk, learn, and interact with others.

The Individuals with Disabilities Education Act (IDEA) says that children with a diagnosed disability should get special education services. The IDEA says that children under the age of three who are at risk of having developmental delays might be eligible for early intervention treatment services even if the child has not received a formal diagnosis. Treatment for particular symptoms, such as speech therapy for language delays, may not require a formal diagnosis.

Although early intervention is extremely important, intervention at any age can be helpful. It is best to get an evaluation early so that any needed interventions can get started. When parents are concerned about a child's development, it can be very challenging for them to figure out the right steps to take. States have created parent centers. These centers help families learn how and where to have their children evaluated and how to find services.[2]

[2] National Center on Birth Defects and Developmental Disabilities (NCBDDD), "Developmental Monitoring and Screening," Centers for Disease Control and Prevention (CDC), April 13, 2023. Available online. URL: www.cdc.gov/ncbddd/actearly/screening.html. Accessed February 23, 2024.

Chapter 8 | Milestone Checklist

Chapter Contents

Skills such as taking a first step, smiling for the first time, and waving "bye-bye" are called "developmental milestones." Children reach milestones in how they play, learn, speak, act, and move.

IMPORTANT MILESTONES: YOUR CHILD BY TWO MONTHS

How your child plays, learns, speaks, acts, and moves offers important clues about your child's development. Developmental milestones are things most children (75 percent or more) can do by a certain age.

- Social/emotional milestones:
  - calms down when spoken to or picked up
  - looks at your face
  - seems happy to see you when you walk up to him or her
  - smiles when you talk to or smile at him or her
- Language/communication milestones:
  - makes sounds other than crying
  - reacts to loud sounds
- Cognitive milestones (learning, thinking, and problem-solving):
  - watches you as you move
  - looks at a toy for several seconds
- Movement/physical development milestones:
  - holds head up when on tummy
  - moves both arms and both legs
  - opens hands briefly
- Other important things to share with the doctor:
  - What are some things you and your child do together?
  - What are some things your child likes to do?
  - Is there anything your child does or does not do that concerns you?
  - Has your child lost any skills he or she once had?
  - Does your child have any special health-care needs, or was he or she born prematurely?

Tips and Activities: What You Can Do for Your Two-Month-Old Child

As your child's first teacher, you can help with his or her learning and brain development. Try these simple tips and activities in a safe way. Talk with your child's doctor and teachers if you have questions or for more ideas on how to help your child's development.

- **Respond positively to your child.** Act excited, smile, and talk to him or her when he or she makes sounds. This teaches him or her to take turns "talking" back and forth in conversation.
- **Enhance your child's language skills.** Talk, read, and sing to your child to help him or her develop and understand language.
- **Spend time cuddling and holding your child.** This will help him or her feel safe and cared for. You will not spoil your child by holding or responding to him or her.

IMPORTANT MILESTONES: YOUR CHILD BY FOUR MONTHS

- Social/emotional milestones:
  - smiles on his or her own to get your attention
  - chuckles (not yet a full laugh) when you try to make him or her laugh
  - looks at you, moves, or makes sounds to get or keep your attention
- Language/communication milestones:
  - makes sounds such as "oooo" and "aahh" (cooing)
  - makes sounds back when you talk to him or her
  - turns head toward the sound of your voice
- Cognitive milestones (learning, thinking, and problem-solving):
  - if hungry, opens his or her mouth when he or she sees the breast or bottle
  - looks at his or her hands with interest
- Movement/physical development milestones:
  - holds head steady without support when you are holding him or her

- holds a toy when you put it in his or her hand
- uses his or her arm to swing at toys
- brings hands to mouth
- pushes up onto elbows/forearms when on tummy

IMPORTANT MILESTONES: YOUR CHILD BY SIX MONTHS

- Social/emotional milestones:
  - knows familiar people
  - likes to look at self in a mirror
  - laughs
- Language/communication milestones:
  - takes turns making sounds with you
  - blows "raspberries" (sticks tongue out and blows)
  - makes squealing noises
- Cognitive milestones (learning, thinking, and problem-solving):
  - puts things into his or her mouth to explore them
  - reaches to grab a toy he or she wants
  - closes lips to show he or she does not want more food
- Movement/physical development milestones:
  - rolls from tummy to back
  - pushes up with straight arms when on tummy
  - leans on hands to support himself or herself when sitting

IMPORTANT MILESTONES: YOUR CHILD BY NINE MONTHS

- Social/emotional milestones:
  - is shy, clingy, or fearful around strangers
  - shows several facial expressions, such as happy, sad, angry, and surprised
  - looks when you call him or her name
  - reacts when you leave (looks, reaches for you, or cries)
  - smiles or laughs when you play peekaboo
- Language/communication milestones:
  - makes a lot of different sounds such as "mamamama" and "babababa"
  - lifts arms up to be picked up

- Cognitive milestones (learning, thinking, and problem-solving):
  - looks for objects when dropped out of sight (such as his or her spoon or toy)
  - bangs two things together
- Movement/physical development milestones:
  - gets to a sitting position by himself or herself
  - moves things from one hand to his or her other hand
  - uses fingers to "rake" food toward himself or herself
  - sits without support

IMPORTANT MILESTONES: YOUR CHILD BY ONE YEAR

- Social/emotional milestones:
  - plays games with you, such as pat-a-cake
- Language/communication milestones:
  - waves "bye-bye"
  - calls a parent "mama" or "dada" or another special name
  - understands "no" (pauses briefly or stops when you say it)
- Cognitive milestones (learning, thinking, and problem-solving):
  - puts something in a container, such as a block in a cup
  - looks for things he or she sees you hide, such as a toy under a blanket
- Movement/physical development milestones:
  - pulls up to stand
  - walks, holding on to furniture
  - drinks from a cup without a lid, as you hold it
  - picks things up between thumb and pointer finger, such as small bits of food

IMPORTANT MILESTONES: YOUR CHILD BY 15 MONTHS

- Social/emotional milestones:
  - copies other children while playing, such as taking toys out of a container when another child does

    - shows you an object he or she likes
    - claps when excited
    - hugs stuffed doll or other toy
    - shows you affection (hugs, cuddles, or kisses you)
- Language/communication milestones:
    - tries to say one or two words besides "mama" or "dada," such as "ba" for ball or "da" for dog
    - looks at a familiar object when you name it
    - follows directions given with both a gesture and words (e.g., he or she gives you a toy when you hold out your hand and say, "Give me the toy")
    - points to ask for something or to get help
- Cognitive milestones (learning, thinking, and problem-solving):
    - tries to use things the right way, such as a phone, cup, or book
    - stacks at least two small objects, such as blocks
- Movement/physical development milestones:
    - takes a few steps on his or her own
    - uses fingers to feed himself or herself some food

IMPORTANT MILESTONES: YOUR CHILD BY 18 MONTHS

- Social/emotional milestones:
    - moves away from you but looks to make sure you are close by
    - points to show you something interesting
    - puts hands out for you to wash them
    - looks at a few pages in a book with you
    - helps you dress him or her by pushing the arm through a sleeve or lifting up the foot
- Language/communication milestones:
    - tries to say three or more words besides "mama" or "dada"
    - follows one-step directions without any gestures, such as giving you the toy when you say, "Give it to me"

- Cognitive milestones (learning, thinking, and problem-solving):
  - copies you doing chores, such as sweeping with a broom
  - plays with toys in a simple way, such as pushing a toy car
- Movement/physical development milestones:
  - walks without holding on to anyone or anything
  - scribbles
  - drinks from a cup without a lid and may spill sometimes
  - feeds himself or herself with his or her fingers
  - tries to use a spoon
  - climbs on and off a couch or chair without help

IMPORTANT MILESTONES: YOUR CHILD BY TWO YEARS

- Social/emotional milestones:
  - notices when others are hurt or upset, such as pausing or looking sad when someone is crying
  - looks at your face to see how to react in a new situation
- Language/communication milestones:
  - points to things in a book when you ask, such as "Where is the bear?"
  - says at least two words together, such as "more milk"
  - points to at least two body parts when you ask him or her to show you
  - uses more gestures than just waving and pointing, such as blowing a kiss or nodding yes
- Cognitive milestones (learning, thinking, and problem-solving):
  - holds something in one hand while using the other hand (e.g., holding a container and taking the lid off)
  - tries to use switches, knobs, or buttons on a toy
  - plays with more than one toy at the same time, such as putting toy food on a toy plate

- Movement/physical development milestones:
  - kicks a ball
  - runs
  - walks (not climbs) up a few stairs with or without help
  - eats with a spoon

IMPORTANT MILESTONES: YOUR CHILD BY 30 MONTHS

- Social/emotional milestones:
  - plays next to other children and sometimes plays with them
  - shows you what he or she can do by saying, "Look at me!"
  - follows simple routines when told, such as helping pick up toys when you say, "It's clean-up time"
- Language/communication milestones:
  - says about 50 words
  - says two or more words together, with one action word, such as "Doggie run"
  - names things in a book when you point and ask, "What is this?"
  - says words such as "I," "me," or "we"
- Cognitive milestones (learning, thinking, and problem-solving):
  - uses things to pretend, such as feeding a block to a doll as if it were food
  - shows simple problem-solving skills, such as standing on a small stool to reach something
  - follows two-step instructions such as "Put the toy down and close the door"
  - shows he or she knows at least one color, such as pointing to a red crayon when you ask, "Which one is red?"
- Movement/physical development milestones:
  - uses hands to twist things, such as turning doorknobs or unscrewing lids
  - takes some clothes off by himself or herself, such as loose pants or an open jacket

- jumps off the ground with both feet
- turns book pages, one at a time, when you read to him or her

IMPORTANT MILESTONES: YOUR CHILD BY THREE YEARS

- Social/emotional milestones:
    - calms down within 10 minutes after you leave him or her, such as at a childcare drop-off
    - notices other children and joins them to play
- Language/communication milestones:
    - talks with you in conversation using at least two back-and-forth exchanges
    - asks "who," "what," "where," or "why" questions, such as "Where is mommy/daddy?"
    - says what action is happening in a picture or book when asked, such as "running," "eating," or "playing"
    - says first name, when asked
    - talks well enough for others to understand most of the time
- Cognitive milestones (learning, thinking, and problem-solving):
    - draws a circle when you show him or her how
    - avoids touching hot objects, such as a stove, when you warn him or her
- Movement/physical development milestones:
    - strings items together, such as large beads or macaroni
    - puts on some clothes by himself or herself, such as loose pants or a jacket
    - uses a fork[1]

---

[1] National Center on Birth Defects and Developmental Disabilities (NCBDDD), "CDC's Developmental Milestones," Centers for Disease Control and Prevention (CDC), June 6, 2023. Available online. URL: www.cdc.gov/ncbddd/actearly/milestones/index.html. Accessed January 2, 2024.

Section 8.2 | **Key Preschool Milestones**

IMPORTANT MILESTONES: YOUR CHILD BY FOUR YEARS

What most babies do by this age:

- Social/emotional milestones:
  - pretends to be something else during play (teacher, superhero, or dog)
  - asks to play with children if none are around, such as "Can I play with Alex?"
  - comforts others who are hurt or sad, such as hugging a crying friend
  - avoids danger, such as not jumping from tall heights at the playground
  - likes to be a "helper"
  - changes behavior based on where he or she is (place of worship, library, and playground)
- Language/communication milestones:
  - says sentences with four or more words
  - says some words from a song, story, or nursery rhyme
  - talks about at least one thing that happened during his or her day, such as "I played soccer"
  - answers simple questions such as "What is a coat for?" or "What is a crayon for?"
- Cognitive milestones (learning, thinking, and problem-solving):
  - names a few colors of items
  - tells what comes next in a well-known story
  - draws a person with three or more body parts
- Movement/physical development milestones:
  - catches a large ball most of the time
  - serves himself or herself food or pours water, with adult supervision
  - unbuttons some buttons
  - holds crayon or pencil between fingers and thumb (not a fist)

Tips and Activities: What You Can Do for Your Four-Year-Old Child

- **Help your child be ready for new places and meeting new people.** For example, you can read stories or role-play (pretend play) to help him or her be comfortable.
- **Read with your child.** Ask him or her what is happening in the story and what he or she thinks might happen next.
- **Help your child learn about colors, shapes, and sizes.** For example, ask about the color, shapes, and size of things he or she sees during the day.

IMPORTANT MILESTONES: YOUR CHILD BY FIVE YEARS

What most babies do by this age:

- Social/emotional milestones:
  - follows rules or takes turns when playing games with other children
  - sings, dances, or acts for you
  - does simple chores at home, such as matching socks or clearing the table after eating
- Language/communication milestones:
  - tells a story he or she heard or made up with at least two events (e.g., a cat was stuck in a tree, and a firefighter saved it)
  - answers simple questions about a book or story after you read or tell it to him or her
  - keeps a conversation going with more than three back-and-forth exchanges
  - uses or recognizes simple rhymes (bat-cat and ball-tall)
- Cognitive milestones (learning, thinking, and problem-solving):
  - counts to 10
  - names some numbers between one and five when you point to them
  - uses words about time, such as "yesterday," "tomorrow," "morning," or "night"

    - pays attention for 5–10 minutes during activities (e.g., during story time or making arts and crafts (screen time does not count))
    - writes some letters in his or her name
    - names some letters when you point to them
- Movement/physical development milestones:
    - buttons some buttons
    - hops on one foot

Tips and Activities: What You Can Do for Your Five-Year-Old Child

- **Your child might start to "talk back" to feel independent and test what happens.** Limit the attention you give to the negative words. Find alternative activities for him or her to do that allow him or her to take the lead and be independent. Make a point of noticing good behavior (e.g., "You stayed calm when I told you it's bedtime").
- **Ask your child what he or she is playing.** Help him or her expand his or her answers by asking "Why?" and "How?" For example, say, "That's a nice bridge you're building. Why did you put it there?"
- **Encourage creative play with toys.** Play with toys that encourage your child to put things together, such as puzzles and building blocks.[2]

[2] National Center on Birth Defects and Developmental Disabilities (NCBDDD), "CDC's Developmental Milestones," Centers for Disease Control and Prevention (CDC), June 6, 2023. Available online. URL: www.cdc.gov/ncbddd/actearly/milestones/index.html. Accessed January 2, 2024.

Chapter 9 | Speech and Language Development

WHAT ARE VOICE, SPEECH, AND LANGUAGE?

Voice, speech, and language are the tools we use to communicate with each other.

- **Voice**. This is the sound we make as air from our lungs is pushed between vocal folds in our larynx, causing them to vibrate.
- **Speech**. This is talking, which is one way to express language. It involves the precisely coordinated muscle actions of the tongue, lips, jaw, and vocal tract to produce the recognizable sounds that make up language.
- **Language**. This is a set of shared rules that allow people to express their ideas in a meaningful way. Language may be expressed verbally or by writing, signing, or making other gestures, such as eye blinking or mouth movements.

HOW DO SPEECH AND LANGUAGE DEVELOP?

The first three years of life, when the brain is developing and maturing, are the most intensive period for acquiring speech and language skills. These skills develop best in a world that is rich with sounds, sights, and consistent exposure to the speech and language of others.

There appear to be critical periods for speech and language development in infants and young children when the brain is best able to absorb language. If these critical periods are allowed to pass without exposure to language, it will be more difficult to learn.

WHAT ARE THE MILESTONES FOR SPEECH AND LANGUAGE DEVELOPMENT?

The first signs of communication occur when an infant learns that a cry will bring food, comfort, and companionship. Newborns also begin to recognize important sounds in their environment, such as the voice of their mother or primary caretaker. As they grow, babies begin to sort out the speech sounds that compose the words of their language. By six months of age, most babies recognize the basic sounds of their native language.

Children vary in their development of speech and language skills. However, they follow a natural progression or timetable for mastering the skills of language.

WHAT IS THE DIFFERENCE BETWEEN A SPEECH DISORDER AND A LANGUAGE DISORDER?

Children who have trouble understanding what others say (receptive language) or difficulty sharing their thoughts (expressive language) may have a language disorder. Developmental language disorder (DLD) is a language disorder that delays the mastery of language skills. Some children with DLD may not begin to talk until their third or fourth year.

Children who have trouble producing speech sounds correctly or who hesitate or stutter when talking may have a speech disorder. Apraxia of speech (AOS) is a speech disorder that makes it difficult to put sounds and syllables together in the correct order to form words.

WHAT SHOULD YOU DO IF YOUR CHILD'S SPEECH OR LANGUAGE APPEARS TO BE DELAYED?

Talk to your child's doctor if you have any concerns. Your doctor may refer you to a speech-language pathologist, who is a health professional trained to evaluate and treat people with speech or language disorders. The speech-language pathologist will talk to you about your child's communication and general development. He or she will also use special spoken tests to evaluate your child. A hearing test is often included in the evaluation because a hearing problem can affect speech and language development.

Depending on the result of the evaluation, the speech-language pathologist may suggest activities you can do at home to stimulate your child's development. They might also recommend a group or individual therapy or suggest further evaluation by an audiologist (a health-care professional trained to identify and measure hearing loss) or a developmental psychologist (a health-care professional with special expertise in the psychological development of infants and children).[1]

[1] "Speech and Language Developmental Milestones," National Institute on Deafness and Other Communication Disorders (NIDCD), October 13, 2022. Available online. URL: www.nidcd.nih.gov/health/speech-and-language. Accessed February 23, 2024.

Chapter 10 | **Addressing Developmental Concerns**

The following tips will help you talk with your child's doctor's office and the evaluation centers.

DOCTOR'S OFFICE

When you call your child's doctor's office, say, "I would like to make an appointment to see the doctor because I am concerned about my child's development."

Be ready to share your specific concerns about your child when you call. If you wrote down notes about your concerns, keep them. Your notes will be helpful during your visit with the doctor.

EARLY INTERVENTION SERVICES OFFICE

When you call your state's early intervention services office (if your child is not yet three years old), say, "I am concerned about my child's development and would like to request an evaluation. Can you help me or let me speak with someone who can?"

- Be ready to share your specific concerns about your child. You will also be asked for some general information about yourself and your child (your name, your child's name and age, where you live, and more).
- Write down who you spoke to, the date, and what was said; you might need this information later.

ELEMENTARY SCHOOL OR BOARD OF EDUCATION

When you call your local elementary school or board of education (if your child is three or older), say, "I am concerned about my child's development and would like to talk with someone about having my child evaluated. Can you help me or let me speak with someone who can?"

- Be ready to share your specific concerns about your child. You will also be asked for some general information about yourself and your child (your name, your child's name and age, where you live, and more).
- Write down who you spoke to, the date, and what was said; you might need this information later.

WHILE YOU WAIT

If you have to wait to get an appointment to see a specialist or start intervention services, know that there are some simple things you can do today and every day to help your child's development.[1]

MAKE THE MOST OF PLAYTIME

Interact with your child as much as possible. Read books, sing songs, play with toys, make crafts, do household chores, and play outside together. Talk to your child: label items, point out interesting things, tell stories, comment about what you see and how you feel, and explain how things work and why things happen. Your child may not always seem to be listening, but he or she may be hearing more than you think.

FIND SUPPORT

Reach out. You are not alone. To find support and information for your family, visit the Family Voices website (https://familyvoices.org) or call 888-835-5669.[2]

---

[1] National Center on Birth Defects and Developmental Disabilities (NCBDDD), "How to Talk to the Doctor about Developmental Concerns," Centers for Disease Control and Prevention (CDC), June 6, 2023. Available online. URL: www.cdc.gov/ncbddd/actearly/concerned-whattosay.html. Accessed February 27, 2024.

[2] National Center on Birth Defects and Developmental Disabilities (NCBDDD), "What to Do While You Wait to See a Developmental Specialist," Centers for Disease Control and Prevention (CDC), June 6, 2023. Available online. URL: www.cdc.gov/ncbddd/actearly/concerned-whileyouwait.html. Accessed February 27, 2024.

Chapter 11 | **Developmental Milestones for Puberty and Adolescence**

GENERAL PHYSICAL CHANGES ADOLESCENTS EXPERIENCE

Although some of the physical changes that happen during adolescence are internal and not visible, others can be seen easily by others. These obvious changes in the body can affect how adults and peers of all sexes view and treat young people.

The changes that occur both inside and outside the body during adolescence happen through a process called "puberty." This process stems from the release of certain hormones (chemicals) in the brain. These hormones released are the same in all adolescents, but differences in hormone levels lead to different results in males and females. The physical changes in adolescents shift them from their childhood bodies to their adult bodies and give them the ability to get pregnant or cause pregnancy. This ability to get pregnant or cause pregnancy is called "fertility."

Anyone who looks at an adolescent male and female side by side will see some clear differences. Still, adolescents of both sexes exhibit many changes in common, most notably growth spurts in height and weight. During these growth spurts, bones and muscles get longer and stronger, which allows adolescents to take on tasks they were not able to do as younger children, such as lifting heavy objects and walking, running, or biking long distances. Many young people will reach their full adult height by the end of puberty. Beyond the growth spurts, other physical changes that happen in both males and females include body odor, acne, and more body hair.

As noted above, many of the physical changes in adolescence are related to fertility. Some adolescents may be embarrassed by these changes at first, but they need to know that these changes happen to everyone. Consider this short list:

- **Females will see changes where fat appears on their bodies**. For example, breasts become fuller, and hips grow wider. Females typically experience their first menstruation (or period) during adolescence. Early on, periods can be irregular and affected by illness, stress, and even exercise.
- **Males' shoulders become broader, and their muscles get bigger**. The penis and testicles also grow, and males will begin to experience erections and ejaculations, both voluntary and involuntary (sometimes happening while asleep). Males' voices also deepen during this time and may crack during the shift.

Beyond developing fertility, these visible sex-specific changes also let others know that a person is no longer a child. While the physical changes that adolescents experience happen to everyone, the timing and order of these changes will vary from person to person.

UNIQUE ISSUES IN PHYSICAL DEVELOPMENT

Although the major physical development milestones of adolescence happen to everyone, the timing of these milestones varies a lot, both between and within the sexes. Some adolescents exhibit physical signs of maturity sooner than their peers, and others exhibit them later. For example, the visible physical changes in males often begin a couple of years after they begin in females. The timing of a female's first period also varies: girls can start their period as early as 8 and as late as 16.

These differences can be hard for adolescents. They may feel self-conscious or worry that they do not fit in if they do not look like others of their age. These variations also can lead to other people treating adolescents in a way that does not match their cognitive or emotional development. For instance, females who develop visible curves or males whose voices change during middle school may be treated more like older teenagers by both their peers and adults, even if they do not have the cognitive or emotional maturity of older teenagers. In contrast, adolescents who exhibit physical changes later than their peers may be treated like younger children, even though they are more mature cognitively and emotionally. Some research suggests that youth who experience faster physical development are more likely to engage in risk-taking behavior than their peers and that teens who develop more slowly than their peers may be more likely to face bullying. Many factors can be responsible for differences in the timing and results of adolescents' physical changes, such as the following:

- **Genes**. A person's genetic makeup can affect the timing of puberty and what the changes look like.
- **Diet/nutrition and exercise before and during adolescence**. Overweight females, for example, are more likely to have their first period and experience breast development at younger ages than their peers.
- **Chronic illnesses**. Conditions such as cystic fibrosis (CF), asthma, diabetes, or bowel problems can contribute to delays in growth and puberty because of nutrient deficiencies, toxin excess, and/or medication side effects.
- **Substance use**. Smoking or using other drugs can harm adolescents' growth and development. Smoking can stunt lung growth and make it harder to grow strong bones.
- **Development in other areas**. Variations in cognitive, emotional, social, and/or moral development can also influence and be influenced by physical changes in adolescence. For instance, those who look different from their peers (e.g., being overweight or underweight) are at a higher risk of being bullied by peers.

HOW PARENTS AND CARING ADULTS CAN SUPPORT PHYSICAL DEVELOPMENT

Here are some ways that parents and other caring adults can support adolescents through these physical changes:

- **Let adolescents know that what they are going through is normal.** Although "normal" development covers a wide range, even older adolescents (and sometimes, their parents) are concerned with "fitting in." Remind teens that despite their concerns, their personal developmental path is okay, even if it is different from that of their peers. People develop at different times, and not all bodies will look the same even when fully developed. Variation is not at all unusual.
- **Encourage adolescents to have a positive view of their bodies.** Beyond reassuring that the timing of changes in the body varies from person to person, parents and caring adults can help adolescents appreciate their own bodies and developmental experiences. Reminding teens that they are valued and accepted no matter how they look can help nurture self-respect and self-esteem in adolescents and counter negative body image issues or other anxieties.
- **Get active with adolescents.** As with healthy eating, parents and caring adults can model physical activity, making it easier for adolescents to avoid becoming "couch potatoes." If able, parents can go on walks or bike rides with their adolescents or just toss around a ball. If a teen is competitive or very social, parents can help the teen to sign up for a sport at school or in a community league. For video game fans, parents can select games that involve physical activity, such as Just Dance.
- **Teach adolescents to avoid drugs.** It is important for parents to talk to adolescents about how smoking and other drug use can hurt their health and keep them from growing strong and to lead by example.
- **Make sure adolescents get enough sleep.** Sleep helps adolescents grow and strengthen their bodies and

perform better in school, sports, and other activities. Strategies for parents include having a "lights out" rule, limiting the number of electronic devices (e.g., cell phone, computer) in a teen's bedroom, and encouraging routines that help adolescents relax at the end of the day, such as reading a book before bed.

- **Show adolescents how to discuss and maintain their health**. Adolescents should receive regular health care, including vaccines and preventive care, such as "well visits." Parents and other adults also can help adolescents by giving them the skills to communicate with doctors and other health-care professionals comfortably and effectively, as well as time alone with health-care providers to discuss health concerns in private. This support matters even more for adolescents who have chronic conditions or disabilities.[1]

DEVELOPMENTAL MILESTONES

This is a time of many physical, mental, emotional, and social changes. Hormones change as puberty begins. Most boys grow facial and pubic hair, and their voices deepen. Most girls grow pubic hair and breasts and start their period. They might be worried about these changes and how they are looked at by others. This also will be a time when your teen might face peer pressure to use alcohol, tobacco products, and drugs, and to have sex. Other challenges can be eating disorders, depression, and family problems. At this age, teens make more of their own choices about friends, sports, studying, and school. They become more independent, with their own personality and interests, although parents are still very important.

[1] Office of Population Affairs (OPA), "Physical Development," U.S. Department of Health and Human Services (HHS), March 19, 2021. Available online. URL: https://opa.hhs.gov/adolescent-health/adolescent-development-explained/physical-development. Accessed February 27, 2024.

Here is some information on how young teens develop:

Emotional/Social Changes

Children in this age group might:

- show more concern about body image, looks, and clothes
- focus on themselves; going back and forth between high expectations and lack of confidence
- experience more moodiness
- show more interest in and influence by peer groups
- express less affection toward parents; sometimes might seem rude or short-tempered
- feel stress from more challenging schoolwork
- develop eating problems
- feel a lot of sadness or depression, which can lead to poor grades at school, alcohol or drug use, unsafe sex, and other problems.

Thinking and Learning

Children in this age group might:

- have more ability for complex thought
- be better able to express feelings through talking
- develop a stronger sense of right and wrong

Positive Parenting Tips

Following are some things you, as a parent, can do to help your child during this time:

- Be honest and direct with your teen when talking about sensitive subjects such as drugs, drinking, smoking, and sex.
- Meet and get to know your teen's friends.
- Show an interest in your teen's school life.
- Help your teen make healthy choices while encouraging him or her to make his or her own decisions.
- Respect your teen's opinions and take into account his or her thoughts and feelings. It is important that he or she knows you are listening to him or her.

- When there is a conflict, be clear about goals and expectations (such as getting good grades, keeping things clean, and showing respect) but allow your teen input on how to reach those goals (such as when and how to study or clean).

CHILD SAFETY FIRST

You play an important role in keeping your child safe—no matter how old he or she is. Here are a few tips to help protect your child:

- **Make sure your teen knows about the importance of wearing seat belts.** Motor vehicle crashes are the leading cause of death among 12–14-year-olds.
- **Encourage your teen to wear a helmet when riding a bike or a skateboard or using inline skates; riding on a motorcycle, snowmobile, or all-terrain vehicle; or playing contact sports.** Injuries from sports and other activities are common.
- **Talk with your teen about the dangers of drugs, drinking, smoking, and risky sexual activity.** Ask him or her what he or she knows and thinks about these issues and share your thoughts and feelings with him or her. Listen to what he or she says and answer him or her questions honestly and directly.
- **Talk with your teen about the importance of having friends who are interested in positive activities.** Encourage him or her to avoid peers who pressure him or her to make unhealthy choices.
- **Know where your teen is and whether an adult is present.** Make plans with him or her for when he or she will call you, where you can find him or her, and what time you expect him or her home.
- **Set clear rules for your teen when he or she is home alone.** Talk about such issues as having friends at the house, how to handle situations that can be dangerous (emergencies, fire, drugs, sex, etc.), and completing homework or household tasks.

HEALTHY BODIES

- **Encourage your teen to be physically active.** He or she might join a team sport or take up an individual sport. Helping with household tasks such as mowing the lawn, walking the dog, or washing the car also will keep your teen active.
- **Mealtime is very important for families.** Eating together helps teens make better choices about the foods they eat, promotes healthy weight, and gives your family members time to talk with each other.
- **Keep television sets out of your teen's bedroom.** Set limits for screen time, including cell phones, computers, video games, and other devices, and develop a family media plan.
- **Ensure your child gets enough sleep.** Make sure your child gets the recommended amount of sleep each night: For teenagers 13–18 years, 8–10 hours per 24 hours (including naps).[2]

---

[2] National Center on Birth Defects and Developmental Disabilities (NCBDDD), "Young Teens (12–14 Years of Age)," Centers for Disease Control and Prevention (CDC), September 23, 2021. Available online. URL: www.cdc.gov/ncbddd/childdevelopment/positiveparenting/adolescence.html. Accessed February 27, 2024.

Chapter 12 | Communicating with Your Child

Chapter Contents

Attention from you and other caregivers is important to your child. In fact, toddlers and preschoolers demand a lot of adult attention. Attention can be both positive and negative.

POSITIVE ATTENTION

Positive attention is used to show your child that he or she has done something you like. Positive attention includes things such as:

- praise
- hugs
- kisses
- pats on the back
- high-fives

NEGATIVE ATTENTION

Negative attention lets your child know you do not like what he or she has done. Negative attention includes things such as:

- scolding
- correcting
- yelling

There are two key things to remember about attention:

- Any attention (positive or negative) your child receives right after his or her behavior increases the chance that the behavior will happen again.
- Negative attention becomes a problem when we use it MORE than positive attention.

Let us take a look at an example.
Examples of positive and negative attention:
You are in the checkout line at the grocery store with your child.

- **Positive attention.** If your child waits by your side, you might say, "Thank you for being patient and staying by me."
- **Negative attention.** If your child runs away, you yell at him or her, "Come back here, now!"

WHEN TO NOT GIVE ATTENTION

Any attention you give after your child's behavior makes the behavior more likely to happen again. So, if you give your child attention after he or she does something you do not like, the misbehavior can increase. You can decrease misbehavior by limiting the negative attention you give. Ignoring is another good way to limit attention for behaviors you do not like.[1]

Attention from parents is very rewarding for children. Attention can be both positive and negative. Positive attention refers to things you do to let your child know you like something he or she did. Negative attention happens when you give your child attention for something you do not like. If your child keeps tugging at your shirt and calling your name, you may tell him or her to "Stop!" In this example, you have given your child attention. You may find yourself giving attention to negative behaviors more than positive behaviors because you are rushed or in a hurry. But for children, negative attention from you is still attention. Ignoring works because it takes away attention from the behaviors you want to decrease. Your child learns that he or she will not receive attention for misbehaving.

WHAT IS IGNORING?

Do not be fooled by the term ignoring. It is a very active process for the parent. Think of ignoring as the opposite of paying attention. When you ignore your child, you do not neglect him or her or stand by while he or she misbehaves. Instead, you take all your attention away from your child and his or her behavior. Ignoring usually helps stop behaviors that your child is using to get your attention. This includes behaviors such as throwing tantrums, whining, and interrupting. When you are ignoring, you do not look at your child or talk to him or her. Ignore all protests or excuses to get your attention. The goal is to decrease behaviors you do not like, or you want your child to stop.

---

[1] "Responding to Behavior," Centers for Disease Control and Prevention (CDC), November 5, 2019. Available online. URL: www.cdc.gov/parents/essentials/toddlersandpreschoolers/communication/goodbehavior.html. Accessed February 28, 2024.

WHY SHOULD YOU IGNORE YOUR CHILD'S MISBEHAVIOR?

Ignoring can help you reduce your child's misbehavior. Remember that children love attention. Negative attention, such as screaming or yelling, can be rewarding to a child. This is especially true if you were not paying attention to your child before the misbehavior started. By giving your child attention during tantrums, you may accidentally reward the behavior and increase the chance it will happen again. When you ignore some misbehaviors, you can make it less likely your child will do the behavior again.

WHAT MISBEHAVIORS SHOULD YOU IGNORE?

Ignoring is usually most effective for behaviors such as whining, crying when nothing is physically wrong or hurting, and tantrums. These misbehaviors are often done for attention. If parents, friends, family, or other caregivers consistently ignore these behaviors, they will eventually stop. Your child may also misbehave in ways that are not meant for attention and put him or her in danger. Dangerous and destructive behaviors should not be ignored. For example, if your child is hurting himself or herself, hurting others, or destroying objects, he or she should not be ignored. These misbehaviors should be stopped immediately. Other discipline and consequences such as time-out should be used.[2]

PRAISE

Praise happens when you give positive attention to your child for good behavior.

Why Is Praise a Good Tool to Use?

Praise lets your child know what behaviors you like. When you praise behaviors you like, your child will do those behaviors more often. Praise can also help your child feel good about himself or herself.

---

[2] "How to Use Ignoring," Centers for Disease Control and Prevention (CDC), October 2, 2017. Available online. URL: www.cdc.gov/parents/essentials/toddlersandpreschoolers/consequences/ignoring.html. Accessed February 28, 2024.

What Type of Praise Works Best?

Specific praise works best because your child knows exactly what you like. This type of praise is called "labeled praise." Unlabeled praise is a general statement that shows approval or affection. Unlabeled praise can help children feel good but does not help improve behavior. It does not let your child know exactly what is liked.

EXAMPLES OF UNLABELED PRAISE AND LABELED PRAISE

Unlabeled praise:

- Great job!
- Super!
- Way to go!

Labeled praise:

- What a great job of putting your toys away!
- You did a super job making your bed!
- Way to go sharing with your brother!

IMITATION

You imitate your child's behavior when you copy or mimic what he or she is doing. This means that you play with the same or a similar toy and attempt to use the toy like your child is using it.

Why Is Imitation a Good Tool to Use?

Any behavior you imitate is likely to be repeated by your child. When you imitate your child's play, you show him or her you are paying attention and like what he or she is doing. Imitation can help a child feel good about himself or herself and gives you a lot of chances to give positive attention.

DESCRIPTION

Descriptions occur when you talk about what your child is doing in as much detail as possible. You describe what your child is doing like a sports reporter might describe what is going on to someone who cannot see the action.

Why Is Description a Good Tool to Use?

Descriptions show your child you are interested in what he or she is doing, and you are giving him or her your full attention. In this way, descriptions can help build self-esteem because it lets your child know you think what he or she is doing is interesting. Descriptions are also helpful in holding your child's attention. This helps increase the length of time your child is able to stick to the task, which prepares your child for the focus he or she needs when he or she begins school. Descriptions can encourage language development because your descriptions give your child words to describe something, which helps build vocabulary, and they can help you teach your child. For example, you can teach your child how to count or name colors by using descriptions.

EXAMPLE: USING DESCRIPTION DURING PLAYTIME

"You're looking at all the pieces and trying to decide which one you want. Oh, you decided to put a green cowboy hat on the potato. Nice job getting the hat on. Now he has a mustache. You picked the green glasses that match the green hat. Those glasses are tough to put on, and I like how hard you are trying. I am glad you stuck with it, and you got those glasses on his face."[3]

Section 12.2 | **Effective Communication through Active Listening**

Active listening is a good way to improve your communication with your child. It lets your child know you are interested in what he or she has to say.

To practice active listening:

- Give your full attention to your child.
- Make eye contact and stop other things you are doing.
- Get down on your child's level.

[3] "Praise, Imitation, and Description," Centers for Disease Control and Prevention (CDC), November 5, 2019. Available online. URL: www.cdc.gov/parents/essentials/toddlersandpreschoolers/communication/goodbehavior-praise.html. Accessed February 28, 2024.

- Reflect on or repeat back what he or she is saying and what he or she may be feeling to make sure you understand.

It can be tempting to brush off our children's problems, especially if we have had a bad day or if we are busy. But our children need to know that we are going to listen to them. This will make it more likely our children will talk with us about their hopes and problems when they are older. Here is an example:

- **Active listening example 1**. Your child's baseball game is at 6:00 p.m. You only have a short time to make dinner, help with homework, and get everyone ready for the game. While the kids play, you quickly start making dinner. Soon, you hear your son crying. He comes and tells you that his brother hit him and called him a bad name. You are tempted to keep making dinner while nodding your head at what your son is saying, but then you decide to show him you are actively listening. You stop what you are doing, turn to him, make eye contact, and summarize what he has told you and how he seems to be feeling. You say, "It sounds like your brother made you feel sad when he hit you and said mean things." By doing this, you have let your child know that he has your full attention. He knows that his emotions and feelings are important to you.

Sometimes a child who is upset may not be able to name the emotion he or she is feeling. Active listening can be a great way to help him or her. Here is an example:

- **Active listening example 2**. You pick up your daughter from preschool. She is crying and tells you that her friend took her favorite toy and stuck out his tongue at her. You show her that you are actively listening when you say, "It seems like you are sad about your friend taking your favorite toy." Your daughter continues to cry and nods her head. She says that she thinks her friend will break the toy. You show her that you are still actively listening by saying, "So you are scared that your friend might break your toy." At this time, your daughter calms down a bit. You and your daughter continue to talk, and she knows that it is okay to be upset. She has begun to learn how to label and cope with her feelings by talking to someone.

USING REFLECTIONS TO SHOW YOU ARE LISTENING

Reflection is one way for you to show you are actively listening to your child. You can do this by repeating back what your child has said or by labeling and summing up how you think he or she feels.

Reflections of Words

When you reflect your child's words, you are giving attention to him or her for his or her use of words. This increases the chance that your child will talk more because he or she wants your attention. You do not have to repeat exactly what your child said, but what you say is usually very similar. You can add detail, shorten, or correct what your child has said. Following is an example.

Reflection example:

Child: "I drawed some sghetti."

Parent Response: "You drew some long spaghetti."

In this example, the parent corrects the grammar, pronounces "spaghetti" for the child and adds detail by describing the spaghetti as "long."

Reflection of Emotions

When you reflect your child's emotions, you watch your child's behavior and describe the emotions he or she seems to be having. This gives your child a word for the emotion and helps him or her learn that it is okay to talk about feelings. Reflection of emotions is not always easy. Here are some tips to make it easier:

- **Take a guess even if you are unsure**. There may be times when you are unsure what your child is feeling. For example, your child may be crying, but you may not know if he or she is angry, scared, or sad. Let him or her know that you are paying attention by saying, "It seems like you are upset" or "It sounds/looks like something is bothering you." Your child may not know himself or herself what he or she is feeling, and by talking, you can figure it out together.

- **Words are not needed all the time**. You can let your child know you are paying attention to how he or she feels by what you do even if you do not say anything. You can just sit with your child while he or she is upset or stay physically close and hold or comfort him or her.
- **You do not always have to agree**. Sometimes it is difficult to summarize or label your child's feelings because you think he or she should be responding in a different way. Telling your child to stop feeling a particular way does not show your child you are trying to understand how he or she feels. Help him or her deal with and understand his or her feelings by talking with your child about it.
- **Talk about other feelings**. Children may have several emotions at the same time. For example, your child might feel sad and afraid at the same time. Show your child you care about what he or she is showing on the outside and maybe feeling on the inside by talking about all the feelings.
- **Do not worry about getting it wrong**. Sometimes when parents are learning active listening skills, they worry that they will incorrectly summarize and label their child's feelings. You should not worry. Children usually correct their parents if their feelings are described incorrectly. If your child corrects you, try again. Reflect on what he or she has said to you and expand on it to give him or her more words and to learn ways to describe his or her feelings.[4]

---

[4] "Active Listening," Centers for Disease Control and Prevention (CDC), November 5, 2019. Available online. URL: www.cdc.gov/parents/essentials/toddlersandpreschoolers/communication/activelistening.html. Accessed February 28, 2024.

Section 12.3 | **Importance of Playtime**

Special playtime is a chance for you to focus on your child's good behaviors and build a strong, nurturing relationship. You can use the time to actively listen and practice praising, imitating, and describing your child's behavior. The more you practice the skills, the easier it is to use them in everyday situations.

TOYS AND ACTIVITIES FOR SPECIAL PLAYTIME

- **Use toys or activities that encourage your child to be creative**. Blocks, crayons, and paper are some toys and supplies that allow your child to use his or her imagination. If a toy moves and plays by itself, it is probably not a good idea to use it during special playtime.
- **Use toys and activities that are safe for your child's age**. Child scissors, plastic pots and pans, and large plastic blocks are good choices for young children. Avoid toys with small detachable parts for very young children.
- **Use toys and activities that are at the right skill level for your child**. With young children, you may want to use larger blocks because they are easier for younger children to hold and put together.
- **Make sure you have enough toys, so you can play with your child**. For example, you might want to have two dolls or trucks for special playtime so that you can easily imitate your child's behavior.

TIPS FOR SPECIAL PLAYTIME

- **Try to spend at least 5–10 minutes each day playing with your child**. Begin with at least five minutes of special playtime. When parents first start using praise, description, imitation, and active listening, they find that it takes a lot of energy and focus. It is hard to use the skills for more than five minutes. You can increase the amount of time you spend with your child in special playtime as your skill level improves. Other positive time with your child in addition to the special playtime is always good for you and your child. For instance, reading before bed or cuddling when watching a favorite show are also important for building a positive relationship with your child.

- **Be consistent with special playtime**. Try to make special playtime with your child happen at the same time each day. You and your child will enjoy it more when you choose a time when you can focus on having fun, you are not distracted by other activities, and when the time is predictable. Even if your child has had a bad day, keep the special playtime. This time will give your child the chance to get praise and attention from you for good behavior. It is a great way to show your child that you always love him or her.
- **Allow your child to lead the play activity**. Young children are told what to do all day. They have few chances to take the lead. If they are given time each day when they get to know the most about the activity and make the decisions, it will help them feel more independent and build confidence.
- **Praise your child's good behaviors**. Let your child know what you like about what he or she is doing. When you praise behaviors you like, your child will do those behaviors more often. Make the praise specific, so your child knows exactly what you like. Use hugs, high-fives, a pat on the head, or a pat on the back to give more power to your praise.
- **Imitate your child's behavior**. Copy or mimic things your child does or things he or she says. Play with the same or a similar toy and attempt to use the toy like your child is using it. When you imitate your child's behavior, your child will do those behaviors more often.
- **Describe what your child is doing**. Talk in as much detail as possible about what your child is doing. This is similar to the way a sports reporter or commentator might

describe what is going on to someone who cannot see the action. This shows your child you are interested in what he or she is doing and giving him or her your full attention.

- **Be enthusiastic**. Show your child you are excited to play with him or her. If you are unsure how to show enthusiasm, think about how your child reacts when he or she gets a new toy that he or she really likes. You want to act that way. Enthusiasm lets your child know you are enjoying your time with him or her. When you have fun, he or she will have fun too.
- **Reflect your child's words and emotions**. Reflect or repeat back what your child says. Watch his or her behavior and reflect what you think he or she is feeling. When you reflect your child's words and feelings, you show him or her you are actively listening and help him or her understand and deal with his or her feelings.
- **Limit questions during special playtime**. When you ask your child something and expect a response, you are asking a question. Your child is asked many questions throughout his or her day such as, "How was school?", "How old are you?", and What are you doing over there?" When we ask questions, we lead the conversation. Our questions may also suggest that we are not really paying attention or that we disagree with what our child is doing. For example, asking, "Would not you rather play with the blocks?" suggests you do not want to play with the toy your child has chosen. Asking "Why are you doing that?" suggests that your child is doing something wrong.
- **Limit directions during special playtime**. Directions tell your child what to do or guide his or her activities. Directions can be obvious requests such as "Hand me that crayon" or less obvious requests such as "How about using the pink now?" Directions take the lead away from your child. Remember, the child should be in the lead during special playtime. If the child does what you tell him or her to do, he or she is not making the decisions about the special playtime activity. And if the child disobeys, conflict

may occur. We want special playtime to be positive for the parent and the child.

- **Limit criticisms during special playtime**. Criticisms show you do not approve of something your child is doing. Criticisms often include words like "No," "Do not," "Stop," "Quit," and "Not." For example, you might say to your child, who is using a blue crayon and describes it as purple: "That is not blue. You are using a purple crayon." Criticism can also be much more obvious: "That was a dumb thing to do" or "You sure sound ugly when you whine like that." If children are criticized often, it can cause self-esteem problems. Criticism does not help to reduce problem behaviors. There are many times during the day when you need to use the words, "Stop," "No," and "Do not." This is okay. Avoiding these words during special playtime helps you and your child have time to focus more on the positive.
- **Ignore minor misbehaviors during special playtime**. Ignore minor challenging behaviors, such as whining that happen during special playtime. If your child is doing something dangerous or destructive, stop the behavior immediately and use a consequence, such as distraction or removal of a privilege. Remember that giving attention after any behavior will cause that behavior to happen more often. When you limit the attention you give to your child after misbehaviors, you can decrease the chance it will happen again.[5]

[5] "Special Playtime," Centers for Disease Control and Prevention (CDC), November 5, 2019. Available online. URL: www.cdc.gov/parents/essentials/toddlersandpreschoolers/communication/specialplaytime.html. Accessed February 28, 2024.

Chapter 13 | Early Intervention in Developmental Delays or Disabilities

Early intervention services can help infants and toddlers with disabilities or delays to learn many key skills and catch up in their development. There is a lot to know about early intervention.

WHAT IS EARLY INTERVENTION?

Early intervention is a system of services that helps babies and toddlers with developmental delays or disabilities. It focuses on helping eligible babies and toddlers learn the basic and brand-new skills that typically develop during the first three years of life, such as:

- **Physical**. Reaching, rolling, crawling, and walking.
- **Cognitive**. Thinking, learning, and solving problems.
- **Communication**. Talking, listening, and understanding.
- **Social/Emotional**. Playing and feeling secure and happy.
- **Self-help**. Eating and dressing.

Examples of Early Intervention Services

If an infant or toddler has a disability or a developmental delay in one or more of these developmental areas, that child will likely be eligible for early intervention services. Those services will be tailored to meet the child's individual needs and may include:

- assistive technology (devices a child might need)
- audiology or hearing services
- speech and language services
- counseling and training for a family
- medical services
- nursing services
- nutrition services
- occupational therapy
- physical therapy
- psychological services

Services may also be provided to address the needs and priorities of the child's family. Family-directed services are meant to help family members understand the special needs of their child and how to enhance his or her development.

Authorized by Law

Early intervention is available in every state and territory of the United States. The Individuals with Disabilities Education Act (IDEA) requires it—Part C of the IDEA, to be precise. That is why you will sometimes hear early intervention referred to as "Part C."

WHO IS ELIGIBLE FOR EARLY INTERVENTION?

Early intervention is intended for infants and toddlers who have a developmental delay or disability. Eligibility is determined by evaluating the child (with parents' consent) to see if the little one does, in fact, have a delay in development or a disability. Eligible children can receive early intervention services from birth through three years of age (and sometimes beyond).

- **For some children, from birth.** Sometimes it is known from the moment a child is born that early intervention services will be essential in helping the child grow and develop. Often this is so for children who are diagnosed at birth with a specific condition or who experience

significant prematurity, very low birth weight, illness, or surgery soon after being born. Even before heading home from the hospital, the child's parents may be given a referral to their local early intervention office.
- **For others, because of delays in development**. Some children have a relatively routine entry into the world but may develop more slowly than others, experience setbacks, or develop in ways that seem very different from other children. For these children, a visit with a developmental pediatrician and a thorough evaluation may lead to an early intervention referral.

Parents do not have to wait for a referral to early intervention. If you are concerned about your child's development, you may contact your local program directly and ask to have your child evaluated. That evaluation is provided free of charge. However, when a child comes to be referred, evaluated, and determined eligible, early intervention services provide vital support so that children with developmental needs can thrive and grow.

WHAT IS A DEVELOPMENTAL DELAY?

The term "developmental delay" is an important one in early intervention. Broadly speaking, it means that a child is delayed in some area of development. There are five areas in which development may be affected:

- cognitive development
- physical development, including vision and hearing
- communication development
- social or emotional development
- adaptive development

Developmental Milestones

Think of all the baby skills that can fall under any one of the developmental areas mentioned previously. Babies and toddlers have a lot of new skills to learn, so it is always of concern when a child's development seems slow or more difficult than would normally be expected.

Definition of "Developmental Delay"

Part C of the IDEA broadly defines the term "developmental delay." But the exact meaning of the term varies from state to state, because each state defines the term for itself, including:

- describing the evaluation and assessment procedures that will be used to measure a child's development in each of the five developmental areas
- specifying the level of delay in functioning (or other comparable criteria) that constitutes a developmental delay in each of the five developmental areas

IF YOU ARE CONCERNED ABOUT A BABY OR TODDLER'S DEVELOPMENT

It is not uncommon for parents and family members to become concerned when their beautiful baby or growing toddler does not seem to be developing according to the normal schedule of "baby" milestones.

"He hasn't rolled over yet."

"The little girl next door is already sitting up on her own!"

"She should be saying a few words by now."

While it is true that children develop differently at their own pace and that the range of what is "normal" development is quite broad, it is hard not to worry and wonder.

What to Do

If you think that your child is not developing at the same pace or in the same way as most children his or her age, it is often a good idea to talk first to your child's pediatrician. Explain your concerns. Tell the doctor what you have observed with your child. Your child may have a disability or a developmental delay, or he or she may be at risk of having a disability or delay. You can also get in touch with your community's early intervention program and ask to have your little one evaluated to see if he or she has a developmental delay or disability. This evaluation is free of charge, will not hurt your child, and looks at his or her basic skills. Based on that evaluation, your child may be eligible for early intervention services, which will be designed to address your child's special needs or delays.

How to Get in Touch with Your Community's Early Intervention Program

There are several ways to connect with the early intervention program in your community. Try any of the following suggestions:

- Contact the Pediatrics branch in a local hospital and ask where you should call to find out about early intervention services in your area.
- Ask your pediatrician for a referral to the local early intervention system.
- Visit the early intervention "contacts" page of the Early Childhood Technical Assistance Center (ECTA) at http://ectacenter.org/contact/ptccoord.asp.

What to Say to the Early Intervention Contact Person

Explain that you are concerned about your child's development and think your child may need early intervention services. Explain that you would like to have your child evaluated under Part C of the IDEA.

Referral

Write down any information the contact person gives you. You will probably be referred either to your community's early intervention program or to what is known as "Child Find." Child Find operates in every state to identify babies and toddlers who need early intervention services because of developmental delays or disabilities. You can use the Parent's Record-Keeping Worksheet (www.parentcenterhub.org/wp-content/uploads/repo_items/recordkeeping.pdf) to keep track of this important information. In general, it is a good idea to write down the names and phone numbers of everyone you talk to as you move through the early intervention process.

THE EVALUATION AND ASSESSMENT PROCESS

Service Coordinator

Once connected with either Child Find or your community's early intervention program, you will be assigned a service coordinator who will explain the early intervention process and help you through the next steps in that process. The service coordinator will serve as your single point of contact with the early intervention system.

Screening and/or Evaluation

One of the first things that will happen is that your child will be evaluated to see if he or she has a developmental delay or disability (In some states, there may be a preliminary step called "screening" to see if there is cause to suspect that a baby or toddler has a disability or developmental delay.). The family's service coordinator will explain what is involved in the screening and/or evaluation and ask for your permission to proceed. You must provide your written consent before screening and/or evaluation may take place.

The evaluation group will be made up of qualified people who have different areas of training and experience. Together, they know about children's speech and language skills, physical abilities, hearing and vision, and other important areas of development. They know how to work with children, even very young ones, to discover if a child has a problem or is developing within normal ranges. Group members may evaluate your child together or individually. As part of the evaluation, the team will observe your child, ask your child to do things, talk to you and your child, and use other methods to gather information. These procedures will help the team find out how your child functions in the five areas of development.

Exceptions for Diagnosed Physical or Mental Conditions

It is important to note that an evaluation of your child will not be necessary if he or she is automatically eligible due to a diagnosed physical or mental condition that has a high probability of resulting in a developmental delay. Such conditions include, but are not limited to, chromosomal abnormalities, genetic or congenital disorders, sensory impairments, inborn errors of metabolism, disorders reflecting disturbance of the nervous system's development, congenital infections, severe attachment disorders, and disorders secondary to exposure to toxic substances, including fetal alcohol syndrome. Many states have policies that further specify what conditions automatically qualify an infant or toddler for early intervention (e.g., Down syndrome and fragile X syndrome (FXS)).

Determining Eligibility

The results of the evaluation will be used to determine your child's eligibility for early intervention services. You and a team of professionals will meet and review all of the data, results, and reports. The people on the team will talk with you about whether your child meets the criteria under the IDEA and state policy for having a developmental delay, a diagnosed physical or mental condition, or being at risk for having a substantial delay. If so, your child is generally found to be eligible for services.

Initial Assessment of the Child

With parental consent, an in-depth assessment will be conducted to determine your child's unique needs and the early intervention services appropriate to address those needs. The initial assessment will include reviewing the results of the evaluation, personal observation of your child, and identifying his or her needs in each developmental area.

Initial Assessment of the Family

With the approval of the family members involved, assessments of family members are also conducted to identify the resources, concerns, and priorities of the family related to enhancing the development of your child. The family-directed assessment is voluntary for each family member participating in the assessment and is based on information gathered through an assessment tool and an interview with those family members who elect to participate.

Who Pays for All This?

Under the IDEA, evaluations and assessments are provided at no cost to parents. They are funded by state and federal monies.

WRITING THE INDIVIDUALIZED FAMILY SERVICE PLAN

Having collected a great deal of information about your child and family, it is now possible for the team (including you as parents) to sit down and write an individualized plan of action for your child and family. This plan is called the "Individualized Family Service Plan" (IFSP). It is a very important document, and you, as parents, are important members of the team that develops it. Each state has specific guidelines for the IFSP. Your service coordinator can explain what the IFSP guidelines are in your state.

Guiding Principles

The IFSP is a written document that, among other things, outlines the early intervention services that your child and family will receive. One guiding principle of the IFSP is that the family is a child's greatest resource and that a young child's needs are closely tied to the needs of his or her family. The best way to support children and meet their needs is to support and build upon the individual strengths of their family. So the IFSP is a whole family plan with the parents as major contributors to its development. The involvement of other team members will depend on what the child needs. These other team members could come from several agencies and may include medical people, therapists, child development specialists, social workers, and others.

What Info Is Included in an Individualized Family Service Plan?

Your child's IFSP must include:

- your child's present physical, cognitive, communication, social/emotional, and adaptive development levels and needs
- family information (with your agreement), including the resources, priorities, and concerns of you, as parents, and other family members closely involved with the child
- the major results or outcomes expected to be achieved for your child and family
- the specific services your child will be receiving

- where in the natural environment (e.g., home and community) the services will be provided (If the services will not be provided in the natural environment, the IFSP must include a statement justifying why not.)
- when and where your son or daughter will receive services
- the number of days or sessions he or she will receive each service and how long each session will last
- who will pay for the services
- the name of the service coordinator overseeing the implementation of the IFSP
- the steps to be taken to support your child's transition out of early intervention and into another program when the time comes

The IFSP may also identify services your family may be interested in, such as financial information or information about raising a child with a disability.

Informed Parental Consent

The IFSP must be fully explained to you, the parents, and your suggestions must be considered. You must give written consent for each service to be provided. If you do not give your consent in writing, your child will not receive that service.

Reviewing and Updating the Individualized Family Service Plan

The IFSP is reviewed every six months and is updated at least once a year. This takes into account that children can learn, grow, and change quickly in just a short period of time.

WHO PAYS FOR THE SERVICES?

Whether or not you, as parents, will have to pay for any services for your child depends on the policies of your state. Check with your service coordinator. Your state's system of payments must be available in writing and given to you, so there are no surprises or unexpected bills later.

What Is Free to Families?

Under Part C of the IDEA, the following services must be provided at no cost to families:

- the Child Find services
- evaluations and assessments
- the development and review of the IFSP
- service coordination

When Services Are Not Free

Depending on your state's policies, you may have to pay for certain other services. You may be charged a "sliding scale" fee, meaning the fees are based on what you earn. Some services may be covered by your health insurance, Medicaid, or Indian Health Services (IHS). The Part C system may ask for your permission to access your public or private insurance in order to pay for the early intervention services your child receives. In most cases, the early intervention system may not use your health-care insurance (private or public) without your express, written consent. If you do not give such consent, the system may not limit or deny you or your child services. Every effort is made to provide services to all infants and toddlers who need help, regardless of family income. Services cannot be denied to a child just because his or her family is not able to pay for them.[1]

[1] Center for Parent Information & Resources (CPIR), "Overview of Early Intervention," U.S. Department of Education (ED), July 2021. Available online. URL: www.parentcenterhub.org/ei-overview. Accessed February 27, 2024.

Part 3 | Birth Defects and Developmental Disabilities

Chapter 14 | **Understanding Birth Defects**

BIRTH DEFECTS ARE COMMON

Birth defects are common, costly, and critical conditions that affect 1 in every 33 babies born in the United States each year. Every 4 ½ minutes, a baby is born with a birth defect in the United States. That means nearly 120,000 babies are affected by birth defects each year. Birth defects are structural changes present at birth that can affect almost any part or parts of the body (e.g., heart, brain, foot). They may affect how the body looks, works, or both. Birth defects can vary from mild to severe. The well-being of each child affected with a birth defect depends mostly on which organ or body part is involved and how much it is affected. Depending on the severity of the defect and what body part is affected, the expected lifespan of a person with a birth defect may or may not be affected.

IDENTIFYING BIRTH DEFECTS

A birth defect can be found before birth, at birth, or any time after birth. Most birth defects are found within the first year of life. Some birth defects (such as cleft lip) are easy to see, but others (such as heart defects or hearing loss) are found using special tests, such as echocardiogram (an ultrasound picture of the heart), x-rays, or hearing tests.

CAUSES OF BIRTH DEFECTS

Birth defects can occur during any stage of pregnancy. Most birth defects occur in the first three months of pregnancy when the organs of the baby are forming. This is a very important stage of development. However, some birth defects occur later in pregnancy. During the last six months of pregnancy, the tissues and organs continue to grow and develop. For some birth defects, such as fetal alcohol syndrome, we know the cause. But for most birth defects, we do not know what causes them. For most birth defects, we think they are caused by a complex mix of factors. These factors include our genes (information inherited from our parents), our behaviors, and things in the environment. But we do not fully understand how these factors might work together to cause birth defects. While we still have more work to do, we have learned a lot about birth defects through past research. For example, some things might increase the chances of having a baby with a birth defect, such as:

- smoking, drinking alcohol, or taking certain drugs during pregnancy
- having certain medical conditions, such as being obese or having uncontrolled diabetes before and during pregnancy
- taking certain medications, such as isotretinoin (a drug used to treat severe acne)
- having someone in your family with a birth defect (To learn more about your risk of having a baby with a birth defect, you can talk with a clinical geneticist or a genetic counselor.)
- having certain infections during pregnancy, such as Zika virus and cytomegalovirus (CMV)
- experiencing fever greater than 101 °F (38.33 °C) or having an elevated body temperature due to heat exposure
- being an older mother, as the risk of chromosomal abnormalities increases with age

Having one or more of these risks does not mean you will have a pregnancy affected by a birth defect. Also, women can have a baby born with a birth defect even when they do not have any of these risks. It is important to talk to your doctor about what you can do to lower your risk.

PREVENTION OF BIRTH DEFECTS

Not all birth defects can be prevented. But there are things that a woman can do before and during pregnancy to increase her chance of having a healthy baby:

- Be sure to see your health-care provider regularly and start prenatal care as soon as you think you might be pregnant.
- Get 400 micrograms (mcg) of folic acid every day, starting at least one month before getting pregnant.
- Do not drink alcohol or smoke.
- Talk to a health-care provider about any medications you are taking or thinking about taking. This includes prescription and over-the-counter (OTC) medications and dietary or herbal supplements. Do not stop or start taking any type of medication without first talking with a doctor.
- Know how to prevent infections during pregnancy.
- Be proactive in identifying and treating fever when ill or after getting a vaccine. Treat fevers higher than 101 °F (38.33 °C) with Tylenol® (or store-brand acetaminophen), and avoid hot tubs, saunas, or other environments that might cause overheating.
- If possible, be sure any medical conditions are under control, before becoming pregnant. Some conditions, such as diabetes, can increase the risk of birth defects.

LIVING WITH A BIRTH DEFECT

Babies who have birth defects often need special care and interventions to survive and to thrive developmentally. State birth defects tracking programs provide one way to identify and refer children as early as possible for services they need. Early intervention is vital to improving outcomes for these babies. If your child has a birth defect, you should ask his or her doctor about local resources and treatment. Geneticists, genetic counselors, and other specialists are another resource.[1]

[1] National Center on Birth Defects and Developmental Disabilities (NCBDDD), "What Are Birth Defects?" Centers for Disease Control and Prevention (CDC), June 28, 2023. Available online. URL: www.cdc.gov/ncbddd/birthdefects/facts.html. Accessed March 11, 2024.

Chapter 15 | **Diagnosis of Birth Defects**

WHY GET TESTED

You may or may not want to know if your baby has a health condition before birth.

If you decide to have a diagnostic test, you can learn more about your baby's condition. You can also learn how to care for your baby after birth. You may need to make plans to give birth in a hospital that can provide your baby with special medical care.

WHO SHOULD BE TESTED

If you receive an abnormal screening test result, your provider will discuss diagnostic test options. These diagnostic tests are also offered to women with higher-risk pregnancies, which may include:

- women who are 35 years of age or older
- women who have had a previous pregnancy affected by a birth defect
- women who have chronic diseases such as lupus, diabetes, or epilepsy
- women who use certain medications

TYPES OF TESTS

High-Resolution Ultrasound

An ultrasound creates pictures of the baby. This type of ultrasound is used to look in more detail for possible birth defects or other concerns with the baby. It is usually completed between 18 and 22 weeks of pregnancy.

Chorionic villus sampling (CVS) testing involves collecting and testing a tiny piece of the placenta, called the "chorionic villus." This test can check for chromosomal or genetic disorders in the baby. It is completed between 10 and 12 weeks of pregnancy.

Amniocentesis

Amniocentesis is a prenatal test that takes amniotic fluid from around your baby in the uterus. The fluid is then tested to measure the baby's protein levels. Cells in the fluid can be tested for chromosomal disorders, such as Down syndrome, and genetic problems, such as cystic fibrosis. Amniocentesis is completed between 15 and 18 weeks of pregnancy.

There are several proteins for which an amniocentesis tests, which can indicate certain birth defects.

- **Alpha-fetoprotein (AFP).** One of the proteins the baby produces. A high level of AFP in the amniotic fluid may indicate a defect with an opening in the tissue. This could be a neural tube defect (NTD; anencephaly or spina bifida) or a body wall defect, such as omphalocele or gastroschisis.
- **Acetylcholinesterase (AChE).** An enzyme that the baby produces. This enzyme can pass from the baby to the amniotic fluid if there is an opening in the neural tube.

AFTER THE BABY IS BORN

Whether your baby is diagnosed during pregnancy or after birth, they may need special care as they grow. Parents can prepare for their child's needs by learning about their child's condition. This knowledge can equip you to make the best possible choices for your child's health. Children with special health care needs can benefit from the medical home approach to care. This personalized approach supports working together to ensure that the medical and nonmedical needs of children and families are met.[1]

---

[1] "Diagnosis of Birth Defects," Centers for Disease Control and Prevention (CDC), May 16, 2024. Available online. URL: www.cdc.gov/birth-defects/screening/diagnosis.html. Accessed June 28, 2024.

Chapter 16 | **Heart Defects**

Chapter Contents

Section 16.1 | **Congenital Heart Defects**

Congenital heart defects (CHDs) are the most common type of birth defect. As medical care and treatment have advanced, babies with CHDs are living longer and healthier lives.

WHAT ARE CONGENITAL HEART DEFECTS?

Congenital heart defects are present at birth and can affect the structure of a baby's heart and its function. They can affect how blood flows through the heart and to the rest of the body. CHDs can vary from mild (such as a small hole in the heart) to severe (such as missing or poorly formed parts of the heart). About one in four babies born with a heart defect has a critical congenital heart defect (CCHD). Babies with a CCHD need surgery or other procedures within the first year of life.

TYPES OF CONGENITAL HEART DEFECTS

The following are examples of different types of CHDs. The types marked with an asterisk (*) are considered CCHDs.

- atrial septal defect (ASD)
- atrioventricular septal defect (AVSD)
- coarctation of the aorta*
- souble outlet right ventricle (DORV)*
- dextro-transposition of the great arteries (d-TGA)*
- Ebstein anomaly*
- hypoplastic left heart syndrome (HLHS)*
- interrupted aortic arch (IAA)*
- pulmonary atresia*
- single ventricle*
- tetralogy of Fallot*
- total anomalous pulmonary venous return (TAPVR)*
- tricuspid atresia*
- truncus arteriosus*
- ventricular septal defect (VSD)

CAUSES OF CONGENITAL HEART DEFECTS

The causes of CHDs in most babies are unknown. Some babies have heart defects because of changes in their individual genes or chromosomes. CHDs are also thought to be caused by a combination of genes and other factors, such as environmental influences, the mother's diet, the mother's health conditions, or the mother's medication use during pregnancy. For example, certain conditions a mother has, such as preexisting diabetes or obesity, have been linked to heart defects in the baby. Smoking during pregnancy, as well as taking certain medications, has also been linked to heart defects.

SIGNS AND SYMPTOMS OF CONGENITAL HEART DEFECTS

Signs and symptoms of CHDs depend on the type and severity of the particular defect. Some defects might have few or no signs or symptoms. Others might cause a baby to exhibit the following symptoms:

- blue-tinted nails or lips
- fast or troubled breathing
- tiredness when feeding
- sleepiness

DIAGNOSIS OF CONGENITAL HEART DEFECTS

Some CHDs may be diagnosed during pregnancy using a special type of ultrasound called a "fetal echocardiogram," which creates ultrasound images of the developing baby's heart. However, some CHDs are not detected until after birth or later in life, during childhood or adulthood. If a health care provider suspects a CHD may be present, the baby can undergo several tests (such as an echocardiogram) to confirm the diagnosis.

TREATMENT FOR CONGENITAL HEART DEFECTS

Treatment for CHDs depends on the type and severity of the defect. Some affected infants and children might need one or more surgeries to repair the heart or blood vessels. Others can be treated without surgery using a procedure called "cardiac catheterization." In this procedure, a long tube called a "catheter" is threaded through the blood vessels into the heart, where a doctor can take measurements and pictures, perform tests, or repair the problem. Sometimes the heart defect cannot be fully repaired, but these procedures can improve blood flow and heart function. It is important to note that even if their heart defect has been repaired, many people with CHDs are not cured and require follow-up care.

LIVING WITH A CONGENITAL HEART DEFECT

As medical care and treatment have advanced, infants with CHDs are living longer and healthier lives. Many children with CHDs are now living into adulthood. It is estimated that more than two million individuals in the United States are living with a CHD. Many people with a CHD lead independent lives with little or no difficulty. Others might develop disabilities over time. Some people with a CHD have genetic problems or other health conditions that increase their risk for disability.

Even with improved treatments, many people with a CHD are not cured, even if their heart defect has been repaired. People with a CHD can develop other health problems over time, depending on their specific heart defect, the number of heart defects they have, and the severity of their heart defect. For example, some other health problems that might develop include irregular heartbeat (arrhythmias), an increased risk of infection in the heart muscle (infective endocarditis), or weakness in the heart (cardiomyopathy). People with a CHD need routine checkups with a cardiologist to stay as healthy as possible. They also might need further operations after initial childhood surgeries. It is important for people with a CHD to visit their doctor regularly and discuss their health, including their specific heart condition, with their doctor.[1]

[1] National Center on Birth Defects and Developmental Disabilities (NCBDDD), "What Are Congenital Heart Defects?" Centers for Disease Control and Prevention (CDC), February 2, 2023. Available online. URL: www.cdc.gov/ncbddd/heartdefects/facts.html. Accessed March 12, 2024.

DATA AND STATISTICS ON CONGENITAL HEART DEFECTS

Congenital heart defects are the most common types of birth defects, and babies born with these conditions are living longer and healthier lives. The statistics about CHDs are as follows:

Number of U.S. Babies Born with Congenital Heart Defects

- CHDs affect nearly 1 percent of—or about 40,000—births per year in the United States.
- The prevalence (the number of babies born with a heart defect compared to the total number of births) of some CHDs, especially mild types, is increasing, while the prevalence of other types has remained stable. The most common type of heart defect is a VSD.
- About one in four babies with a CHD has a CCHD. Infants with CCHDs generally need surgery or other procedures in their first year of life.
- The prevalence of all types of CHDs, including CCHDs, varies by state and by type of defect.[2]

Section 16.2 | Critical Congenital Heart Defects

About one in every four babies born with a heart defect has a critical congenital heart defect (CCHD). Babies with a CCHD need surgery or other procedures within the first year of life.

WHAT ARE CRITICAL CONGENITAL HEART DEFECTS?

In the United States, about 7,200 babies born each year have CCHDs. Typically, these types of heart defects lead to low levels of oxygen in a newborn and may be identified using pulse oximetry screening at least 24 hours after birth. Babies with a CCHD

[2] National Center on Birth Defects and Developmental Disabilities (NCBDDD), "Data and Statistics on Congenital Heart Defects," Centers for Disease Control and Prevention (CDC), September 19, 2023. Available online. URL: www.cdc.gov/ncbddd/heartdefects/data.html. Accessed March 12, 2024.

need surgery or other procedures within the first year of life. Other heart defects can be just as severe as CCHDs and may also require treatment soon after birth.

IMPORTANCE OF NEWBORN SCREENING FOR CRITICAL CONGENITAL HEART DEFECTS

Some CHDs may be diagnosed during pregnancy using a special type of ultrasound called a "fetal echocardiogram," which creates pictures of the developing baby's heart. However, some heart defects are not found during pregnancy. In these cases, heart defects may be detected at birth or as the child ages.

Some babies born with a CCHD appear healthy at first and may be sent home before their heart defect is detected. These babies are at risk of having serious complications within the first few days or weeks of life and often require emergency care. Newborn screening (NBS) is a tool that can identify some of these babies so they can receive prompt care and treatment. Timely care may prevent disability or death early in life.

HOW NEWBORN SCREENING FOR CRITICAL CONGENITAL HEART DEFECTS IS DONE

Newborn screening for CCHDs involves a simple bedside test called "pulse oximetry." This test estimates the amount of oxygen in a baby's blood. Low levels of oxygen in the blood can be a sign of a CCHD. The test is done using a machine called a "pulse oximeter," with sensors placed on the baby's skin. The test is painless and takes only a few minutes. Pulse oximetry screening does not replace a complete history and physical examination, which can sometimes detect a CCHD before oxygen levels in the blood become low. Pulse oximetry screening, therefore, should be used along with the physical examination.

TIMING OF CRITICAL CONGENITAL HEART DEFECTS SCREENING

Screening is done when a baby is at least 24 hours of age or as late as possible if the baby is to be discharged from the hospital before reaching 24 hours of age.

PULSE OXIMETRY SCREENING RESULTS

Pulse oximetry screening is most likely to detect seven of the CCHDs. These seven defects are hypoplastic left heart syndrome (HLHS), pulmonary atresia, tetralogy of Fallot, total anomalous pulmonary venous return (TAPVR), transposition of the great arteries, tricuspid atresia, and truncus arteriosus. Other heart defects can be just as severe as these seven and also require treatment soon after birth. However, pulse oximetry screening may not detect these heart defects as consistently as the seven listed previously.

Pass

If the baby passes the screen (also called a "negative" or "in-range" result), it means that the baby's test results did not show signs of a low level of oxygen in the blood. A baby that passes the screen is unlikely to have a CCHD. However, not all babies with a CCHD will have a low level of oxygen in the blood that is detected during NBS. Thus, it is possible for a baby who passes the screen to still have a CCHD or other CHD.

Fail

If the baby fails the screen (also known as a "positive" or "out-of-range" result), it means that the baby's test results showed low levels of oxygen in the blood, which could be a sign of a CCHD. This does not always mean that the baby has a CCHD, but it could mean that more testing is needed. There may be other causes, such as breathing problems, for low levels of oxygen in the blood. The baby's doctor might recommend that the baby be screened again or have more specific tests, such as an echocardiogram (an ultrasound picture of the heart), to diagnose a CCHD.[3]

[3] National Center on Birth Defects and Developmental Disabilities (NCBDDD), "Critical Congenital Heart Defects," Centers for Disease Control and Prevention (CDC), January 24, 2022. Available online. URL: www.cdc.gov/ncbddd/heartdefects/cchd-facts.html. Accessed March 12, 2024.

Section 16.3 | Septal Defects of the Heart

WHAT IS AN ATRIAL SEPTAL DEFECT?

An atrial septal defect is a birth defect of the heart in which there is a hole in the wall (septum) that divides the upper chambers (atria) of the heart. A hole can vary in size and may close on its own or may require surgery. An atrial septal defect is one type of congenital heart defect (CHD). Congenital means present at birth. As a baby's heart develops during pregnancy, there are normally several openings in the wall dividing the upper chambers of the heart (atria). These usually close during pregnancy or shortly after birth.

If one of these openings does not close, a hole is left, and it is called an "atrial septal defect." The hole increases the amount of blood that flows through the lungs, and over time, it may cause damage to the blood vessels in the lungs. Damage to the blood vessels in the lungs may cause problems in adulthood, such as high blood pressure (HBP) in the lungs and heart failure. Other problems may include abnormal heartbeat and an increased risk of stroke.

Occurrence of Atrial Septal Defect

In a study in Atlanta, the Centers for Disease Control and Prevention (CDC) estimated that 13 of every 10,000 babies born had an atrial septal defect. This means about 5,240 babies are born each year in the United States with an atrial septal defect. In other words, about 1 in every 769 babies born in the United States each year is born with an atrial septal defect.

Causes and Risk Factors of Atrial Septal Defect

The causes of heart defects, such as atrial septal defect, among most babies are unknown. Some babies have heart defects because of changes in their genes or chromosomes. These types of heart defects are also thought to be caused by a combination of genes and other risk factors, such as things the mother comes in contact with in the environment, what the mother eats or drinks, or the medicines the mother uses.

Diagnosis of Atrial Septal Defect

An atrial septal defect may be diagnosed during pregnancy or after the baby is born. In many cases, it may not be diagnosed until adulthood.

DURING PREGNANCY

During pregnancy, there are screening tests (prenatal tests) to check for birth defects and other conditions. An atrial septal defect might be seen during an ultrasound (which creates pictures of the body), but it depends on the size of the hole and its location. If an atrial septal defect is suspected, a specialist will need to confirm the diagnosis.

After the Baby Is Born

An atrial septal defect is present at birth, but many babies do not have any signs or symptoms. Signs and symptoms of a large or untreated atrial septal defect may include the following:

- frequent respiratory or lung infections
- difficulty breathing
- tiring when feeding (infants)
- shortness of breath when being active or exercising
- skipped heartbeats or a sense of feeling the heartbeat
- a heart murmur, or a whooshing sound that can be heard with a stethoscope
- swelling of legs, feet, or stomach area
- stroke

It is possible that an atrial septal defect might not be diagnosed until adulthood. One of the most common ways an atrial septal defect is found is by detecting a murmur when listening to a person's heart with a stethoscope. If a murmur is heard or other signs or symptoms are present, the health-care provider might request one or more tests to confirm the diagnosis. The most common test is an echocardiogram, which is an ultrasound of the heart.

Treatments for Atrial Septal Defect

Treatment for an atrial septal defect depends on the age at diagnosis, the number or seriousness of symptoms, the size of the hole, and the presence of other conditions. Sometimes surgery is needed to repair the hole. Sometimes medications are prescribed to help treat symptoms. There are no known medications that can repair the hole. If a child is diagnosed with an atrial septal defect, the health-care provider may want to monitor it for a while to see if the hole closes on its own. During this period, the health care provider might treat symptoms with medicine. A health-care provider may recommend closing the atrial septal defect for a child with a large atrial septal defect, even if there are few symptoms, to prevent problems later in life. Closure may also be recommended for an adult who has many or severe symptoms. Closure of the hole may be done during cardiac catheterization or open-heart surgery. After these procedures, follow-up care will depend on the size of the defect, the person's age, and whether the person has other birth defects.[4]

WHAT IS A VENTRICULAR SEPTAL DEFECT?

A ventricular septal defect (VSD) is a birth defect of the heart in which there is a hole in the wall (septum) that separates the two lower chambers (ventricles) of the heart. This wall is also called the "ventricular septum." A VSD happens during pregnancy if the wall that forms between the two ventricles does not fully develop, leaving a hole. A VSD is one type of CHD. Congenital means present at birth. In a baby without a CHD, the right side of the heart pumps oxygen-poor blood from the heart to the lungs, and the left side of the heart pumps oxygen-rich blood to the rest of the body.

In babies with a VSD, blood often flows from the left ventricle through the VSD to the right ventricle and into the lungs. This extra blood being pumped into the lungs forces the heart and lungs to work harder. Over time, if not repaired, this defect can increase the

[4] National Center on Birth Defects and Developmental Disabilities (NCBDDD), "Facts about Atrial Septal Defect," Centers for Disease Control and Prevention (CDC), June 21, 2023. Available online. URL: www.cdc.gov/ncbddd/heartdefects/atrialseptaldefect.html. Accessed March 12, 2024.

risk for other complications, including heart failure, HBP in the lungs (called "pulmonary hypertension"), irregular heart rhythms (called "arrhythmia"), or stroke.

Occurrence of Ventricular Septal Defects

In a study in Atlanta, the CDC estimated that 42 of every 10,000 babies born had a VSD. This means about 16,800 babies are born each year in the United States with a VSD. In other words, about 1 in every 240 babies born in the United States each year is born with a VSD.

Causes and Risk Factors of Ventricular Septal Defects

The causes of heart defects, such as a VSD, among most babies are unknown. Some babies have heart defects because of changes in their genes or chromosomes. Heart defects are also thought to be caused by a combination of genes and other risk factors, such as things the mother comes in contact with in the environment, what the mother eats or drinks, or the medicines the mother uses.

Diagnosis of Ventricular Septal Defects

A VSD is usually diagnosed after a baby is born. The size of the VSD will influence what symptoms, if any, are present and whether a doctor hears a heart murmur during a physical examination. Signs of a VSD might be present at birth or might not appear until well after birth. If the hole is small, it usually will close on its own, and the baby might not show any signs of the defect. However, if the hole is large, the baby might have symptoms, including:

- shortness of breath
- fast or heavy breathing
- sweating
- tiredness while feeding
- poor weight gain

During a physical examination, the doctor might hear a distinct whooshing sound, called a "heart murmur." If the doctor hears a heart murmur or other signs are present, the doctor can request one or more tests to confirm the diagnosis. The most common test is an echocardiogram, which is an ultrasound of the heart that can show problems with the structure of the heart, reveal how large the hole is, and indicate how much blood is flowing through the hole.

Treatments for Ventricular Septal Defects

Treatments for a VSD depend on the size of the hole and the problems it might cause. Many VSDs are small and close on their own. If the hole is small and not causing any symptoms, the doctor will check the infant regularly to ensure there are no signs of heart failure and that the hole closes on its own. If the hole does not close on its own or if it is large, further actions might need to be taken.

Depending on the size of the hole, symptoms, and general health of the child, the doctor might recommend either cardiac catheterization or open-heart surgery to close the hole and restore normal blood flow. After surgery, the doctor will schedule regular follow-up visits to ensure that the VSD remains closed. Most children who have a VSD that closes (either on its own or with surgery) live healthy lives.

MEDICINES

Some children will need medications to help strengthen the heart muscle, lower their blood pressure, and help the body get rid of extra fluid.

NUTRITION

Some babies with a VSD become tired while feeding and do not eat enough to gain weight. To ensure healthy weight gain, a special high-calorie formula might be prescribed. Some babies become extremely tired while feeding and might need to be fed through a feeding tube.[5]

---

[5] National Center on Birth Defects and Developmental Disabilities (NCBDDD), "Facts about Ventricular Septal Defect," Centers for Disease Control and Prevention (CDC), January 24, 2022. Available online. URL: www.cdc.gov/ncbddd/heartdefects/ventricularseptaldefect.html. Accessed March 12, 2024.

WHAT IS ATRIOVENTRICULAR SEPTAL DEFECT?

An atrioventricular septal defect (AVSD) is a heart defect affecting the valves between the heart's upper and lower chambers and the walls between the chambers. An AVSD is a heart defect in which there are holes between the chambers of the right and left sides of the heart, and the valves that control the flow of blood between these chambers may not be formed correctly. This condition is also called "atrioventricular canal" (AV canal) defect or endocardial cushion defect. In AVSD, blood flows where it normally should not go. The blood may also have a lower than normal amount of oxygen, and extra blood can flow to the lungs. This extra blood being pumped into the lungs forces the heart and lungs to work hard and may lead to congestive heart failure. There are two general types of AVSD that can occur, depending on which structures are not formed correctly:

- **Complete AVSD**. A complete AVSD occurs when there is a large hole in the center of the heart that allows blood to flow between all four chambers. This hole occurs where the septa (walls) separating the two top chambers (atria) and two bottom chambers (ventricles) normally meet. There is also one common atrioventricular valve in the center of the heart instead of two separate valves—the tricuspid valve on the right side of the heart and the mitral valve on the left side. This common valve often has leaflets (flaps) that may not be formed correctly or do not close tightly. A complete AVSD arises during pregnancy when the common valve fails to separate into the two distinct valves (tricuspid and mitral valves) and when the septa (walls) that split the upper and lower chambers of the heart do not grow all the way to meet in the center of the heart.
- **Partial or incomplete AVSD**. A partial or incomplete AVSD manifests when the heart exhibits some, but not all, defects found in a complete AVSD. There is usually a hole in the atrial wall or in the ventricular wall near the center of the heart. A partial AVSD usually has both

mitral and tricuspid valves, but one of the valves (usually mitral) may not close completely, allowing blood to leak backward from the left ventricle into the left atrium.

Occurrence of Atrioventricular Septal Defect

The CDC estimates that about 2,118 babies (1 in 1,859 babies) are born with AVSD every year in the United States.

Causes and Risk Factors of Atrioventricular Septal Defect

The causes of CHDs, such as AVSD, among most babies are unknown. Some babies have heart defects because of changes in their genes or chromosomes. In particular, AVSD is common in babies with Down syndrome, a genetic condition that involves an extra chromosome 21 (also called "trisomy 21"). CHDs are also thought to be caused by the combination of genes and other risk factors, such as things the mother comes in contact with in her environment, what she eats or drinks, or certain medications she uses during pregnancy.

Diagnosis of Atrioventricular Septal Defect

Atrioventricular septal defect may be diagnosed during pregnancy or soon after the baby is born.

DURING PREGNANCY

During pregnancy, there are screening tests (also called "prenatal tests") to check for birth defects and other conditions. AVSD may be diagnosed during pregnancy with an ultrasound test (which creates pictures of the baby using sound waves), but whether or not the defect can be seen with the ultrasound test depends on the size or type (partial or complete) of the AVSD. The health-care provider can request a fetal echocardiogram to confirm the diagnosis if AVSD is suspected. A fetal echocardiogram is an ultrasound of the baby's heart that shows more detail than the routine prenatal ultrasound test. It can reveal problems with the heart's structure and function.

AFTER THE BABY IS BORN

During an infant's physical examination, a complete AVSD may be suspected. Using a stethoscope, a doctor often detects a heart murmur (an abnormal "whooshing" sound caused by blood flowing through the abnormal hole). However, not all heart murmurs are present at birth. Babies with a complete AVSD typically manifest signs of problems within the first few weeks after birth. Symptoms may include:

- breathing problems
- pounding heart
- weak pulse
- ashen or bluish skin color
- poor feeding, slow weight gain
- tiring easily
- swelling of the legs or belly

For partial AVSDs, if the holes between the chambers of the heart are not large, the signs and symptoms may not occur in the newborn or infancy periods. In these cases, people with partial AVSD might not be diagnosed for years. Symptoms which might indicate that a child's complete AVSD or partial AVSD is getting worse include the following:

- **Arrhythmia.** It is an abnormal heart rhythm. It can cause the heart to beat too fast, too slow, or erratically. When the heart does not beat properly, it cannot pump blood effectively.
- **Congestive heart failure.** When the heart cannot pump enough blood and oxygen to meet the needs of the body.
- **Pulmonary hypertension.** A type of HBP that affects the arteries in the lungs and the right side of the heart.

The health-care provider can request one or more tests to confirm the diagnosis of AVSD. The most common test is an echocardiogram. This ultrasound of the heart can show structural problems, such as holes between the chambers of the right and left side of the heart and any irregular blood flow. An electrocardiogram (ECG or

EKG), which measures the heart's electrical activity, chest x-rays, and other medical tests may also be used to make the diagnosis. Because many babies with Down syndrome have an AVSD, all infants with Down syndrome should have an echocardiogram to check for an AVSD or other heart defects.

Treatments for Atrioventricular Septal Defect

All AVSDs, both partial and complete, usually require surgery. During surgery, any holes in the chambers are closed using patches. If the mitral valve does not close completely, it is repaired or replaced. For a complete AVSD, the common valve is separated into two distinct valves—one on the right side and one on the left side.

The age at which surgery is performed depends on the child's health and the specific structure of the AVSD. If possible, surgery should be done before there is permanent damage to the lungs from excessive blood flow. Medication may be used to treat congestive heart failure, but it is only a short-term measure until the infant is strong enough for surgery.

Infants who undergo surgical repairs for AVSD are not cured and might face lifelong complications. The most common of these complications is a leaky mitral valve, where the valve does not close completely, allowing blood to flow backward. This condition can cause the heart to work harder to supply enough blood to the rest of the body and may require surgical repair. A child (or adult) with an AVSD will need regular follow-up visits with a cardiologist to monitor progress, avoid complications, and check for other health conditions that might develop as the child gets older. With proper treatment, most babies with AVSD grow up to lead healthy, productive lives.[6]

---

[6] National Center on Birth Defects and Developmental Disabilities (NCBDDD), "Facts about Atrioventricular Septal Defect (AVSD)," Centers for Disease Control and Prevention (CDC), February 2, 2023. Available online. URL: www.cdc.gov/ncbddd/heartdefects/avsd.html. Accessed March 12, 2024.

Section 16.4 | Valve and Blood Vessel Defects

WHAT IS COARCTATION OF THE AORTA?

Coarctation of the aorta is a birth defect in which a part of the aorta is narrower than usual. If the narrowing is severe and undiagnosed, the baby may have serious problems and may need surgery or other procedures soon after birth. For this reason, coarctation of the aorta is often considered a critical congenital heart defect (CCHD). The defect occurs when a baby's aorta does not form correctly during pregnancy.

The narrowing of the aorta usually occurs in the section of the blood vessel just after the arteries branch off to supply blood to the head and arms, near the patent ductus arteriosus. However, sometimes the narrowing occurs before or after the ductus arteriosus. In some babies with coarctation, it is believed that some tissue from the wall of the ductus arteriosus blends into the tissue of the aorta. When the tissue tightens and the ductus arteriosus closes normally after birth, this extra tissue may also tighten and narrow the aorta.

The narrowing, or coarctation, blocks normal blood flow to the body. This can back up flow into the left ventricle of the heart, making the muscles in this ventricle work harder to get blood out of the heart. Since the narrowing of the aorta is usually located after arteries branch to the upper body, coarctation in this region can lead to normal or high blood pressure (HBP) pulsing of blood in the head and arms, and low blood pressure and weak pulses in the legs and lower body. If the condition is very severe, enough blood may not be able to get through to the lower body. The extra work on the heart can cause the walls of the heart to become thicker to pump harder. This eventually weakens the heart muscle. If the aorta is not widened, the heart may weaken enough that it leads to heart failure. Coarctation of the aorta often occurs with other congenital heart defects (CHDs).

Occurrence of Coarctation of the Aorta

The Centers for Disease Control and Prevention (CDC) estimates that about 2,200 babies are born with coarctation of the aorta each year in the United States. In other words, about 1 in every

1,800 babies born in the United States each year is born with coarctation of the aorta.

Causes and Risk Factors of Coarctation of the Aorta

The causes of heart defects, including coarctation of the aorta, among most babies are unknown. Some babies have heart defects because of changes in their genes or chromosomes. Heart defects, such as coarctation of the aorta, are also thought to be caused by a combination of genes and other risk factors, such as things the mother comes in contact with in the environment, what the mother eats or drinks, or medicines the mother uses.

Diagnosis of Coarctation of the Aorta

Coarctation of the aorta is usually diagnosed after the baby is born. How early in life the defect is diagnosed typically depends on the severity of the symptoms. Newborn screening (NBS) using pulse oximetry during the first few days of life may or may not detect coarctation of the aorta. In babies with a more serious condition, early signs usually include the following:

- pale skin
- irritability
- heavy sweating
- difficulty breathing

Detection of the defect is often made during a physical exam. In infants and older individuals, the pulse will be noticeably weaker in the legs or groin than in the arms or neck, and a heart murmur—an abnormal whooshing sound caused by disrupted blood flow—may be heard through a doctor's stethoscope. Older children and adults with coarctation of the aorta often have HBP in the arms. Once suspected, an echocardiogram is the most commonly used test to confirm the diagnosis.

Treatments for Coarctation of the Aorta

No matter the age at which the defect is diagnosed, the narrow aorta will need to be widened once symptoms are present. This can be done with surgery or a procedure called "balloon angioplasty," which is performed during a cardiac catheterization. A balloon angioplasty uses a thin, flexible tube called a "catheter," which is inserted into a blood vessel and directed to the aorta. When the catheter reaches the narrow area, a balloon at the tip is inflated to expand the blood vessel. Sometimes a mesh-covered tube (stent) is inserted to keep the vessel open. The stent is often used to initially widen the aorta or re-widen it if it narrows again after surgery. During surgery to correct a coarctation, the narrow portion is removed, and the aorta is reconstructed or patched to allow normal blood flow through the aorta.

Even after surgery, children with coarctation of the aorta often have HBP that is treated with medication. It is important for children and adults with coarctation of the aorta to follow up regularly with a cardiologist (a heart doctor) to monitor their progress and check for other health conditions that might develop as they get older.[7]

WHAT IS PULMONARY ATRESIA?

Pulmonary atresia is a birth defect of the pulmonary valve, which controls blood flow from the right ventricle (lower right chamber of the heart) to the main pulmonary artery (the blood vessel that carries blood from the heart to the lungs). Pulmonary atresia occurs when this valve does not form at all, preventing blood from flowing from the right ventricle to the lungs. Because a baby with pulmonary atresia may need surgery or other procedures soon after birth, this birth defect is considered a CCHD.

In a baby without a CHD, the right side of the heart pumps oxygen-poor blood from the heart to the lungs through the pulmonary artery. The blood that returns from the lungs is oxygen-rich and can then be pumped to the rest of the body. In babies with pulmonary atresia, the pulmonary valve that usually controls blood flow through the pulmonary artery is not formed, preventing blood from flowing directly from the right ventricle to the lungs.

[7] National Center on Birth Defects and Developmental Disabilities (NCBDDD), "Facts about Coarctation of the Aorta," Centers for Disease Control and Prevention (CDC), February 2, 2023. Available online. URL: www.cdc.gov/ncbddd/heartdefects/coarctationofaorta.html. Accessed March 12, 2024.

Causes and Risk Factors of Pulmonary Atresia

The causes of heart defects, such as pulmonary atresia, among most babies are unknown. Some babies have heart defects because of changes in their genes or chromosomes. Heart defects are also thought to result from a combination of genes and other factors, such as the things the mother comes in contact with in the environment, what the mother eats or drinks, or certain medicines she uses.

Diagnosis of Pulmonary Atresia

Pulmonary atresia may be diagnosed during pregnancy or soon after a baby is born.

DURING PREGNANCY

During pregnancy, there are screening tests (also called "prenatal tests") to check for birth defects and other conditions. Pulmonary atresia might be detected during an ultrasound (which creates pictures of the body). Some findings from the ultrasound may lead the health-care provider to suspect that the baby has pulmonary atresia. If so, the health-care provider can request a fetal echocardiogram to confirm the diagnosis. This test can show problems with the structure of the heart and how well the heart is functioning.

AFTER THE BABY IS BORN

Babies born with pulmonary atresia will show symptoms at birth or very soon afterward. They may have a bluish-looking skin color, called "cyanosis," because their blood does not carry enough oxygen. Infants with pulmonary atresia can have additional symptoms such as:

- problems breathing
- ashen or bluish skin color
- poor feeding
- extreme sleepiness

During a physical examination, a doctor can see the symptoms, such as bluish skin or problems breathing. Using a stethoscope, a doctor will check for a heart murmur (an abnormal "whooshing" sound caused by blood not flowing properly). However, it is not uncommon for a heart murmur to be absent right at birth.

If a doctor suspects a problem, they can request one or more tests to confirm the diagnosis of pulmonary atresia. The most common test is an echocardiogram, an ultrasound of the baby's heart that can show problems with the structure of the heart, such as holes in the walls between chambers, and any irregular blood flow. Cardiac catheterization (inserting a thin tube into a blood vessel and guiding it to the heart) can also confirm the diagnosis by examining the inside of the heart and measuring blood pressure and oxygen levels. An electrocardiogram (ECG or EKG), which measures the heart's electrical activity, and other medical tests may also be used for diagnosis.

Treatments for Pulmonary Atresia

Most babies with pulmonary atresia will need medication to keep the ductus arteriosus open after birth. Keeping this blood vessel open will help with blood flow to the lungs until the pulmonary valve can be repaired. Treatment for pulmonary atresia depends on its severity.

- In some cases, blood flow can be improved by using cardiac catheterization (inserting a thin tube into a blood vessel and guiding it to the heart). During this procedure, doctors can expand the valve using a balloon, or they may need to place a stent (a small tube) to keep the ductus arteriosus open.
- In most cases of pulmonary atresia, a baby may need surgery soon after birth. During surgery, doctors widen or replace the pulmonary valve and enlarge the passage to the pulmonary artery. If a baby has a ventricular septal defect (VSD), the doctor will also place a patch over the VSD to close the hole between the two lower chambers of the heart. These actions will improve blood flow to the lungs and the rest of the body. If a baby with pulmonary atresia has an underdeveloped right ventricle, he or she might need staged surgical

procedures, similar to those used for hypoplastic left heart syndrome (HLHS).

Most babies with pulmonary atresia will need regular follow-up visits with a cardiologist to monitor their progress and check for other health conditions that might develop as they get older. As adults, they may need more surgery or medical care for other possible problems.[8]

WHAT IS TRUNCUS ARTERIOSUS?

Truncus arteriosus, also known as "common truncus," is a rare heart defect in which a single common blood vessel comes out of the heart instead of the usual two vessels (the main pulmonary artery and aorta). Truncus arteriosus is a birth defect of the heart. It occurs when the blood vessel coming out of the heart in the developing baby fails to separate completely during development, leaving a connection between the aorta and pulmonary artery.

There are several types of truncus, depending on how the arteries remain connected. There is usually a hole between the bottom two chambers of the heart (ventricles) called a "VSD." Because a baby with this defect may need surgery or other procedures soon after birth, truncus arteriosus is considered a CCHD. Congenital means present at birth. In a baby without a CHD, the right side of the heart pumps oxygen-poor blood through the pulmonary artery to the lungs.

The left side of the heart pumps oxygen-rich blood through the aorta to the rest of the body. In babies with a truncus arteriosus, oxygen-poor blood and oxygen-rich blood are mixed together as blood flows to the lungs and the rest of the body. As a result, too much blood goes to the lungs, and the heart works harder to pump blood to the rest of the body. Also, instead of having both an aortic valve and a pulmonary valve, babies with truncus arteriosus have a single common valve (truncal valve) controlling blood flow out

[8] National Center on Birth Defects and Developmental Disabilities (NCBDDD), "Facts about Pulmonary Atresia," Centers for Disease Control and Prevention (CDC), January 24, 2022. Available online. URL: www.cdc.gov/ncbddd/heartdefects/pulmonaryatresia.html. Accessed March 12, 2024.

of the heart. The truncal valve is often abnormal. The valve can be thickened and narrowed, which can block the blood as it leaves the heart. It can also leak, causing blood that leaves the heart to leak back into the heart across the valve.

Causes and Risk Factors of Truncus Arteriosus

The causes of heart defects, such as truncus arteriosus, among most babies are unknown. Some babies have CHDs because of changes in their genes or chromosomes. CHDs are also thought to be caused by the combination of genes and other risk factors, such as things the mother comes in contact with in her environment, what the mother eats or drinks, or certain medications she uses.

Diagnosis of Truncus Arteriosus

Truncus arteriosus may be diagnosed during pregnancy or soon after the baby is born.

DURING PREGNANCY

During pregnancy, there are screening tests (also called "prenatal tests") to check for birth defects and other conditions. Some heart defects might be seen during an ultrasound (which creates pictures of the body). If a health-care provider suspects a baby might have truncus arteriosus, the health-care provider can request a fetal echocardiogram to confirm the diagnosis. A fetal echocardiogram is a more detailed ultrasound of the baby's heart. This test can show problems with the structure of the heart, such as a single large vessel coming from the heart, and how the heart is working with this defect.

AFTER A BABY IS BORN

Infants with truncus arteriosus are usually in distress in the first few days of life because of the high amount of blood going to the lungs, which makes the heart work harder. They can have a bluish-looking skin color, called "cyanosis," because their blood does not carry enough oxygen. Infants with truncus arteriosus or other conditions causing cyanosis can have symptoms such as:

- problems breathing
- pounding heart
- weak pulse
- ashen or bluish skin color
- poor feeding
- extreme sleepiness

If a health-care provider suspects a baby might have truncus arteriosus, they can request an echocardiogram to confirm the diagnosis. An echocardiogram is an ultrasound of the heart that can show problems with the structure of the heart, such as the single large vessel coming from the heart or misshapen truncal valve. It can also show how the heart is working (or not) with this defect, such as if the blood is leaking back into the heart or if it is moving through a hole between the ventricles. Echocardiograms are also useful for helping the doctor follow the child's health over time.

Treatment for Truncus Arteriosus

MEDICATIONS

Some babies with truncus arteriosus will also need medicines to help strengthen the heart muscle, lower their blood pressure, and help their body get rid of extra fluid.

NUTRITION

Some babies with truncus arteriosus might become tired while feeding and might not eat enough to gain weight. To make sure babies have a healthy weight gain, a special high-calorie formula might be prescribed. Some babies become extremely tired while feeding and might need to be fed through a feeding tube.

SURGERY

Surgery is needed to repair the heart and blood vessels. This is usually done in the first few months of life. Options for repair depend on how sick the child is and the specific structure of the defect. The goal of the surgery to repair truncus arteriosus is to create a separate flow of oxygen-poor blood to the lungs and oxygen-rich blood to the body. Usually, surgery to repair this defect involves the following steps:

- Close the hole between the bottom chambers of the heart (VSD), usually with a patch.
- Use the original single blood vessel to create a new aorta to carry oxygen-rich blood from the left ventricle out to the body.
- Use an artificial tube (conduit) with an artificial valve to connect the right ventricle to the arteries going to the lungs to carry oxygen-poor blood to the lungs.

Most babies with truncus arteriosus survive the surgical repair but may need more surgery or other procedures as they get older. For example, the artificial tube does not grow, so it will need to be replaced as the child grows. There may also be blockages to blood flow which may need to be relieved, or problems with the truncal valve. Thus, a person born with truncus arteriosus will need regular follow-up visits with a cardiologist to monitor their progress and avoid complications or other health problems.[9]

Section 16.5 | **Tetralogy of Fallot**

WHAT IS TETRALOGY OF FALLOT?

Tetralogy of Fallot is a birth defect that affects normal blood flow through the heart. It happens when a baby's heart does not form correctly as the baby grows and develops in the mother's womb

[9] National Center on Birth Defects and Developmental Disabilities (NCBDDD), "Facts about Truncus Arteriosus," Centers for Disease Control and Prevention (CDC), February 3, 2023. Available online. URL: www.cdc.gov/ncbddd/heartdefects/truncusarteriosus.html. Accessed March 12, 2024.

during pregnancy. Tetralogy of Fallot is made up of the following four defects of the heart and its blood vessels:

- **A hole in the wall between the two lower chambers—or ventricles—of the heart.** This condition is also called a "ventricular septal defect" (VSD).
- **A narrowing of the pulmonary valve and main pulmonary artery.** This condition is also called "pulmonary stenosis."
- **The aortic valve, which opens to the aorta, is enlarged and seems to open from both ventricles, rather than from the left ventricle only, as in a normal heart.** In this defect, the aortic valve sits directly on top of the VSD.
- **The muscular wall of the lower right chamber of the heart (right ventricle) is thicker than normal.** This is also called "ventricular hypertrophy."

Because a baby with tetralogy of Fallot may need surgery or other procedures soon after birth, this birth defect is considered a critical congenital heart defect (CCHD). Congenital means present at birth. This heart defect can reduce the oxygen in the blood that flows to the rest of the body. Infants with tetralogy of Fallot can have a bluish-looking skin color, called "cyanosis," because their blood does not carry enough oxygen. At birth, infants might not have blue-looking skin but might later develop sudden episodes of bluish skin during crying or feeding. These episodes are called "tet spells." Infants with tetralogy of Fallot or other conditions causing cyanosis can have problems including:

- a higher risk of getting an infection of the layers of the heart called "endocarditis"
- a higher risk of having irregular heart rhythms, called "arrhythmia"
- dizziness, fainting, or seizures because of the low oxygen levels in their blood
- delayed growth and development

OCCURRENCE OF TETRALOGY OF FALLOT

The Centers for Disease Control and Prevention (CDC) estimates that each year about 1,660 babies in the United States are born with tetralogy of Fallot. In other words, about 1 in every 2,518, babies born in the United States each year is born with tetralogy of Fallot.

CAUSES AND RISK FACTORS OF TETRALOGY OF FALLOT

The causes of heart defects (such as tetralogy of Fallot) among most babies are unknown. Some babies have heart defects because of changes in their genes or chromosomes. Heart defects such as tetralogy of Fallot are also thought to be caused by a combination of genes and other risk factors, such as the things the mother or fetus comes in contact with in the environment, what the mother eats or drinks, or the medicines she uses.

DIAGNOSIS OF TETRALOGY OF FALLOT

Tetralogy of Fallot may be diagnosed during pregnancy or soon after a baby is born.

During Pregnancy

During pregnancy, there are screening tests (also called "prenatal tests") to check for birth defects and other conditions. Tetralogy of Fallot might be detected during an ultrasound (which creates pictures of the body). Some findings from the ultrasound may lead the health-care provider to suspect that a baby has tetralogy of Fallot. If so, the health-care provider can request a fetal echocardiogram to confirm the diagnosis. A fetal echocardiogram is an ultrasound of the heart of the fetus. This test can show problems with the structure of the heart and how the heart is functioning with this defect.

After a Baby Is Born

Tetralogy of Fallot is usually diagnosed after a baby is born, often after the infant has an episode of turning blue during crying or feeding (a tet spell). Some findings on a physical exam may make the health-care provider think a baby may have tetralogy of Fallot, including bluish-looking skin or a heart murmur (a "whooshing" sound caused by blood not flowing properly through the heart). However, it is not uncommon for a heart murmur to be absent right at birth. The health-care provider can request one or more tests to confirm the diagnosis. The most common test is an echocardiogram. An echocardiogram is an ultrasound of the heart that can show problems with the structure of the heart and how the heart is working (or not) with this defect. Echocardiography is also useful for helping the doctor follow the child's health over time. Tetralogy of Fallot is a CCHD that may be detected with newborn screening (NBS) using pulse oximetry (also known as "pulse ox"). Pulse oximetry is a simple bedside test to estimate the amount of oxygen in a baby's blood. Low levels of oxygen in the blood can be a sign of a CCHD. NBS using pulse oximetry can identify some infants with a CCHD, such as tetralogy of Fallot before they show any symptoms.

TREATMENT FOR TETRALOGY OF FALLOT

Tetralogy of Fallot can be treated by surgery soon after the baby is born. During surgery, doctors widen or replace the pulmonary valve and enlarge the passage to the pulmonary artery. They will also place a patch over the VSD to close the hole between the two lower chambers of the heart. These actions will improve blood flow to the lungs and the rest of the body. Most infants will live active, healthy lives after surgery. However, they will need regular follow-up visits with a cardiologist to monitor their progress and check for other health conditions that might develop as they get older. As adults, they may need more surgery or medical care for other possible problems.[10]

---

[10] National Center on Birth Defects and Developmental Disabilities (NCBDDD), "Facts about Tetralogy of Fallot," Centers for Disease Control and Prevention (CDC), February 3, 2023. Available online. URL: www.cdc.gov/ncbddd/heartdefects/tetralogyoffallot.html. Accessed March 12, 2024.

Chapter 17 | **Neural Tube Defects**

Neural tube defects (NTDs) are abnormalities that can occur in the brain, spinal cord, or spine of a developing fetus. Very early in the development of a fetus, certain cells form a tube (called the "neural tube") that will later become the spinal cord, the brain, and the nearby structures that protect them, including the backbone (also called the "spinal column" or "vertebrae"). As development progresses, the top of the tube becomes the brain, and the remainder becomes the spinal cord. An NTD occurs when this tube does not close completely somewhere along its length, resulting in a hole in the spinal column or another type of problem. These defects occur in the first month of pregnancy, often before a woman even knows that she is pregnant. Because they are present at birth, they are categorized as birth defects.[1]

WHAT IS SPINA BIFIDA?

Spina bifida is a condition that affects the spine and is usually apparent at birth. It is a type of NTD. Spina bifida can happen anywhere along the spine if the neural tube does not close all the way. When the neural tube does not close all the way, the backbone that protects the spinal cord does not form and close as it should. This often results in damage to the spinal cord and nerves. Spina

[1] "Neural Tube Defects (NTDs)," *Eunice Kennedy Shriver* National Institute of Child Health and Human Development (NICHD), August 17, 2018. Available online. URL: www.nichd.nih.gov/health/topics/ntds. Accessed March 12, 2024.

bifida might cause physical and intellectual disabilities that range from mild to severe (see Figure 17.1). The severity depends on:

- the size and location of the opening in the spine
- whether part of the spinal cord and nerves are affected

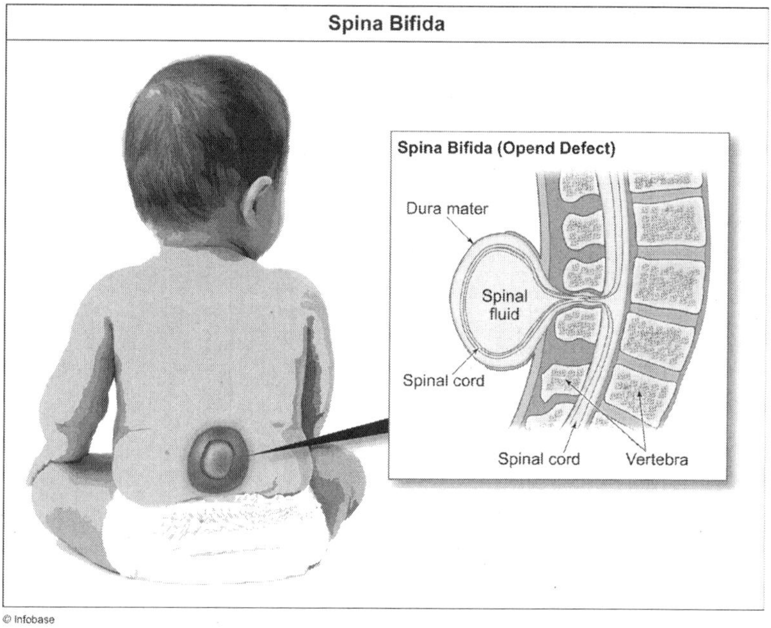

Figure 17.1. Spina Bifida

Infobase

Types of Spina Bifida

The three most common types of spina bifida are as follows:

- **Myelomeningocele.** When people talk about spina bifida, most often they are referring to myelomeningocele. Myelomeningocele is the most serious type of spina bifida. With this condition, a sac of fluid comes through an opening in the baby's back. Part of the spinal cord and nerves are in this sac and are damaged. This type of spina bifida causes moderate-to-severe disabilities, such as problems affecting how the person goes to the bathroom, loss of feeling in the person's legs or feet, and not being able to move the legs.

- **Meningocele**. Another type of spina bifida is meningocele. With meningocele, a sac of fluid comes through an opening in the baby's back. But the spinal cord is not in this sac. There is usually little or no nerve damage. This type of spina bifida can cause minor disabilities.
- **Spina bifida occulta**. Spina bifida occulta is the mildest type of spina bifida. It is sometimes called "hidden spina bifida." With it, there is a small gap in the spine but no opening or sac on the back. The spinal cord and the nerves are usually normal. Many times, spina bifida occulta is not discovered until late childhood or adulthood. This type of spina bifida usually does not cause any disabilities.

Causes of Spina Bifida

All the causes of spina bifida are not well known. The role that genetics and the environment play in causing spina bifida needs to be studied further.

Diagnosis of Spina Bifida

Spina bifida can be diagnosed during pregnancy or after the baby is born. Spina bifida occulta might not be diagnosed until late childhood or adulthood or might never be diagnosed.

DURING PREGNANCY

During pregnancy, there are screening tests (prenatal tests) to check for spina bifida and other birth defects. Talk with your doctor about any questions or concerns you have about this prenatal testing.

AFTER THE BABY IS BORN

In some cases, spina bifida might not be diagnosed until after the baby is born. Sometimes a hairy patch of skin or a dimple on the baby's back is first noticed after birth. A doctor can use an image scan, such as an x-ray, magnetic resonance imaging (MRI), or computed tomography (CT), to get a clearer view of the baby's spine and the bones in the back. Sometimes spina bifida is not diagnosed until after birth because the mother did not receive prenatal care or the ultrasound did not show clear pictures of the affected part of the spine.

Treatments for Spina Bifida

Not all people born with spina bifida have the same needs, so treatment will be different for each person. Some people have problems that are more serious than others. People with myelomeningocele and meningocele will need more treatments than people with spina bifida occulta.

Prevention of Spina Bifida

There are ways for women to reduce the risk of having a baby with spina bifida both before and during her pregnancy. If you are pregnant or could get pregnant, use the following tips to help prevent your baby from having spina bifida:

- Take 400 micrograms (mcg) of folic acid every day. If you have already had a pregnancy affected by spina bifida, you may need to take a higher dose of folic acid before pregnancy and during early pregnancy. Talk to your doctor to discuss what is best for you.
- Talk to your doctor or pharmacist about any prescription and over-the-counter (OTC) drugs, vitamins, and dietary or herbal supplements you are taking.
- If you have a medical condition—such as diabetes or obesity—be sure it is under control before you become pregnant.
- Avoid overheating your body, as might happen if you use a hot tub or sauna.
- Treat any fever you have right away with Tylenol® (or store-brand acetaminophen).[2]

[2] National Center on Birth Defects and Developmental Disabilities (NCBDDD), "What Is Spina Bifida?" Centers for Disease Control and Prevention (CDC), October 4, 2023. Available online. URL: www.cdc.gov/ncbddd/spinabifida/facts.html. Accessed March 12, 2024.

WHAT IS ANENCEPHALY?

Anencephaly is a serious birth defect in which a baby is born without parts of the brain and skull. It is a type of NTD. As the neural tube forms and closes, it helps develop the baby's brain and skull (upper part of the neural tube), spinal cord, and backbones (lower part of the neural tube). Anencephaly occurs if the upper part of the neural tube does not close completely. This often results in a baby being born without the front part of the brain (forebrain) and the thinking and coordinating part of the brain (cerebrum). The remaining parts of the brain are often not covered by bone or skin.

How Many Babies Are Born with Anencephaly?

Researchers estimate that about 1 in every 4,600 babies is born with anencephaly in the United States.

Causes of Anencephaly

The causes of anencephaly among most infants are unknown. Some babies have anencephaly because of a change in their genes or chromosomes. Anencephaly might also be caused by a combination of genes and other factors, such as the things the mother comes in contact with in the environment, what the mother eats or drinks, or certain medicines she uses during pregnancy.

Diagnosis of Anencephaly

Anencephaly can be diagnosed during pregnancy or after the baby is born.

DURING PREGNANCY

During pregnancy, there are screening tests (prenatal tests) to check for birth defects and other conditions. Anencephaly would result in an abnormal result on a blood or serum screening test, or it might be seen during an ultrasound (which creates pictures of the body).

AFTER THE BABY IS BORN

In some cases, anencephaly might not be diagnosed until after the baby is born. Anencephaly is immediately seen at birth.

Treatments for Anencephaly

There is no known cure or standard treatment for anencephaly. Almost all babies born with anencephaly will die shortly after birth.

Prevention of Anencephaly

Getting enough folic acid before and during early pregnancy can help prevent NTDs, such as anencephaly. If you are pregnant or could get pregnant, take 400 mcg of folic acid every day. If you have already had a pregnancy affected by an NTD, you can speak with your doctor about taking a higher dose of folic acid before pregnancy and during early pregnancy.

- Since the United States began fortifying grains with folic acid, there has been a 28 percent decline in pregnancies affected by NTDs (spina bifida and anencephaly).
- In order to get the recommended 400 mcg of folic acid every day, a woman of reproductive age can take a supplement containing folic acid or eat foods fortified with folic acid, or both, depending on her dietary habits.[3]

[3] National Center on Birth Defects and Developmental Disabilities (NCBDDD), "Facts about Anencephaly," Centers for Disease Control and Prevention (CDC), June 28, 2023. Available online. URL: www.cdc.gov/ncbddd/birthdefects/anencephaly.html. Accessed March 12, 2024.

Chapter 18 | Microcephaly

Microcephaly is a condition where a baby's head is much smaller than expected. During pregnancy, a baby's head grows because the brain grows. Microcephaly can occur if the brain has not developed properly during pregnancy or has stopped growing after birth, resulting in a smaller head size. Microcephaly can be an isolated condition, occurring with no other major birth defects, or it can occur in combination with other major birth defects.

WHAT IS SEVERE MICROCEPHALY?

Severe microcephaly is a more serious, extreme form of this condition where a baby's head is much smaller than expected. It can result from improper brain development during pregnancy or from brain damage that occurred at some point during pregnancy.

OTHER PROBLEMS

Babies with microcephaly can have a range of other problems, depending on how severe their microcephaly is. Microcephaly has been linked with the following problems:

- seizures
- developmental delay, such as problems with speech or other developmental milestones (such as sitting, standing, and walking)
- intellectual disability (decreased ability to learn and function in daily life)
- problems with movement and balance
- feeding problems, such as difficulty swallowing
- hearing loss
- vision problems

These problems can range from mild to severe and are often lifelong. Because the baby's brain is small and underdeveloped, babies with severe microcephaly can have more of these problems, or have more difficulty with them, than babies with milder microcephaly. Severe microcephaly can also be life-threatening. Because it is difficult to predict at birth what problems a baby will have from microcephaly, babies with microcephaly often need close follow-up through regular checkups with a health-care provider to monitor their growth and development.

HOW MANY BABIES ARE BORN WITH MICROCEPHALY?

Microcephaly is not a common condition. Researchers estimate that about 1 in every 800–5,000 babies is born with microcephaly in the United States.

CAUSES AND RISK FACTORS OF MICROCEPHALY

The causes of microcephaly in most babies are unknown. Some babies have microcephaly because of changes in their genes. Other causes of microcephaly, including severe microcephaly, can include the following exposures during pregnancy:

- certain infections during pregnancy, such as rubella, toxoplasmosis, or cytomegalovirus (CMV)
- severe malnutrition, meaning a lack of nutrients or not getting enough food
- exposure to harmful substances, such as alcohol, certain drugs, or toxic chemicals
- interruption of the blood supply to the baby's brain during development

Some babies with microcephaly have been reported among mothers who were infected with Zika virus while pregnant.

DIAGNOSIS OF MICROCEPHALY

Microcephaly can be diagnosed during pregnancy or after the baby is born.

During Pregnancy

During pregnancy, microcephaly can sometimes be diagnosed with an ultrasound test (which creates pictures of the body). To see microcephaly during pregnancy, the ultrasound test should be done late in the second trimester or early in the third trimester.

After the Baby Is Born

To diagnose microcephaly after birth, a health-care provider will measure the distance around a newborn baby's head, also called the "head circumference," during a physical exam. The provider then compares this measurement to population standards by sex and age. Microcephaly is defined as a head circumference measurement that is smaller than a certain value for babies of the same age and sex. This value is usually more than two standard deviations (SDs) below the average or less than the third percentile. This means the baby's head is extremely small compared to babies of the same age and sex.

Microcephaly can be determined by measuring the head circumference after birth. Although head circumference measurements may be influenced by molding and other factors related to delivery, they should be taken on the first day of life because commonly used birth head circumference reference charts by age and sex are based on measurements taken before 24 hours of age. The most important factor is that the head circumference is carefully measured and documented. If measurement within the first 24 hours of life is not done, the head circumference should be measured as soon as possible after birth. If the health-care provider suspects the baby has microcephaly, he or she can request one or more tests to help confirm the diagnosis. For example, special tests such as magnetic resonance imaging (MRI) can provide critical information on the structure of the baby's brain and can help determine if the newborn had an infection during pregnancy. These tests can also help the health-care provider look for other problems that might be present.

TREATMENTS FOR MICROCEPHALY

Microcephaly is a lifelong condition. There is no known cure or standard treatment for microcephaly. Because microcephaly can range from mild to severe, treatment options can range as well. Babies with mild microcephaly often do not experience any other problems besides small head size. These babies will need routine checkups to monitor their growth and development.

For more severe microcephaly, babies will need care and treatment focused on managing their other health problems. Developmental services early in life will often help babies with microcephaly improve and maximize their physical and intellectual abilities. These services, known as "early intervention," can include speech, occupational, and physical therapies. Sometimes medications are also needed to treat seizures or other symptoms.[1]

[1] National Center on Birth Defects and Developmental Disabilities (NCBDDD), "Facts about Microcephaly," Centers for Disease Control and Prevention (CDC), June 28, 2023. Available online. URL: www.cdc.gov/ncbddd/birthdefects/microcephaly.html. Accessed March 12, 2024.

Chapter 19 | **Upper and Lower Limb Reduction Defects**

WHAT ARE LIMB REDUCTION DEFECTS?

Upper and lower limb reduction defects occur when a part of or the entire arm (upper limb) or leg (lower limb) of a fetus fails to form completely during pregnancy. The defect is referred to as a "limb reduction" because a limb is reduced from its normal size or is missing.

OTHER PROBLEMS

Babies and children with limb reduction defects will face various issues and difficulties, but the extent of these will depend on the location and size of the reduction. Some potential difficulties and problems include the following:

- difficulties with normal development, such as motor skills
- needing assistance with daily activities, such as self-care
- limitations with certain movements, sports, or activities
- potential emotional and social issues because of physical appearance

HOW MANY BABIES ARE BORN WITH LIMB REDUCTION DEFECTS?

Researchers estimate that about 1 in every 1,900 babies is born with a limb reduction defect in the United States. Some of these babies will have both upper and lower limb reduction defects.

CAUSES AND RISK FACTORS OF LIMB REDUCTION DEFECTS

The cause of limb reduction defects is unknown. However, research has shown that certain behaviors or exposures during pregnancy can increase the risk of having a baby with a limb reduction defect. These include the following:

- exposure of the mother to certain chemicals or viruses while she is pregnant
- exposure of the mother to certain medications
- possible exposure of the mother to tobacco smoking (although more research is needed)

The Centers for Disease Control and Prevention (CDC) works with many researchers to study risk factors that can increase the chance of having a baby with limb reduction defects, as well as the outcomes of babies with the defect.

TREATMENT FOR LIMB REDUCTION DEFECTS

Specific treatment for limb reduction defects will be determined by the child's doctor, based on things such as the child's age, the extent and type of defect, and the child's tolerance for certain medications, procedures, and therapies.

Treatment can vary for each child. Potential treatments include the following:

- prosthetics (artificial limbs)
- orthotics (splints or braces)
- surgery
- rehabilitation (physical or occupational therapy)

It is important to remember that some babies and children with limb reductions will have some difficulties and limitations throughout life, but with proper treatment and care, they can live long, healthy, and productive lives.[1]

[1] National Center on Birth Defects and Developmental Disabilities (NCBDDD), "Facts about Upper and Lower Limb Reduction Defects," Centers for Disease Control and Prevention (CDC), June 28, 2023. Available online. URL: www.cdc.gov/ncbddd/actearly/pdf/parents_pdfs/VisionLossFactSheet.pdf. Accessed March 12, 2024.

Chapter 20 | **Cleft Lip and Cleft Palate**

Cleft lip and cleft palate are birth defects that occur when a baby's lip or mouth does not form properly during pregnancy. Together, these birth defects are commonly called "orofacial clefts."

WHAT IS A CLEFT LIP?

The lip forms between the fourth and seventh weeks of pregnancy. As a baby develops, body tissue and special cells from each side of the head grow toward the center of the face and join together to form the facial features, such as the lips and mouth. A cleft lip occurs if the tissue that makes up the lip does not join completely before birth, resulting in an opening in the upper lip. The opening can be a small slit or a large gap that extends through the lip into the nose. A cleft lip can be on one or both sides of the lip or in the middle, which is very rare. Children with a cleft lip can also have a cleft palate.

WHAT IS CLEFT PALATE?

The roof of the mouth (palate) is formed between the sixth and ninth weeks of pregnancy. A cleft palate happens if the tissue that makes up the roof of the mouth does not join together completely during pregnancy. For some babies, both the front and back parts of the palate are open. For other babies, only part of the palate is open.

OTHER PROBLEMS

Children with a cleft lip with or without a cleft palate or a cleft palate alone often have problems with feeding and speaking clearly and can have ear infections. They might also have hearing problems and problems with their teeth.

HOW MANY BABIES ARE BORN WITH CLEFT LIP/CLEFT PALATE?

- About 1 in every 1,600 babies is born with cleft lip with cleft palate in the United States.
- About 1 in every 2,800 babies is born with cleft lip without cleft palate in the United States.
- About 1 in every 1,700 babies is born with cleft palate in the United States.

CAUSES AND RISK FACTORS OF CLEFT LIP/CLEFT PALATE

The causes of orofacial clefts in most infants are unknown. Some children have a cleft lip or cleft palate due to changes in their genes. Cleft lip and cleft palate are thought to be caused by a combination of genes and other factors, such as things the mother comes in contact with in her environment, what the mother eats or drinks, or certain medications she uses during pregnancy. The Centers for Disease Control and Prevention (CDC) has reported important findings from research studies about factors that increase the chance of having a baby with an orofacial cleft:

- **Smoking**. Women who smoke during pregnancy are more likely to have a baby with an orofacial cleft than women who do not smoke.
- **Diabetes**. Women with diabetes diagnosed before pregnancy have an increased risk of having a child with a cleft lip with or without cleft palate, compared to women who did not have diabetes.
- **Use of certain medicines**. Women who used certain medicines to treat epilepsy, such as topiramate or valproic acid, during the first trimester (the first three months) of pregnancy have an increased risk of having a baby with cleft lip with or without cleft palate, compared to women who did not take these medicines.

If you are pregnant or thinking about becoming pregnant, talk with your doctor about ways to increase your chances of having a healthy baby.

DIAGNOSIS OF CLEFT LIP/CLEFT PALATE

Orofacial clefts, especially cleft lip with or without cleft palate, can be diagnosed during pregnancy by a routine ultrasound. They can also be diagnosed after the baby is born, especially cleft palate. However, sometimes certain types of cleft palate (e.g., submucous cleft palate and bifid uvula) might not be diagnosed until later in life.

MANAGEMENT AND TREATMENT OF CLEFT LIP/CLEFT PALATE

Services and treatment for children with orofacial clefts can vary depending on the severity of the cleft, the child's age and needs, and the presence of associated syndromes or other birth defects, or both. Surgery to repair a cleft lip usually occurs in the first few months of life and is recommended within the first 12 months. Surgery to repair a cleft palate is recommended within the first 18 months or earlier if possible. Many children will need additional surgical procedures as they get older. Surgical repair can improve the look and appearance of a child's face and might also improve breathing, hearing, and speech and language development. Children born with orofacial clefts might need other types of treatments and services, such as special dental or orthodontic care or speech therapy. With treatment, most children with orofacial clefts do well and lead a healthy life. Some children with orofacial clefts may have issues with self-esteem if they are concerned with visible differences between themselves and other children. Parent-to-parent support groups can prove to be useful for families of babies with birth defects of the head and face, such as orofacial clefts.[1]

[1] National Center on Birth Defects and Developmental Disabilities (NCBDDD), "Facts about Cleft Lip and Cleft Palate," Centers for Disease Control and Prevention (CDC), June 28, 2023. Available online. URL: www.cdc.gov/ncbddd/birthdefects/cleftlip.html. Accessed March 12, 2024.

Chapter 21 | Intellectual and Developmental Disabilities

Chapter Contents

Section 21.1 | **Facts about Intellectual Disability**

WHAT IS INTELLECTUAL DISABILITY?

Intellectual disability is a term used when there are limits to a person's ability to learn at an expected level and function in daily life. Levels of intellectual disability vary greatly in children. Children with intellectual disability might have a hard time letting others know their wants and needs and taking care of themselves. Intellectual disability can cause a child to learn and develop more slowly than other children of the same age. It might take longer for a child with an intellectual disability to learn to speak, walk, dress, or eat without help, and they could have trouble learning in school.

Intellectual disability can be caused by a problem that starts any time before a child turns 18 years old—even before birth. It can be caused by injury, disease, or a problem in the brain. For many children, the cause of their intellectual disability is not known. Some of the most commonly known causes of intellectual disability—such as Down syndrome, fetal alcohol syndrome, fragile X syndrome (FXS), genetic conditions, birth defects, and infections—happen before birth. Others happen while a baby is being born or soon after birth. Still, other causes of intellectual disability do not occur until a child is older; these might include serious head injury, stroke, or certain infections.

WHAT ARE SOME OF THE SIGNS OF INTELLECTUAL DISABILITY?

Usually, the more severe the degree of intellectual disability, the earlier the signs can be noticed. However, it might still be hard to predict how young children will be affected later in life. There are many signs of intellectual disability. For example, children with intellectual disability may:

- sit up, crawl, or walk later than other children
- learn to talk later or have trouble speaking
- find it hard to remember things
- have trouble understanding social rules
- have trouble seeing the results of their actions
- have trouble solving problems

WHAT CAN YOU DO IF YOU THINK YOUR CHILD MAY HAVE AN INTELLECTUAL DISABILITY?

Talk with your child's doctor or nurse. If you or your doctor thinks there could be a problem, you can take your child to see a developmental pediatrician or other specialist, and you can contact your local early intervention agency (for children under the age of three) or public school (for children aged three and older). To find out whom to speak to in your area, you can contact the parent center in your state at www.parentcenterhub.org/find-your-center. To help your child reach his or her full potential, it is very important to get help as early as possible.[1]

Section 21.2 | **Down Syndrome**

WHAT IS DOWN SYNDROME?

Down syndrome is a condition in which a person has an extra chromosome. Chromosomes are small "packages" of genes in the body that determine how a baby's body forms and functions as it grows during pregnancy and after birth. Typically, a baby is born with 46 chromosomes. Babies with Down syndrome have an extra copy of one of these chromosomes, chromosome 21. The medical term for having an extra copy of a chromosome is "trisomy." Down syndrome is also referred to as "trisomy 21." This extra copy changes how the baby's body and brain develop, causing both mental and physical challenges. People with Down syndrome usually have an intelligence quotient (IQ; a measure of intelligence) in the mildly to moderately low range and are slower to speak than other children. Some common physical features of Down syndrome include:

- a flattened face, especially the bridge of the nose
- almond-shaped eyes that slant up
- a short neck

[1] National Center on Birth Defects and Developmental Disabilities (NCBDDD), "Facts about Intellectual Disability," Centers for Disease Control and Prevention (CDC), May 10, 2022. Available online. URL: www.cdc.gov/ncbddd/developmentaldisabilities/facts-about-intellectual-disability.html. Accessed March 12, 2024.

- small ears
- a tongue that tends to stick out of the mouth
- tiny white spots on the iris (colored part) of the eye
- small hands and feet
- a single line across the palm of the hand (palmar crease)
- small pinky fingers that sometimes curve toward the thumb
- poor muscle tone or loose joints
- shorter in height as children and adults

HOW MANY BABIES ARE BORN WITH DOWN SYNDROME?

Down syndrome remains the most common chromosomal condition diagnosed in the United States. Each year, about 6,000 babies born in the United States have Down syndrome. This means that Down syndrome occurs in about 1 in every 700 babies.

TYPES OF DOWN SYNDROME

There are three types of Down syndrome. People often cannot tell the difference between each type without looking at the chromosomes because the physical features and behaviors are similar.

- **Trisomy 21**. About 95 percent of people with Down syndrome have trisomy 21. With this type of Down syndrome, each cell in the body has three separate copies of chromosome 21 instead of the usual two copies.
- **Translocation Down syndrome**. This type accounts for a small percentage of people with Down syndrome (3%). This occurs when an extra part or a whole extra chromosome 21 is present, but it is attached or "translocated" to a different chromosome rather than being a separate chromosome 21.
- **Mosaic Down syndrome**. This type affects about 2 percent of the people with Down syndrome. Mosaic means mixture or combination. For children with mosaic Down syndrome, some of their cells have three copies of chromosome 21, but other cells have the typical two copies

of chromosome 21. Children with mosaic Down syndrome may have the same features as other children with Down syndrome. However, they may have fewer features of the condition due to the presence of some (or many) cells with a typical number of chromosomes.

CAUSES AND RISK FACTORS OF DOWN SYNDROME

The extra chromosome 21 leads to the physical features and developmental challenges that can occur among people with Down syndrome. Researchers know that Down syndrome is caused by an extra chromosome, but the exact reasons for its occurrence and the factors involved are still unknown. One factor that increases the risk of having a baby with Down syndrome is the mother's age. Women who are 35 years or older when they become pregnant are more likely to have a pregnancy affected by Down syndrome than women who become pregnant at a younger age. However, the majority of babies with Down syndrome are born to mothers less than 35 years old because there are many more births among younger women.

DIAGNOSIS OF DOWN SYNDROME

There are two basic types of tests available to detect Down syndrome during pregnancy: screening tests and diagnostic tests. A screening test can tell a woman and her health-care provider whether her pregnancy has a lower or higher chance of having Down syndrome. Screening tests do not provide an absolute diagnosis, but they are safer for the mother and the developing baby. Diagnostic tests can typically determine whether a baby will have Down syndrome, but they carry more risk for the mother and the developing baby. Neither screening nor diagnostic tests can predict the full effect of Down syndrome on a baby; no one can predict this.

SCREENING TESTS FOR DOWN SYNDROME

Screening tests often include a combination of a blood test, which measures the amount of various substances in the mother's blood (e.g., maternal serum alpha-fetoprotein (MS-AFP), triple screen, quad screen), and an ultrasound, which creates a picture of the baby. During an ultrasound, the technician looks at the fluid behind the baby's neck; extra fluid in this region could indicate a genetic problem. These screening tests can help determine the baby's risk of Down syndrome. Rarely, screening tests can give an abnormal result even when there is nothing wrong with the baby. Sometimes the test results are normal but miss an existing problem.

DIAGNOSTIC TESTS FOR DOWN SYNDROME

Diagnostic tests are usually performed after a positive screening test to confirm a Down syndrome diagnosis. The following are different types of diagnostic tests:

- **Chorionic villus sampling (CVS).** Examines material from the placenta.
- **Amniocentesis.** Examines the amniotic fluid (the fluid from the sac surrounding the baby).
- **Percutaneous umbilical blood sampling (PUBS).** Examines blood from the umbilical cord.

These tests look for changes in the chromosomes that would indicate a Down syndrome diagnosis.

OTHER HEALTH PROBLEMS OF DOWN SYNDROME

Many people with Down syndrome have common facial features and no other major birth defects. However, some people with Down syndrome might have one or more major birth defects or other medical problems. Some of the more common health problems among children with Down syndrome are as follows:

- hearing loss
- obstructive sleep apnea, which is a condition where the person's breathing temporarily stops while asleep
- ear infections
- eye diseases
- heart defects present at birth

Health-care providers routinely monitor children with Down syndrome for these conditions.

TREATMENTS FOR DOWN SYNDROME

Down syndrome is a lifelong condition. Services early in life will often help babies and children with Down syndrome improve their physical and intellectual abilities. Most of these services focus on helping children with Down syndrome develop to their full potential. These services include speech, occupational, and physical therapy, and they are typically offered through early intervention programs in each state. Children with Down syndrome may also need extra help or attention in school, although many children are included in regular classes.[2]

Section 21.3 | **Cerebral Palsy**

WHAT IS CEREBRAL PALSY?

Cerebral palsy (CP) is a group of disorders that affect a person's ability to move and maintain balance and posture. CP is the most common motor disability in childhood. "Cerebral" means having to do with the brain, and "palsy" means weakness or problems with using the muscles. CP is caused by abnormal brain development or damage to the developing brain that affects a person's ability to control their muscles. The symptoms of CP vary from person to person. A person with severe CP might need to use special equipment to walk or might not be able to walk at all and might need lifelong care. A person with mild CP might walk a little awkwardly but might not need any special help. CP does not get worse over time, though the exact symptoms can change over a person's lifetime. All people with CP have problems with movement and posture. Many also have related conditions such as intellectual disability, seizures, problems with vision, hearing, or speech, changes in the spine (such as scoliosis), or joint problems (such as contractures).

[2] National Center on Birth Defects and Developmental Disabilities (NCBDDD), "Facts about Down Syndrome," Centers for Disease Control and Prevention (CDC), October 10, 2023. Available online. URL: www.cdc.gov/ncbddd/birthdefects/downsyndrome.html. Accessed March 12, 2024.

TYPES OF CEREBRAL PALSY

Doctors classify CP according to the main type of movement disorder involved. Depending on which areas of the brain are affected, one or more of the following movement disorders can occur:

- stiff muscles (spasticity)
- uncontrollable movements (dyskinesia)
- poor balance and coordination (ataxia)

There are four main types of CP.

Spastic Cerebral Palsy

The most common type of CP is spastic CP, which affects about 80 percent of people with CP. People with spastic CP have increased muscle tone, meaning their muscles are stiff, and as a result, their movements can be awkward. Spastic CP is usually described by the parts of the body affected:

- **Spastic diplegia/diparesis**. In this type of CP, muscle stiffness is mainly in the legs, with the arms less affected or not affected at all. People with spastic diplegia might have difficulty walking because tight hip and leg muscles cause their legs to pull together, turn inward, and cross at the knees (also known as "scissoring").
- **Spastic hemiplegia/hemiparesis**. This type of CP affects only one side of a person's body; usually, the arm is more affected than the leg.
- **Spastic quadriplegia/quadriparesis**. Spastic quadriplegia is the most severe form of spastic CP and affects all four limbs, the trunk, and the face. People with spastic quadriplegia usually cannot walk and often have other developmental disabilities such as intellectual disability, seizures, or problems with vision, hearing, or speech.

Dyskinetic Cerebral Palsy (Also Includes Athetoid, Choreoathetoid, and Dystonic Cerebral Palsies)

People with dyskinetic CP have problems controlling the movement of their hands, arms, feet, and legs, making it difficult to sit and walk.

The movements are uncontrollable and can be slow and writhing or rapid and jerky. Sometimes the face and tongue are affected, making it hard to suck, swallow, and talk. A person with dyskinetic CP has muscle tone that can change (varying from too tight to too loose) not only from day to day but even during a single day.

Ataxic Cerebral Palsy

People with ataxic CP have problems with balance and coordination. They might be unsteady when they walk and have difficulty with quick movements or movements that require a lot of control, such as writing. They might also have trouble controlling their hands or arms when reaching for something.

Mixed Cerebral Palsy

Some people have symptoms of more than one type of CP. The most common type of mixed CP is spastic-dyskinetic CP.

EARLY SIGNS OF CEREBRAL PALSY

The signs of CP vary greatly because there are many different types and levels of disability. The main sign that a child might have CP is a delay in reaching motor or movement milestones (such as rolling over, sitting, standing, or walking). Following are some other signs of possible CP. It is important to note that some children without CP might also have some of these signs:

In a Baby Younger than Six Months of Age

- His or her head lags when you pick him or her up while he or she is lying on his back.
- He or she feels stiff.
- He or she feels floppy.
- When held cradled in your arms, he or she seems to overextend his or her back and neck, constantly acting as if he or she is pushing away from you.
- When you pick him or her up, his or her legs get stiff, and they cross or scissor.

In a Baby Older than Six Months of Age

- He or she does not roll over in either direction.
- He or she cannot bring his or her hands together.
- He or she has difficulty bringing his or her hands to his or her mouth.
- He or she reaches out with only one hand while keeping the other fisted.

In a Baby Older than Ten Months of Age

- He or she crawls in a lopsided manner, pushing off with one hand and leg while dragging the opposite hand and leg.
- He or she scoots around on his or her buttocks or hops on his or her knees but does not crawl on all fours.

Tell your child's doctor or nurse if you notice any of these signs.

CAUSES AND RISK FACTORS OF CEREBRAL PALSY

Cerebral palsy is caused by abnormal development of the brain or damage to the developing brain, which affects a child's ability to control their muscles. There are several possible causes of abnormal development or damage. People used to think that CP was mainly caused by a lack of oxygen during the birth process. Now, scientists believe this accounts for only a small number of CP cases.

The abnormal development of the brain or damage that leads to CP can occur before birth, during birth, within a month after birth, or during the first year of a child's life while the brain is still developing. CP related to abnormal brain development or damage that occurred before or during birth is called "congenital CP." The majority of CP cases (85–90%) are congenital. In many cases, the specific cause is not known. A small percentage of CP cases are caused by abnormal brain development or damage that occurs more than 28 days after birth. This is called "acquired CP" and is usually associated with an infection (such as meningitis) or head injury.

SCREENING AND DIAGNOSIS OF CEREBRAL PALSY

Diagnosing CP at an early age is important to the well-being of children and their families. The diagnosis process can involve several steps:

Developmental Monitoring

Developmental monitoring (also called "surveillance") means tracking a child's growth and development over time. If any concerns about the child's development are raised during monitoring, a developmental screening test should be given as soon as possible.

Developmental Screening

During developmental screening, a short test is given to see if the child has specific developmental delays, such as motor or movement delays. If the results of the screening test are cause for concern, the doctor will make referrals for developmental and medical evaluations.

Developmental and Medical Evaluations

The goal of a developmental evaluation is to diagnose the specific type of disorder that affects a child.

TREATMENTS AND INTERVENTION SERVICES FOR CEREBRAL PALSY

There is no cure for CP, but treatment can improve the lives of those who have the condition. It is important to begin a treatment program as early as possible. After a CP diagnosis is made, a team of health professionals works with the child and family to develop a plan to help the child reach their full potential. Common treatments include medicines, surgery, braces, and physical, occupational, and speech therapy. No single treatment is best for all children with CP. Before deciding on a treatment plan, it is important to talk with the child's doctor to understand all the risks and benefits.

Intervention Services

Both early intervention and school-aged services are available through our nation's special education law, the Individuals with

Disabilities Education Act (IDEA). Part C of IDEA deals with early intervention services for children from birth to 36 months of age, while Part B applies to services for school-aged children from 3 to 22 years of age. Even if your child has not been diagnosed with CP, they may be eligible for IDEA services.

IF YOU ARE CONCERNED

If you think your child is not meeting movement milestones or might have CP, contact your doctor or nurse and share your concerns. If you or your doctor remains concerned, ask for a referral to a specialist who can do a more in-depth evaluation of your child and assist in making a diagnosis. At the same time, call your state's public early childhood system to request a free evaluation to find out if your child qualifies for intervention services. This is sometimes called a "Child Find" evaluation. You do not need to wait for a doctor's referral or a medical diagnosis to make this call. Where to call for a free evaluation from the state depends on your child's age.

- If your child is not yet three years old, contact your local early intervention system. You can find the right contact information for your state by calling the Early Childhood Technical Assistance Center (ECTA) at 919-962-2001 or visiting the ECTA website at www.ectacenter.org/contact/ptccoord.asp.
- If your child is three years of age or older, contact your local public school system. Even if your child is not yet old enough for kindergarten or enrolled in a public school, call your local elementary school or board of education and ask to speak with someone who can help you have your child evaluated.
- If you are not sure whom to contact, you can call the ECTA at 919-962-2001 or visit the ECTA website at www.ectacenter.org/contact/ptccoord.asp.[3]

[3] National Center on Birth Defects and Developmental Disabilities (NCBDDD), "What Is Cerebral Palsy?" Centers for Disease Control and Prevention (CDC), February 28, 2024. Available online. URL: www.cdc.gov/ncbddd/cp/facts.html. Accessed March 12, 2024.

Section 21.4 | Autism Spectrum Disorder

WHAT IS AUTISM SPECTRUM DISORDER?

Autism spectrum disorder (ASD) is a developmental disability caused by differences in the brain. Some people with ASD have a known difference, such as a genetic condition. Other causes are not yet known. Scientists believe there are multiple causes of ASD that act together to alter typical developmental patterns.

People with ASD may behave, communicate, interact, and learn in ways that differ from most other people. There is often nothing about their appearance that sets them apart from others. The abilities of people with ASD can vary significantly. For example, some individuals with ASD may have advanced conversation skills, while others may be nonverbal. Some people with ASD need extensive help in their daily lives, while others can work and live with little to no support.

ASD begins before the age of three and can last throughout a person's life, although symptoms may improve over time. Some children show ASD symptoms within the first 12 months of life. In others, symptoms may not appear until 24 months of age or later. Some children with ASD gain new skills and meet developmental milestones until around 18–24 months of age, then they stop gaining new skills or lose the skills they once had.

As children with ASD become adolescents and young adults, they may have difficulties developing and maintaining friendships, communicating with peers and adults, or understanding what behaviors are expected in school or on the job. They may come to the attention of health-care providers because they also have conditions such as anxiety, depression, or attention deficit hyperactivity disorder (ADHD), which occur more often in people with ASD than in those without ASD.

SIGNS AND SYMPTOMS OF AUTISM SPECTRUM DISORDER

People with ASD often have problems with social communication and interaction, as well as restricted or repetitive behaviors or interests. They may also have different ways of learning, moving, or paying attention. These characteristics can make life very challenging. It is important to note that some people without ASD might also have some of these symptoms.

DIAGNOSIS OF AUTISM SPECTRUM DISORDER

Diagnosing ASD can be difficult since there is no medical test, such as a blood test, to diagnose the disorder. Doctors look at the child's behavior and development to make a diagnosis. ASD can sometimes be detected at 18 months of age or younger. By the age of two, a diagnosis by an experienced professional can be considered reliable. However, many children do not receive a final diagnosis until they are much older. Some people are not diagnosed until they are adolescents or adults. This delay means that people with ASD might not get the early help they need.

TREATMENT FOR AUTISM SPECTRUM DISORDER

Treatments for ASD seek to reduce symptoms that interfere with daily functioning and quality of life (QOL). ASD affects each person differently, meaning that people with ASD have unique strengths and challenges and different treatment needs. Treatment plans usually involve multiple professionals and are catered to the individual.

RISK FACTORS OF AUTISM SPECTRUM DISORDER

There is not just one cause of ASD. Many different factors have been identified that may make a child more likely to have ASD, including environmental, biological, and genetic factors. The available evidence suggests that the following may put children at greater risk for developing ASD:

- having a sibling with ASD
- having certain genetic or chromosomal conditions, such as fragile X syndrome (FXS) or tuberous sclerosis (TS)
- experiencing complications at birth
- being born to older parents

HOW OFTEN AUTISM SPECTRUM DISORDER OCCURS

The Centers for Disease Control and Prevention's (CDC) Autism and Developmental Disabilities Monitoring (ADDM) Network has been estimating the number of eight-year-old children with ASD in the United States since 2000. ASD occurs in all racial, ethnic, and socioeconomic groups and is more than four times more common among boys than girls.

IF YOU ARE CONCERNED

As a parent, you already have what it takes to help your young child learn and grow. The CDC has developed materials to help you track your child's developmental milestones and share that progress, or any concerns, with your child's doctor at every checkup. Contact your child's doctor if you think your child might have ASD or if you have any other concerns about the way your child plays, learns, speaks, or acts. If you are still concerned, ask the doctor for a referral to a specialist who can do a more in-depth evaluation of your child. Specialists who can do a more in-depth evaluation and make a diagnosis include the following:

- **Developmental pediatricians**. Doctors who have special training in child development and children with special needs.
- **Child neurologists**. Doctors who work on the brain, spine, and nerves.
- **Child psychologists or psychiatrists**. Doctors who know about the human mind.

At the same time, call your state's public early childhood system to request a free evaluation, sometimes called a "Child Find evaluation," to find out if your child qualifies for intervention services.[4]

[4] National Center on Birth Defects and Developmental Disabilities (NCBDDD), "What Is Autism Spectrum Disorder?" Centers for Disease Control and Prevention (CDC), December 9, 2022. Available online. URL: www.cdc.gov/ncbddd/autism/facts.html. Accessed March 12, 2024.

Section 21.5 | **Sensory Impairment: Hearing and Vision**

WHAT IS HEARING LOSS IN CHILDREN?

Hearing loss can affect a child's ability to develop speech, language, and social skills. The earlier children with hearing loss start getting services, the more likely they are to reach their full potential. If you think a child might have hearing loss, ask the child's doctor for a hearing screening as soon as possible. Do not wait! Hearing loss can occur when any part of the ear is not functioning properly, including the outer ear, middle ear, inner ear, hearing (acoustic) nerve, and auditory system.

Signs and Symptoms of Hearing Loss

The signs and symptoms of hearing loss are different for each child. If you think your child might have hearing loss, ask the child's doctor for a hearing screening as soon as possible. Do not wait! Even if a child has passed a hearing screening before, it is important to look out for the following signs:

SIGNS IN BABIES

- Does not startle at loud noises.
- Does not turn to the source of a sound after six months of age.
- Does not say single words, such as "dada" or "mama," by one year of age.
- Turns the head when he or she sees you but not if you only call out his or her name. This is sometimes mistaken for not paying attention or just ignoring but could be the result of a partial or complete hearing loss.
- Seems to hear some sounds but not others.

SIGNS IN CHILDREN

- Speech is delayed.
- Speech is not clear.
- Does not follow directions. This is sometimes mistaken for not paying attention or just ignoring but could be the result of a partial or complete hearing loss.

- Often says, "Huh?"
- Turns the television (TV) volume up too high.

Babies and children should reach milestones in how they play, learn, communicate, and act. A delay in any of these milestones could be a sign of hearing loss or other developmental problem.

Causes and Risk Factors of Hearing Loss

Hearing loss can occur at any time in life—from before birth to adulthood. The following are some factors that can increase the chance of a child having hearing loss:

About one in two cases of hearing loss in babies is due to genetic causes. Some babies with a genetic cause for their hearing loss might have family members who also have hearing loss. About one in three babies with genetic hearing loss has a "syndrome." This means they have other conditions in addition to hearing loss, such as Down syndrome or Usher syndrome.

One in four cases of hearing loss in babies is due to maternal infections during pregnancy, complications after birth, or head trauma. For example, the child:

- was exposed to infection before birth
- spent five days or more in a hospital neonatal intensive care unit (NICU) or had complications while in the NICU
- needed a special procedure, such as a blood transfusion, to treat bad jaundice
- has head, face, or ears shaped or formed in a different way than usual
- has a condition, such as a neurological disorder, that may be associated with hearing loss
- had an infection around the brain and spinal cord called "meningitis"
- received a bad injury to the head that required a hospital stay

Screening and Diagnosis of Hearing Loss

Hearing screening can determine if a child might have hearing loss. Hearing screening is easy and not painful. In fact, babies are often asleep while being screened. It takes a very short time—usually only a few minutes.

BABIES

All babies should have a hearing screening no later than one month of age. Most babies have their hearing screened while still in the hospital. If a baby does not pass a hearing screening, it is very important to get a full hearing test as soon as possible, but no later than three months of age.

CHILDREN

Children should have their hearing tested before they enter school or any time there is a concern about the child's hearing. Children who do not pass the hearing screening need to get a full hearing test as soon as possible.

Treatments and Intervention Services for Hearing Loss

No single treatment or intervention is the answer for every person or family. Good treatment plans will include close monitoring, follow-ups, and any necessary changes along the way. There are many different types of communication options for children with hearing loss and their families. Some of these options include:

- learning other ways to communicate, such as sign language
- technology to help with communication, such as hearing aids and cochlear implants
- medicine and surgery to correct some types of hearing loss
- family support services

Prevention of Hearing Loss

The following are tips for parents to help prevent hearing loss in their children:

- Have a healthy pregnancy.
- Make sure your child gets all the regular childhood vaccines.
- Keep your child away from high noise levels, such as from very loud toys. Visit the website of the National Institutes of Health (NIH; www.nidcd.nih.gov/health/hearing/pages/noise.aspx) to learn more about preventing noise-induced hearing loss.

Get Help!

- If you think that your child might have hearing loss, ask the child's doctor for a hearing screening as soon as possible. Do not wait!
- If your child does not pass a hearing screening, ask the child's doctor for a full hearing test as soon as possible.
- If your child has hearing loss, talk to the child's doctor about treatment and intervention services.

If you are a parent and suspect your child has hearing loss, trust your instincts and speak with your child's doctor.[5]

WHAT IS VISION LOSS?

Vision loss means that a person's eyesight is not corrected to a "normal" level. Vision loss can vary greatly among children and can be caused by many factors.

What Causes Loss of Vision?

Vision loss can be caused by damage to the eye itself, by the eye being shaped incorrectly, or by a problem in the brain. Babies can

[5] National Center on Birth Defects and Developmental Disabilities (NCBDDD), "What Is Hearing Loss in Children?" Centers for Disease Control and Prevention (CDC), August 4, 2023. Available online. URL: www.cdc.gov/ncbddd/hearingloss/facts.html. Accessed March 12, 2024.

be born unable to see, and vision loss can occur at any time during a person's life.

When Should Your Child Be Checked?

Your child should be checked for vision problems by an ophthalmologist, optometrist, pediatrician, or other trained specialist from newborn to three months, six months to one year, about three years, and about five years. Having your child's vision checked is especially important if someone in your family has had vision problems.

What Are Some Signs of Vision Loss?

A child with vision loss might:

- close or cover one eye
- squint the eyes or frown
- complain that things are blurry or hard to see
- have trouble reading or doing other close-up work or hold objects close to eyes in order to see, blink more than usual, or seem cranky when doing close-up work (such as looking at books)

One eye of a child with vision loss could look out or cross. One or both eyes could be watery, and one or both of the child's eyelids could also look red-rimmed, crusted, or swollen.

What Can You Do If You Think Your Child May Have Vision Loss?

Talk with your child's doctor or nurse. If you or your doctor thinks there could be a problem, you can take your child to see an ophthalmologist, optometrist, or other specialist, and you can contact your local early intervention agency (for children under the age of three) or public school (for children aged three and older). To find out whom to speak to in your area, contact the National Information Center for Children and Youth with Disabilities (NICHCY) at www.nichcy.org/states.htm or call the Centers for Disease Control and Prevention (CDC) at 800-232-4636. Treating vision problems early may protect your child's sight, and teaching children with severe vision loss how to function as early as possible can help them reach their full potential.[6]

Section 21.6 | Learning Disorders

Many children may struggle in school with some topics or skills from time to time. When children try hard and still struggle with a specific set of skills over time, it could be a sign of a learning disorder. Having a learning disorder means that a child has difficulty in one or more areas of learning, even when overall intelligence or motivation is not affected. Some of the symptoms of learning disorders are:

- difficulty telling right from left
- reversing letters, words, or numbers, after first or second grade
- difficulties recognizing patterns or sorting items by size or shape
- difficulty understanding and following instructions or staying organized
- difficulty remembering what was just said or what was just read
- lacking coordination when moving around
- difficulty doing tasks with the hands, such as writing, cutting, or drawing
- difficulty understanding the concept of time

Examples of learning disorders include the following:

- **Dyslexia**. Difficulty with reading.
- **Dyscalculia**. Difficulty with math.
- **Dysgraphia**. Difficulty with writing.

[6] National Center on Birth Defects and Developmental Disabilities (NCBDDD), "What Is Autism Spectrum Disorder?" Centers for Disease Control and Prevention (CDC), December 9, 2022. Available online. URL: www.cdc.gov/ncbddd/autism/facts.html. Accessed March 12, 2024.

Children with learning disorders may feel frustrated that they cannot master a subject despite trying hard and may act out, act helpless, or withdraw. Learning disorders can also be present with emotional or behavioral disorders, such as attention deficit hyperactivity disorder (ADHD), or anxiety. The combination of problems can make it particularly hard for a child to succeed in school. Properly diagnosing each disorder is crucial so that the child can get the right kind of help for each.

WHAT EVERY PARENT SHOULD KNOW

Children with specific learning disabilities are eligible for special education services or accommodations at school under the Individuals with Disabilities in Education Act (IDEA) and an antidiscrimination law known as "Section 504." The U.S. Department of Education (ED) issued a "Dear Colleague" letter providing clarification to both parents and practitioners about ensuring a high-quality education for children with specific learning disabilities, including children with dyslexia, dyscalculia, and dysgraphia.

THE ROLE OF HEALTH-CARE PROVIDERS

Health-care providers can play an important part in collaborating with schools to help a child with learning disorders or other disabilities get the special services they need. The American Academy of Pediatrics (AAP) describes the roles that health-care providers can have in helping children with disabilities, including learning disorders:

- identifying children in need of early intervention or special education services
- sharing relevant information with early intervention or school personnel
- meeting with early intervention or school personnel and parents or guardians
- using early intervention or school information in medical diagnostic or treatment plans
- working within an early intervention, school, or school-based health clinic

- working at an administrative level to improve school functioning around children with special needs[7]

WHAT CAUSES LEARNING DISABILITIES?

Researchers do not know all of the possible causes of learning disabilities, but they have found a range of risk factors during their work to find potential causes. Research shows that risk factors may be present from birth and tend to run in families. In fact, children who have a parent with a learning disability are more likely to develop a learning disability themselves. To better understand learning disabilities, researchers are studying how children's brains learn to read, write, and develop math skills. Researchers are working on interventions to help address the needs of those who struggle with reading the most, including those with learning disabilities, to improve learning and overall health.

Factors that affect a fetus developing in the womb, such as alcohol or drug use, can put a child at higher risk for a learning problem or disability. Other factors in an infant's environment may play a role, too. These can include poor nutrition or exposure to lead in water or in paint. Young children who do not receive the support they need for their intellectual development may show signs of learning disabilities once they start school. Sometimes a person may develop a learning disability later in life due to injury. Possible causes in such a case include dementia or a traumatic brain injury (TBI).[8]

WHAT ARE THE TREATMENTS FOR LEARNING DISABILITIES?

Learning disabilities have no cure, but early intervention can lessen their effects. People with learning disabilities can develop ways

---

[7] National Center on Birth Defects and Developmental Disabilities (NCBDDD), "Learning Disorders in Children," Centers for Disease Control and Prevention (CDC), July 26, 2022. Available online. URL: www.cdc.gov/ncbddd/developmentaldisabilities/learning-disorder.html. Accessed April 17, 2024.

[8] "What Causes Learning Disabilities?" *Eunice Kennedy Shriver* National Institute of Child Health and Human Development (NICHD), September 11, 2018. Available online. URL: www.nichd.nih.gov/health/topics/learning/conditioninfo/causes. Accessed March 12, 2024.

to cope with their disabilities. Getting help earlier increases the chance of success in school and later in life. If learning disabilities remain untreated, a child may begin to feel frustrated, which can lead to low self-esteem and other problems. Experts can help a child learn skills by building on the child's strengths and finding ways to compensate for the child's weaknesses. Interventions vary depending on the nature and extent of the disability.

SPECIAL EDUCATION SERVICES

Children diagnosed with learning disabilities can receive special education services. The Individuals with Disabilities Education Act (IDEA) requires that public schools provide free special education support to children with disabilities. In most states, each child is entitled to these services beginning at the age of three and extending through high school or until the age of 21, whichever comes first. The rules of the IDEA for each state are available from the Early Childhood Technical Assistance Center (ECTAC). The IDEA requires that children be taught in the least restrictive environment appropriate for them. This means the teaching environment should meet a child's needs and skills while minimizing restrictions to typical learning experiences.

INDIVIDUALIZED EDUCATION PROGRAM

Children who qualify for special education services will receive an Individualized Education Program (IEP). This personalized and written education plan:

- lists goals for the child
- specifies the services the child will receive
- lists the specialists who will work with the child

QUALIFYING FOR SPECIAL EDUCATION

To qualify for special education services, a child must be evaluated by the school system and meet federal and state guidelines. Parents and caregivers can contact their school principal or special education coordinator to find out how to have their child evaluated. Parents can also review these resources:

- Center for Parent Information and Resources (CPIR; www.parentcenterhub.org), which offers information about Parent Training and Information Centers (PTIs) and Community Parent Resource Centers (CPRC; www.parentcenterhub.org/the-parent-center-network).
- IDEA Parent Guide (www.ncld.org/archives/reports-and-studies/idea-parent-guide-2).

INTERVENTIONS FOR SPECIFIC LEARNING DISABILITIES

The following are just a few of the ways schools help children with specific learning disabilities.

Dyslexia

- **Intensive teaching techniques**. These can include specific, step-by-step, and very methodical approaches to teaching reading with the goal of improving both spoken language and written language skills. These techniques are generally more intensive in terms of how often they occur and how long they last and often involve small group or one-on-one instruction.
- **Classroom modifications**. Teachers can give students with dyslexia extra time to finish tasks and provide taped tests that allow the child to hear the questions instead of reading them.
- **Use of technology**. Children with dyslexia may benefit from listening to audiobooks or using word-processing programs.

Dysgraphia

- **Special tools**. Teachers can offer oral exams, provide a notetaker, or allow the child to videotape reports instead of writing them. Computer software can facilitate children being able to produce written text.
- **Use of technology**. A child with dysgraphia can be taught to use word-processing programs, including those

incorporating speech-to-text translation, or an audio recorder instead of writing by hand.
- **Reducing the need for writing.** Teachers can provide notes, outlines, and preprinted study sheets.

Dyscalculia

- **Visual techniques.** Teachers can draw pictures of word problems and show the students how to use colored pencils to differentiate parts of problems.
- **Memory aids.** Rhymes and music can help a child remember math concepts.
- **Computers.** A child with dyscalculia can use a computer for drills and practice.[9]

Section 21.7 | **Language and Speech Disorders**

Children are born ready to learn a language, but they need to learn the language or languages that their family and environment use. Learning a language takes time, and children vary in how quickly they master milestones in language and speech development. Typically, developing children may have trouble with some sounds, words, and sentences while they are learning. However, most children can use language easily around five years of age.

HELPING CHILDREN LEARN LANGUAGE

Parents and caregivers are the most important teachers during a child's early years. Children learn language by listening to others speak and by practicing. Even young babies notice when others repeat and respond to the noises and sounds they make. Children's

[9] "What Are the Treatments for Learning Disabilities?" *Eunice Kennedy Shriver* National Institute of Child Health and Human Development (NICHD), September 11, 2018. Available online. URL: www.nichd.nih.gov/health/topics/learning/conditioninfo/treatment. Accessed March 12, 2024.

language and brain skills get stronger if they hear many different words. Parents can help their child learn in many different ways, such as:

- responding to the first sounds, gurgles, and gestures a baby makes
- repeating what the child says and adding to it
- talking about the things that a child sees
- asking questions and listening to the answers
- looking at or reading books
- telling stories
- singing songs and sharing rhymes

This can happen both during playtime and during daily routines. Parents can also observe the following:

- how their child hears and talks and compare it with typical milestones for communication skills
- how their child reacts to sounds and have their hearing tested if they have concerns

WHAT TO DO IF THERE ARE CONCERNS

Some children struggle with understanding and speaking, and they need help. They may not master the language milestones at the same time as other children, and it may be a sign of a language or speech delay or disorder. Language development has different parts, and children might have problems with one or more of the following:

- Understanding what others say (receptive language). This could be due to:
    - not hearing the words (hearing loss)
    - not understanding the meaning of the words
- Communicating thoughts using language (expressive language). This could be due to:
    - not knowing the words to use
    - not knowing how to put words together
    - knowing the words to use but not being able to express them

Language and speech disorders can exist together or by themselves. Examples of problems with language and speech development include the following:

- Speech disorders:
    - difficulty with forming specific words or sounds correctly
    - difficulty with making words or sentences flow smoothly, such as stuttering or stammering
- Language delay: The ability to understand and speak develops more slowly than is typical.
- Language disorders:
    - aphasia (difficulty understanding or speaking parts of language due to a brain injury or how the brain works)
    - auditory processing disorder (difficulty understanding the meaning of the sounds that the ear sends to the brain)

Language or speech disorders can occur with other learning disorders that affect reading and writing. Children with language disorders may feel frustrated that they cannot understand others or make themselves understood, and they may act out, act helpless, or withdraw. Language or speech disorders can also be present with emotional or behavioral disorders, such as attention deficit hyperactivity disorder (ADHD), or anxiety. Children with developmental disabilities, including autism spectrum disorder, may also have difficulties with speech and language. The combination of challenges can make it particularly hard for a child to succeed in school. Properly diagnosing a child's disorder is crucial so that each child can get the right kind of help.[10]

[10] National Center on Birth Defects and Developmental Disabilities (NCBDDD), "Language and Speech Disorders in Children," Centers for Disease Control and Prevention (CDC), May 11, 2022. Available online. URL: www.cdc.gov/ncbddd/developmentaldisabilities/language-disorders.html. Accessed March 12, 2024.

WHY DO PEOPLE STUTTER?

Stuttering affects more people than you might think. Roughly 3 million Americans have this speech disorder that makes speaking smoothly difficult. Scientists are learning about what causes people to stutter, and genes tell a big part of the story. "People with stuttering know exactly what they want to say. They are just unable to say it at the rate they would like," says Dr. Dennis Drayna, a National Institutes of Health (NIH) expert on the genetics of communication disorders. Stuttering often involves speech sounds that are repeated or held for too long—often when starting words or sentences. It affects about 1 in 20 children. Most will outgrow the disorder on their own or with the help of a professional called a "speech-language pathologist."

"However, about 20–25 percent of children who stutter will continue into adulthood," says Drayna. This condition is known as "persistent developmental stuttering." Overall, about 1 percent of adults stutter, and it is much more common in men than women. For those who stutter, communicating with others can be difficult. It can cause anxiety about speaking and lead them to avoid talking. This, in turn, can affect relationships, self-esteem, and quality of life. It is common for people who stutter to be able to speak without stuttering when in a low-stress environment. They may have no problem speaking fluently with a pet or baby, for example. Singing or speaking together in a group can also lessen stuttering. But stuttering often gets worse if they are feeling tired or anxious.

Researchers are still working to fully understand what causes stuttering. But they do know that it often runs in families. "It is 15 times more likely that a sibling of a person who stutters will stutter than a random person in the population," explains Drayna. By studying families with multiple people who stutter, Drayna has identified several genes that can cause stuttering. Mutations in these genes have now been found in people around the world who stutter. These studies suggest that genes likely play a role for many people who stutter.

All the genes identified so far are involved in a process inside the cell called "intracellular trafficking." This process helps direct things in the cell to their proper locations. Problems with intracellular trafficking have recently been recognized in other neurological disorders, such as Parkinson and Alzheimer disease. But more research is needed to understand how it affects speech and stuttering.

Scientists are also using brain imaging scans to better understand brain activity in people who stutter. This may help show why some children outgrow stuttering and hopefully lead to better treatments one day. For now, treatment for stuttering involves therapy with a speech-language pathologist. Many of the current therapies aim to make speech smoother. Some work to change the thoughts that can bring on or worsen stuttering. Electronic devices are also available to help those who stutter manage their speech. While stuttering can be an obstacle, there are many resources to help overcome it.[11]

Section 21.8 | **Tourette Syndrome**

Tourette syndrome (TS) is a condition of the nervous system. TS causes people to have "tics." Tics are sudden twitches, movements, or sounds that people do repeatedly. People who have tics cannot stop their body from doing these things. For example, a person might keep blinking over and over. Or, a person might make a grunting sound unwillingly. Having tics is a little bit like having hiccups. Even though you might not want to hiccup, your body does it anyway. Sometimes people can stop themselves from doing a certain tic for a while, but it is hard. Eventually, the person has to do the tic. Depending on the type of tics a person has and how long the tics last, a person might be diagnosed with TS or another type of tic disorder.

[11] National Center on Birth Defects and Developmental Disabilities (NCBDDD), "Language and Speech Disorders in Children," Centers for Disease Control and Prevention (CDC), May 11, 2022. Available online. URL: www.cdc.gov/ncbddd/developmentaldisabilities/language-disorders.html. Accessed March 12, 2024.

TYPES OF TICS

The following are two types of tics:

- **Motor tics.** These are movements of the body. Examples of motor tics include blinking, shrugging the shoulders, or jerking an arm.
- **Vocal tics.** These are sounds that a person makes with his or her voice. Examples of vocal tics include humming, clearing the throat, or yelling out a word or phrase. Tics can be either simple or complex:
    - **Simple tics.** These involve just a few parts of the body. Examples of simple tics include squinting the eyes or sniffing.
    - **Complex tics.** These usually involve several different parts of the body and can have a pattern. An example of a complex tic is bobbing the head while jerking an arm and then jumping up.

RISK FACTORS AND CAUSES OF TOURETTE SYNDROME

Doctors and scientists do not know the exact cause of TS. Research suggests that it is an inherited genetic condition. That means it is passed on from the parent to the child through genes.

SYMPTOMS OF TOURETTE SYNDROME

The main symptoms of TS are tics. A person can have tics ranging from simple, temporary tics lasting a few weeks or months to having many complex tics that are long-lasting. Symptoms of TS usually begin when a child is 5–10 years of age. The first symptoms are often motor tics that occur in the head and neck area. The types of tics and how often a person has tics change a lot over time. Even though the symptoms might appear, disappear, and reappear, these conditions are considered chronic.

In most cases, tics decrease during adolescence and early adulthood, and sometimes disappear entirely. However, many people with TS experience tics into adulthood, and in some cases, tics can become worse during adulthood. Although the media often portray people with TS as involuntarily shouting out swear words (called “coprolalia”) or constantly repeating the words of other people (called “echolalia”), these symptoms are rare and are not required for a diagnosis of TS.

DIAGNOSING TOURETTE SYNDROME

There is no single test, such as a blood test, to diagnose TS. Health professionals look at the person’s symptoms to diagnose TS and other tic disorders. The tic disorders differ from each other in terms of the type of tic present (motor or vocal, or a combination of both) and how long the symptoms have lasted. TS can be diagnosed if a person has both motor and vocal tics and has had tic symptoms for at least a year.

TREATMENT FOR TOURETTE SYNDROME

Although there is no cure for TS, there are treatments available to help manage the tics. Many people with TS have tics that do not get in the way of their daily lives and, therefore, do not need any treatment. However, medication and behavioral treatments are available if tics cause pain or injury; interfere with school, work, or social life; or cause stress.

OTHER CONCERNS AND CONDITIONS

Tourette syndrome often occurs with other conditions. Most children diagnosed with TS also have been diagnosed with at least one additional mental, behavioral, or developmental disorder, such as attention deficit hyperactivity disorder (ADHD), anxiety, or obsessive-compulsive disorder (OCD). It is important to find out if a person with TS has any other conditions and treat those conditions properly.[12]

---

[12] National Center on Birth Defects and Developmental Disabilities (NCBDDD), “What Is Tourette Syndrome?” Centers for Disease Control and Prevention (CDC), May 31, 2023. Available online. URL: www.cdc.gov/ncbddd/tourette/facts.html. Accessed March 1, 2024.

Part 4 | **Childhood Illnesses and Conditions**

Chapter 22 | Respiratory Illnesses

Chapter Contents

Section 22.1 | Common Cold

Sneezing, stuffy, and runny nose? You might have a cold. Colds are one of the most frequent reasons for missed school and work. Every year, adults have an average of two to three colds, and children have even more.

CAUSES OF THE COMMON COLD

More than 200 viruses can cause a cold, but rhinoviruses are the most common type. Viruses that cause colds can spread from person to person through the air and close personal contact.

SYMPTOMS OF THE COMMON COLD

Symptoms of a cold usually peak within two to three days and can include the following:

- sneezing
- stuffy nose
- runny nose
- sore throat
- coughing
- mucus dripping down your throat (postnasal drip)
- watery eyes
- fever (although most people with colds do not have a fever)

When viruses that cause colds first infect the nose and sinuses, the nose produces clear mucus. This helps wash the viruses from the nose and sinuses. After two or three days, the mucus may change to a white, yellow, or green color. This is normal and does not mean you need an antibiotic. Some symptoms, especially runny or stuffy nose and cough, can last for up to 10–14 days. These symptoms should improve over time.

RISK FACTORS OF THE COMMON COLD

Many factors can increase your risk of catching a cold, including the following:

- close contact with someone who has a cold
- season (colds are more common during the fall and winter, but it is possible to get a cold any time of the year)
- age (infants and young children have more colds per year than adults)

WHEN TO SEEK MEDICAL CARE FOR THE COMMON COLD

See a doctor if you have:

- trouble breathing or fast breathing
- dehydration
- fever that lasts longer than four days
- symptoms that last more than 10 days without improvement
- symptoms, such as fever or cough. that improve but then return or worsen
- worsening of chronic medical conditions

This list is not all-inclusive. Please see a doctor for any symptom that is severe or concerning. Colds can have similar symptoms to the flu, and it can be difficult (or even impossible) to tell the difference between them based on symptoms alone.

TREATMENT FOR THE COMMON COLD

Your doctor can determine if you have a cold by asking about your symptoms and examining you. Your doctor may also need to order laboratory tests. There is no cure for a cold. It will get better on its own—without antibiotics. Antibiotics will not help you get better if you have a cold. When antibiotics are not needed, they will not help you, and their side effects could still cause harm. Side effects can range from mild reactions, such as a rash, to more serious health problems. These problems can include severe allergic reactions, antibiotic-resistant infections, and *Clostridioides difficile* or

C. difficile (*C. diff*) infection. *C. diff* causes diarrhea that can lead to severe colon damage and death.

HOW TO FEEL BETTER

The following are some ways you can feel better while your body fights off a cold:

- Get plenty of rest.
- Drink plenty of fluids.
- Use a clean humidifier or cool mist vaporizer.
- Use saline nasal spray or drops.
  - For young children, use a rubber suction bulb to clear mucus.
- Breathe in steam from a bowl of hot water or shower.
- Use throat lozenges or cough drops (do not give lozenges to children younger than four years of age).
- Use honey to relieve cough for adults and children at least one year of age or older.

Ask your doctor or pharmacist about over-the-counter (OTC) medicines that can help you feel better. Always use OTC medicines as directed. Remember, OTC medicines may provide temporary relief of symptoms, but they will not cure your illness.

OVER-THE-COUNTER MEDICINE AND CHILDREN

Carefully read and follow instructions on OTC medicine product labels before giving medicines to children. Some OTC medicines are not recommended for children of certain ages.

- Pain relievers:
  - **Children younger than six months**. Only give acetaminophen.
  - **Children six months or older**. It is okay to give acetaminophen or ibuprofen.
  - **Never give aspirin to children because it can cause Reye syndrome**. Reye syndrome is a very serious but rare illness that can harm the liver and brain.

- Cough and cold medicines:
    - **Children younger than four years old**. Do not use OTC cough and cold medicines in young children unless a doctor specifically tells you to. Cough and cold medicines can result in serious and sometimes life-threatening side effects in young children.
    - **Children four years or older**. Discuss with your child's doctor if OTC cough and cold medicines are safe to give to your child.

Ask your doctor or pharmacist about the right dosage of OTC medicines for your child's age and size. Also, tell your child's doctor and pharmacist about all prescription and OTC medicines they are taking.

PREVENTION OF THE COMMON COLD

You can help prevent colds by doing your best to stay healthy and keep others healthy, including the following:

- Clean your hands.
- Avoid close contact with people who have colds or other upper respiratory infections.
- Cover your mouth and nose when coughing or sneezing.
- Avoid touching your eyes, nose, and mouth with unwashed hands.
- Do not smoke and avoid secondhand smoke.
- Stay at home while you are sick and keep children out of school or daycare while they are sick.[1]

[1] "Common Cold," Centers for Disease Control and Prevention (CDC), June 27, 2023. Available online. URL: www.cdc.gov/antibiotic-use/colds.html. Accessed March 12, 2024.

Section 22.2 | Flu

Influenza (flu) is a contagious respiratory disease caused by influenza viruses. Flu can be more dangerous than the common cold for children. Each year, flu places a large burden on the health and well-being of children and their families. Annual flu vaccination offers the best protection against flu and its potentially serious complications in children. Parents can help children fight the flu by getting themselves and their children vaccinated against the flu each year.

SYMPTOMS OF FLU

Flu symptoms include fever, cough, sore throat, runny or stuffy nose, body aches, headache, and fatigue. Some people may also have vomiting and diarrhea, which are more common in children than in adults. People may be infected with flu and have symptoms without a fever.

TREATMENT FOR FLU

Your child's health care provider can help decide whether your child should take antiviral drugs if they become sick with the flu. Antiviral drugs for children come in the form of pills, liquid, inhaled powder, or intravenous solution. They fight the flu by keeping flu viruses from reproducing in the body. Antiviral drugs must be prescribed by a doctor—they are not available over the counter (OTC).

EMERGENCY WARNING SIGNS OF FLU

Children experiencing these warning signs should obtain medical care right away.

In Children

- fast breathing or trouble breathing
- bluish lips or face
- ribs pulling in with each breath

- chest pain
- severe muscle pain (child refuses to walk)
- dehydration (no urine for eight hours, dry mouth, no tears when crying)
- not alert or interacting when awake
- seizures
- fever above 104 °F (40 °C) that is not controlled by fever-reducing medicine
- in children less than 12 weeks, any fever
- fever or cough that improves but then returns or worsens
- worsening of chronic medical conditions

In Adults

- difficulty breathing or shortness of breath
- persistent pain or pressure in the chest or abdomen
- persistent dizziness, confusion, inability to arouse
- seizures
- not urinating
- severe muscle pain
- severe weakness or unsteadiness
- fever or cough that improves but then returns or worsens
- worsening of chronic medical conditions

These lists are not all-inclusive. Please consult your medical provider for any other symptoms that are severe or concerning.

Children younger than five years old, especially those younger than two, are at higher risk of developing serious flu-related complications. Children of any age with certain chronic health conditions are also at higher risk. During the 2022–2023 flu season, 66 percent of children aged 0–17 years hospitalized with flu had at least one underlying health condition, such as asthma, neurologic disease, obesity, or immune suppression.

While not at higher risk, children five years and older can spread the flu to their higher-risk family members, such as infants younger than six months old, adults 65 years and older, or people of any age who have certain chronic health conditions. It is important to vaccinate everyone six months and older in your family against the flu each year to help protect those most at risk. A flu vaccine offers the best defense against flu and its potentially serious complications and can also reduce the spread of flu to others.

In children, annual flu vaccination has been shown to:

- reduce flu illnesses, doctor's visits for flu, and missed school days
- reduce the risk of flu-related hospitalization and death

FLU CAN BE DANGEROUS FOR CHILDREN

Flu illness is more dangerous than the common cold for children. Each year, millions of children get sick with seasonal flu; thousands of children are hospitalized, and some children die from the flu. Children commonly need medical care because of the flu, especially children younger than five years old.

- Complications from flu among children in this age group can include:
  - pneumonia (an illness where the lungs get infected and inflamed)
  - dehydration (when a child's body loses too much water and salts, often because fluid losses are greater than fluid intake)
  - worsening of long-term medical problems such as heart disease or asthma
  - brain dysfunction, such as encephalopathy
  - sinus problems and ear infections
  - in rare cases, flu complications can lead to death
- Flu seasons vary in severity; however, every year, children are at risk.
  - The Centers for Disease Control and Prevention (CDC) estimates that from the 2010–2011 season to the 2019–2020 season, flu-related hospitalizations among children younger than five years old each flu season have ranged from 6,000 to 27,000 annually in the United States.
  - While relatively rare, some children die from the flu each year. From the 2004–2005 season to the 2019–2020 season, flu-related deaths in children reported to the

CDC during regular flu seasons have ranged from 37 to 199 deaths. (During the 2009 H1N1 pandemic, 358 flu-related deaths in children were reported to the CDC from April 2009 to September 2010.)

- Importantly, among reported flu-related deaths in children, about 80 percent occurred in children who were not fully vaccinated.
- Also of note, even though each flu death in a child is supposed to be reported to the CDC, it is likely that not all flu-related deaths in children are captured and that the actual number of deaths is higher. The CDC has developed statistical models that account for the underreporting of flu-related deaths in children to estimate the actual number of deaths. During 2019–2020, for example, 199 flu-related deaths in children were reported to the CDC, but statistical modeling suggests approximately 434 deaths may have occurred.

VACCINATION IS THE BEST PROTECTION AGAINST FLU

The best way to prevent flu and its potentially serious complications is by getting an annual flu vaccine. Even when flu vaccination does not prevent illness entirely, it has been shown in several studies to reduce the severity of illness in people who get vaccinated but still get sick.

The CDC recommends that everyone six months and older get a seasonal flu vaccine each year. Keep in mind that vaccination is especially important for certain people who are at higher risk of developing serious flu complications or who are in close contact with people at higher risk. This includes children at higher risk of developing serious complications from flu illness and adults who are close contacts of those children.

Flu vaccines are updated each season to protect against the four influenza viruses that research indicates will be most common during the upcoming season. This season's flu vaccine has been updated from last season.

TYPES OF FLU VACCINES FOR CHILDREN

The CDC recommends annual flu vaccination for everyone six months and older with any licensed, age-appropriate flu vaccine.

There are many vaccine options:

- Flu shots are given as an injection (with a needle) and are approved for use in people six months and older. (Indications vary by vaccine.)
- The nasal spray vaccine (also known as the "live attenuated influenza vaccine" or "LAIV4") is approved for use in nonpregnant, healthy people aged 2 through 49 years. However, there is a precaution against the use of the nasal spray flu vaccine (LAIV) in people with certain underlying medical conditions. More information can be found about the nasal spray flu vaccine.

Your child's health-care provider will know which vaccines are right for your child.

WHEN SHOULD CHILDREN GET A FLU VACCINE

Children should be vaccinated every flu season for the best protection against flu. For most people who need only one dose of flu vaccine for the season, September and October are generally good times to be vaccinated. Ideally, everyone six months and older should be vaccinated by the end of October. Some children need two doses of flu vaccine. For those children, it is recommended to get the first dose as soon as the vaccine is available—even if this is in July or August—because the second dose needs to be given at least four weeks after the first. Vaccination during July and August can also be considered for children who need only one dose. However, getting vaccinated later can still be protective, as long as flu viruses are spreading—even into January or later. Since it takes about two weeks after vaccination for the body to develop antibodies against flu virus infection, it is best to get vaccinated so they are protected before flu begins spreading in their community.

Special Vaccination Instructions for Children Aged Six Months through Eight Years Old

- Some children six months to eight years old need two doses of flu vaccine.
- Children in this age group getting vaccinated for the first time, those who have previously received only one dose of flu vaccine, and those whose flu vaccination history is unknown should get two doses of vaccine this season.
- For those children, it is recommended they get the first dose as soon as the vaccine is available because the second dose needs to be given at least four weeks after the first.
- Your child's health-care provider can tell you if your child needs two doses.

Other Preventive Actions

In addition to getting a flu vaccine, children and caregivers should take the same everyday preventive actions the CDC recommends for everyone, including avoiding people who are sick, washing hands often, and covering coughs.[2]

Section 22.3 | Human Parainfluenza

Human parainfluenza viruses (HPIVs) commonly cause respiratory infections in infants and young children. Patients usually recover on their own. However, HPIVs can also cause more severe illnesses, such as croup or pneumonia. The flu vaccine will not protect you against HPIV infections.

[2] "Flu Vaccines Are Important for Children," Centers for Disease Control and Prevention (CDC), March 22, 2024. Available online. URL: www.cdc.gov/flu/highrisk/children.htm#vaccination1. Accessed March 25, 2024.

SYMPTOMS AND ILLNESSES OF HUMAN PARAINFLUENZA VIRUSES

Human parainfluenza viruses commonly cause upper and lower respiratory illnesses in infants, young children, older adults, and people with weakened immune systems, but anyone can get infected. Symptoms generally appear two to six days after infection. Signs and symptoms are similar to the common cold and can include the following:

- fever
- runny nose
- cough
- sneezing
- sore throat

Other symptoms of HPIV illness may include the following:

- ear pain
- irritability
- decreased appetite

HPIVs can also cause more serious illnesses in children, including:

- croup (infection of the vocal cords (larynx), windpipe (trachea), and sometimes into the bronchial tubes (bronchi)
- bronchitis (infection of the main air passages that connect the windpipe to the lungs)
- bronchiolitis (infection in the smallest air passages in the lungs)
- pneumonia (an infection of the lungs)

Symptoms of more serious illnesses may include the following:

- barking cough
- hoarseness
- stridor (noisy or high-pitched sound with breathing)
- wheezing

TRANSMISSION: HOW HUMAN PARAINFLUENZA VIRUSES SPREAD

Human parainfluenza viruses usually spread from an infected person to others through:

- the air by coughing and sneezing
- close personal contact, such as touching or shaking hands
- touching objects or surfaces that have HPIVs on them, then touching your mouth, nose, or eyes

People can get HPIV infections any time of the year, but infections are more common in the spring, summer, and fall.

TREATMENT OF HUMAN PARAINFLUENZA VIRUSES

There is no specific antiviral treatment for HPIV illness. Most people with HPIV illness will recover on their own. However, to relieve symptoms, you can:

- take acetaminophen, ibuprofen, and other over-the-counter (OTC) medications for pain and fever (Caution: aspirin should not be given to children.)
- use a room humidifier or take a hot shower to help ease a sore throat and cough

People who are sick should:

- drink plenty of liquids
- stay home and rest

Antibiotics are not effective against HPIVs. Antibiotics are only effective against bacteria. If you are concerned about your or your child's symptoms, you should contact your health-care provider.

PREVENTION OF HUMAN PARAINFLUENZA VIRUSES

There is no vaccine to protect you against infection caused by HPIVs. However, researchers are trying to develop vaccines. You may be able to reduce your risk of HPIVs and other respiratory viral infections by taking everyday actions to help stop the spread of germs:

- washing your hands often with soap and water for at least 20 seconds (if soap and water are not available, use an alcohol-based hand rub)

- avoiding touching your eyes, nose, or mouth
- avoiding close contact with people who are sick

Frequent handwashing is especially important in childcare settings. Breastfeeding may protect babies from HPIVs during their first few months of life. That is because mothers may have antibodies (protective proteins) in their breast milk to fight infection. If you are sick with a common cold illness or cough that may be caused by HPIVs, you can help protect others by:

- staying home while you are sick
- avoiding close contact with others
- covering your mouth and nose when you cough or sneeze
- keeping objects and surfaces clean and disinfected

You may also consider wearing a well-fitted mask. Children aged two years and older can wear masks or respirators to protect themselves and others from HPIVs.

HUMAN PARAINFLUENZA VIRUS SEASONS

In the United States, HPIVs commonly cause respiratory tract illnesses. There are four types of HPIVs and two subtypes that circulate at different times of the year.

- **HPIV-1 infections often cause croup in children**. There are usually more cases in the fall of every other year.
- **HPIV-2 infections can also cause croup**. HPIV-2 infections occur more commonly in the fall of every other year during the years when HPIV-1 is low. It is less frequently detected than HPIV-1 and HPIV-3.
- **HPIV-3 infections usually occur in the spring and early summer months each year**. However, HPIV-3 infections can occur throughout the year, particularly when HPIV-1 and HPIV-2 are not in season.
- **HPIV-4 (subtypes 4a and 4b)**. Seasonal patterns are not as well characterized but appear to occur in fall and winter each year.[3]

[3] "Human Parainfluenza Viruses (HPIVs)," Centers for Disease Control and Prevention (CDC), November 18, 2022. Available online. URL: www.cdc.gov/parainfluenza/index.html. Accessed March 13, 2024.

Section 22.4 | Respiratory Syncytial Virus Infection

Respiratory syncytial virus (RSV) is a common respiratory virus that usually causes mild, cold-like symptoms. Most people recover in a week or two, but RSV can be serious. Infants and older adults are more likely to develop severe RSV and need hospitalization. If you are pregnant, you can get an RSV vaccine between 32 and 36 weeks of pregnancy to protect your infant after birth, or a preventive antibody can be given to your baby after birth.

SYMPTOMS OF RESPIRATORY SYNCYTIAL VIRUS

People infected with RSV usually show symptoms within four to six days after getting infected. Symptoms of RSV infection usually include the following:

- runny nose
- decrease in appetite
- coughing
- sneezing
- fever
- wheezing

These symptoms usually appear in stages and not all at once. In very young infants with RSV, the only symptoms may be irritability, decreased activity, and breathing difficulties. Almost all children will have had an RSV infection by their second birthday.

RESPIRATORY SYNCYTIAL VIRUS CARE

Antiviral medication is not routinely recommended to fight infection. Most RSV infections go away on their own in a week or two. However, RSV can cause severe illness in some people.

Take Steps to Relieve Symptoms

Manage fever and pain with over-the-counter (OTC) fever reducers and pain relievers, such as acetaminophen or ibuprofen (Never give aspirin to children.). Drink enough fluids. It is important for people with RSV infection to drink enough fluids to prevent dehydration (loss of body fluids). Talk to your health-care provider before giving your child nonprescription cold medicines. Some medicines contain ingredients that are not good for children.

Respiratory Syncytial Virus Can Cause More Serious Health Problems

Respiratory syncytial virus can also cause more severe infections such as bronchiolitis, an inflammation of the small airways in the lung, and pneumonia, an infection of the lungs. It is the most common cause of bronchiolitis and pneumonia in children younger than one year of age. Healthy adults and infants infected with RSV do not usually need to be hospitalized. However, some people with RSV infection, especially older adults and infants younger than six months of age, may need to be hospitalized if they are having trouble breathing or are dehydrated. In the most severe cases, a person may require additional oxygen, IV fluids (if they cannot eat or drink enough), or intubation (having a breathing tube inserted through the mouth and down to the airway) with mechanical ventilation (a machine to help a person breathe). In most of these cases, hospitalization only lasts a few days.

RESPIRATORY SYNCYTIAL VIRUS TRANSMISSION

Respiratory syncytial virus can spread when:

- an infected person coughs or sneezes
- you get virus droplets from a cough or sneeze in your eyes, nose, or mouth
- you have direct contact with the virus, such as kissing the face of a child with RSV
- you touch a surface that has the virus on it, such as a doorknob, and then touch your face before washing your hands

People are typically infected with RSV for the first time as an infant or toddler, and nearly all children are infected before their second birthday. However, repeat infections may occur throughout life, and people of any age can be infected. People infected with RSV are usually contagious for three to eight days and may become contagious a day or two before they start showing signs of illness. However, some infants and people with weakened immune systems can continue to spread the virus even after they stop showing symptoms, for as long as four weeks. Children are often exposed to and infected with RSV outside the home, such as in school or childcare centers. They can then transmit the virus to other members of the family.

RSV can survive for many hours on hard surfaces such as tables and crib rails. It typically lives on soft surfaces such as tissues and hands for shorter amounts of time. In most regions of the United States and other areas with similar climates, the RSV season generally starts during the fall and peaks in the winter. The timing and severity of RSV season in a given community can vary from year to year.

PEOPLE AT HIGH RISK FOR SEVERE RESPIRATORY SYNCYTIAL VIRUS INFECTION

Most people who get an RSV infection will have mild illness and will recover in a week or two. Some people, however, are more likely to develop severe RSV infection and may need to be hospitalized. Examples of severe infections include bronchiolitis (an inflammation of the small airways in the lung) and pneumonia. RSV can also make chronic health problems worse. For example, people with asthma may experience asthma attacks as a result of RSV infection, and people with congestive heart failure may experience more severe symptoms triggered by RSV. The following groups of people are more likely to get serious complications if they get sick with RSV:

Respiratory Syncytial Virus in Infants and Young Children

Respiratory syncytial virus can be dangerous for infants and young children. Each year in the United States, an estimated 58,000–80,000 children younger than five years are hospitalized due to RSV infection. Children at greatest risk for severe illness from RSV include the following:

- premature infants

- infants up to 12 months, especially those six months and younger
- children younger than two years with chronic lung disease or congenital (present from birth) heart disease
- children with weakened immune systems
- children who have neuromuscular disorders, including those who have difficulty swallowing or clearing mucus secretions

Following are the preventive options to protect babies from severe RSV. The CDC recommends you use one of these two tools to protect your baby from getting very sick with RSV:

- an RSV vaccine is given during pregnancy
- an RSV immunization is given to infants and older babies
- most infants will not need both

RESPIRATORY SYNCYTIAL VIRUS VACCINES FOR PREGNANT PEOPLE

An RSV vaccine is recommended for those who are 32–36 weeks pregnant from September through January in most of the continental United States. Some areas, where RSV season is slightly different, may have adjustments to the months when the RSV vaccine is recommended. These vaccines provide protection against severe RSV illness in the recipient's baby for up to six months after birth. The protection provided to the baby wanes over time.

RESPIRATORY SYNCYTIAL VIRUS IMMUNIZATION FOR BABIES

The RSV antibodies can help protect babies and young children from severe disease from an RSV infection. They provide an extra layer of defense that helps fight RSV infections and protect children from getting very sick. The protection these antibodies provide wanes over time. A preventive antibody is not a treatment for a child who already has an RSV infection.

RSV antibody immunization is recommended for all infants who are younger than eight months and born during or entering their first RSV season. Most infants whose mothers received an

RSV vaccine do not need to also get an RSV antibody. Additionally, a dose of RSV antibody is recommended for children between the ages of 8 and 19 months entering their second RSV season who are in at least one of these groups:

- children who have chronic lung disease from being born premature and are requiring medical therapy for their lung disease
- children who are severely immunocompromised
- children with cystic fibrosis who have severe disease
- American Indian and Alaska Native children

SEVERE RESPIRATORY SYNCYTIAL VIRUS

Virtually all children get an RSV infection by the time they are two years old. Most of the time, RSV will cause a mild, cold-like illness, but it can also cause severe illnesses such as:

- bronchiolitis (inflammation of the small airways in the lung)
- pneumonia (infection of the lungs)

Some children are at increased risk of severe RSV disease, including those who were born prematurely or who have chronic lung or heart disease or a weakened immune system. Two to three out of every 100 infants with an RSV infection may need to be hospitalized. Those who are hospitalized may require oxygen, IV fluids (if they are not eating and drinking), and mechanical ventilation (a machine to help with breathing). Most improve with this type of supportive care and are discharged in a few days.

SYMPTOMS OF RESPIRATORY SYNCYTIAL VIRUS

RSV may not be severe when it first starts; however, it can become more severe a few days into the illness. Early symptoms of RSV may include the following:

- runny nose
- eating or drinking less
- cough, which may progress to wheezing or difficulty breathing

RESPIRATORY SYNCYTIAL VIRUS IN VERY YOUNG INFANTS

Infants who get an RSV infection almost always show symptoms. This is different from adults, who can sometimes get RSV infections without experiencing symptoms. In very young infants (less than six months old), the symptoms of RSV infection may include the following:

- irritability
- decreased activity
- eating or drinking less
- apnea (pauses in breathing for more than 10 seconds)
- fever may not always occur with RSV infections

Call your health-care provider if you or your child is having difficulty breathing, not drinking enough fluids, or experiencing worsening symptoms.

EVERYDAY PREVENTIVE MEASURES CAN HELP LIMIT THE SPREAD OF RESPIRATORY SYNCYTIAL VIRUS

Respiratory syncytial virus season typically starts in the fall and peaks in the winter in most regions of the United States. Like other respiratory viruses, you can help limit the spread of RSV by following these preventive measures:

- **Wash your hands often**. Wash your hands often with soap and water for at least 20 seconds, and help young children do the same. If soap and water are not available, use an alcohol-based hand sanitizer. Washing your hands will help protect you from germs.
- **Avoid touching your face with unwashed hands**. Avoid touching your eyes, nose, and mouth with unwashed hands. Germs spread this way.
- **Avoid close contact with sick people**. Avoid close contact, such as kissing, and sharing cups or eating utensils with people who have cold-like symptoms.
- **Cover your coughs and sneezes**. Cover your mouth and nose with a tissue or your upper shirt sleeve when coughing or sneezing. Throw the tissue in the trash afterward.

- **Clean frequently touched surfaces.** Clean surfaces and objects that people frequently touch, such as toys, doorknobs, and mobile devices. When people infected with RSV touch surfaces and objects, they can leave behind germs. Also, when they cough or sneeze, droplets containing germs can land on surfaces and objects.
- **Stay home when you are sick.** If possible, stay home from work, school, and public areas when you are sick. This will help protect others from catching your illness.

RESPIRATORY SYNCYTIAL VIRUS PREVENTION

Respiratory syncytial virus is a common respiratory virus that typically causes mild, cold-like symptoms. However, it can pose serious risks for babies, toddlers, and older adults. The Centers for Disease Control and Prevention (CDC) have recommended several new immunizations to protect those most vulnerable to severe RSV illness: infants, toddlers, and adults aged 60 and older. For individuals less likely to experience severe RSV illness, everyday preventive actions can help reduce the spread of the virus.

Respiratory Syncytial Virus Immunizations to Protect Infants and Toddlers

There are two ways to protect your baby from severe RSV illness. One is through an RSV vaccine administered during pregnancy. The other method involves an RSV immunization that provides antibodies to your baby after birth. If you receive the RSV vaccine during pregnancy, your baby will be protected and likely will not need an RSV immunization later on. These are the two options available to safeguard your baby.

- **Get an RSV vaccine if you are 32–36 weeks pregnant during RSV season.** The vaccine is recommended from September through January in most of the United States, as RSV is typically a fall and winter virus. The timing of the RSV season can vary depending on location, and state, local, or territorial health departments may recommend different administration schedules for their respective areas.

- **Get an RSV antibody immunization for your baby if they are younger than eight months and born during, or entering their first RSV season.** In rare cases, a health-care provider may decide that an RSV immunization is necessary for an infant, even if the mother received an RSV vaccine.

Children between the ages of 8 and 19 months entering their second RSV season are recommended to receive a dose of RSV antibody if they belong to at least one of these groups:

- children who have chronic lung disease from being born prematurely
- children who are severely immunocompromised
- children with cystic fibrosis who have severe disease
- American Indian and Alaska Native children

Everyday Preventive Measures to Limit the Spread of Respiratory Syncytial Virus

You can take everyday preventive measures to help reduce the spread of RSV and other respiratory illnesses.

- Stay home when sick.
- Cover your coughs and sneezes with a tissue or your shirt sleeve, not your hands.
- Wash your hands often with soap and water for at least 20 seconds.
- Avoid touching your face with unwashed hands.
- Avoid close contact with others, such as kissing, shaking hands, and sharing cups and eating utensils.
- Clean frequently touched surfaces such as doorknobs and mobile devices.[4]

[4] "Respiratory Syncytial Virus Infection (RSV)," Centers for Disease Control and Prevention (CDC), November 7, 2023. Available online. URL: www.cdc.gov/rsv/index.html. Accessed March 13, 2024.

Section 22.5 | Strep Throat

Several viruses and bacteria can cause acute pharyngitis. *Streptococcus pyogenes*, also known as "group A *Streptococcus*" or "group A strep," specifically causes the condition known as "strep throat."

ETIOLOGY

Group A strep pharyngitis is an infection of the oropharynx caused by *S. pyogenes*. These are gram-positive cocci that grow in chains and exhibit ß-hemolysis (complete hemolysis) on blood agar plates. They are classified as group A in the Lancefield classification system for ß-hemolytic *Streptococcus* and are commonly referred to as "group A streptococci."

CLINICAL FEATURES

Group A strep pharyngitis is an acute condition characterized by:

- sudden onset of sore throat
- painful swallowing (odynophagia)
- fever

Other symptoms may include headache, abdominal pain, nausea, and vomiting, particularly among children. Patients with group A strep pharyngitis typically do not exhibit cough, runny nose (rhinorrhea), hoarseness, oral ulcers, or conjunctivitis, which strongly suggests a viral cause. On clinical examination, patients with group A strep pharyngitis usually present with:

- pharyngeal and tonsillar erythema
- tonsillar hypertrophy with or without exudates
- palatal petechiae
- anterior cervical lymphadenopathy

Patients with group A strep pharyngitis may also develop a scarlatiniform rash, leading to a syndrome known as "scarlet fever" or "scarlatina." Respiratory disease caused by group A strep infection in children under three years of age rarely presents as acute pharyngitis. Instead, these children typically experience mucopurulent rhinitis followed by fever, irritability, and anorexia, referred to as "streptococcal fever" or "streptococcosis." In contrast to typical acute group A strep pharyngitis, this presentation in young children is subacute, with high fever being uncommon.

TRANSMISSION OF STREP THROAT

Group A strep pharyngitis is primarily spread through direct person-to-person transmission, typically via saliva or nasal secretions from an infected person. Those with symptomatic pharyngitis are much more likely to transmit the bacteria than asymptomatic carriers. Crowded environments such as schools, day care centers, or military facilities facilitate transmission. While rare, foodborne outbreaks have occurred due to improper food handling. Transmission via fomites like household items (e.g., plates, toys) is highly unlikely. Humans are the main reservoir for group A strep, and there is no evidence suggesting pets can transmit the bacteria to humans. Effective antibiotic treatment for at least 24 hours generally eliminates the ability to transmit group A strep. Individuals with group A strep pharyngitis or scarlet fever should refrain from attending work, school, or daycare until:

- they are afebrile
- at least 12–24 hours after starting appropriate antibiotic therapy*

**Per the* American Academy of Pediatrics (AAP) Red Book 2021–2024, *children with group A strep pharyngitis should not return to school or a childcare setting until well appearing and at least 12 hours after beginning appropriate antibiotic therapy. In certain scenarios, such as an infection in a health-care worker or in a group A strep outbreak setting, staying home for at least 24 hours after beginning appropriate antibiotics should be considered.*

INCUBATION PERIOD

The incubation period of group A strep pharyngitis is approximately two to five days.

RISK FACTORS OF STREP THROAT

Group A strep pharyngitis can affect individuals of all ages, though it is most prevalent among children aged 5 to 15 years. It is rare in children younger than three years old. Close contact with someone with group A strep pharyngitis is the most common risk factor. Adults who are at increased risk for group A strep pharyngitis include:

- parents of school-aged children
- adults who are often in contact with children

Crowded environments such as schools, military barracks, and day care centers increase the risk of disease spread.

DIAGNOSIS AND TESTING OF STREP THROAT

The differential diagnosis of acute pharyngitis includes numerous viral and bacterial pathogens. Viruses are the primary cause of pharyngitis across all age groups. Experts estimate that group A strep, the most prevalent bacterial cause, accounts for 20–30 percent of pharyngitis cases in children and approximately 5–15 percent in adults. Diagnosis of viral pharyngitis can often be established based on history and clinical examination when typical viral symptoms are present. These symptoms include:

- cough
- rhinorrhea
- hoarseness
- oral ulcers
- conjunctivitis

Patients displaying clear viral symptoms typically do not require testing for group A strep. However, clinicians cannot differentiate between viral and group A strep pharyngitis based solely on clinical examination in the absence of viral symptoms. Therefore, either a rapid antigen-detection test (RADT) or throat culture is necessary to confirm group A strep pharyngitis. RADTs are highly specific for group A strep but have varying sensitivities compared to throat culture, which remains the gold standard diagnostic test.

SPECIAL CONSIDERATIONS

Clinicians should confirm group A strep pharyngitis in children older than three years of age to guide treatment decisions effectively. Administering antibiotics to children with confirmed group A strep pharyngitis can lower their risk of developing sequelae such as acute rheumatic fever (ARF). Routine testing for group A strep pharyngitis is not indicated for:

- children younger than three years of age
- adults

Acute rheumatic fever is uncommon in these age groups. Clinicians can use a positive RADT as confirmation of group A strep pharyngitis in children. However, if a child with symptoms of pharyngitis has a negative RADT, clinicians should follow up with a throat culture. Clinicians should have a process in place to contact the family and start antibiotics if the subsequent throat culture is positive.

TREATMENT OF STREP THROAT

The use of a recommended antibiotic regimen to treat group A strep pharyngitis:

- shortens the duration of symptoms
- reduces the likelihood of transmission to family members, classmates, and other close contacts
- prevents the development of complications, including acute rheumatic fever

When left untreated, the symptoms of group A strep pharyngitis typically resolve on their own. However, untreated infections increase the risk of acute rheumatic fever and suppurative complications such as peritonsillar abscess and mastoiditis. Patients of any age with a positive RADT or throat culture should receive antibiotics. Clinicians should avoid prescribing antibiotics for viral pharyngitis.

CARRIAGE

Asymptomatic carriers of group A strep typically do not require treatment. These individuals have positive throat cultures or are RADT positive but do not exhibit clinical symptoms or an immune response to group A strep antigens in laboratory tests. Compared to those with symptomatic pharyngitis, carriers are much less likely to transmit group A strep to others and are unlikely to develop suppurative or nonsuppurative complications.

Some individuals with recurrent episodes of acute pharyngitis, showing evidence of group A strep via RADT or throat culture, may actually have recurrent viral pharyngitis alongside streptococcal carriage. Repeated antibiotic use in this subset of patients is unnecessary. However, clinically or laboratory identifying carriers can be challenging. The guidelines from the Infectious Diseases Society of America and the Red Book provide guidance on identifying carriers and their management.

PROGNOSIS AND COMPLICATIONS OF STREP THROAT

Rarely, suppurative and nonsuppurative complications can occur following group A strep pharyngitis. Suppurative complications arise from the spread of group A strep from the pharynx to nearby structures. These complications can include:

- peritonsillar abscess
- retropharyngeal abscess
- cervical lymphadenitis
- mastoiditis

Other focal infections or sepsis are even rarer. Acute rheumatic fever (ARF) is a nonsuppurative sequela of group A strep pharyngitis. Poststreptococcal glomerulonephritis is another nonsuppurative sequela of either group A strep pharyngitis or skin infections. These complications manifest after the resolution of the initial infection and typically involve sites distant from the initial group A strep infection site. They are believed to result from the immune response rather than direct infection by group A strep.

PREVENTION OF STREP THROAT

Good hand hygiene and respiratory etiquette can effectively reduce the spread of all types of group A strep infection. It is crucial to practice thorough hand hygiene after coughing, sneezing, before preparing food, or eating. Proper respiratory etiquette includes covering your cough or sneeze. Administering antibiotics to an infected person for at least 24 hours generally eliminates their ability to transmit the bacteria. Therefore, individuals with group A strep pharyngitis should refrain from attending work, school, or daycare until:

- they are afebrile
- at least 24 hours after starting appropriate antibiotic therapy.[5]

Section 22.6 | **Whooping Cough**

Whooping cough (pertussis) can cause serious illness in individuals of all ages but is most dangerous for babies. Vaccination is the best way to protect against pertussis. Ensure that you and your loved ones are up-to-date with your whooping cough vaccines.

CAUSES OF WHOOPING COUGH

Whooping cough, also known as "pertussis," is a highly contagious respiratory illness caused by a bacterium called "*Bordetella pertussis*." This disease exclusively affects humans. *Bordetella pertussis* bacteria attach to the cilia—tiny hair-like extensions lining part of the upper respiratory system. These bacteria release toxins (poisons) that damage the cilia and lead to swelling of the airways.

[5] "Group A Streptococcal (GAS) Disease," Centers for Disease Control and Prevention (CDC), June 27, 2022. Available online. URL: www.cdc.gov/groupastrep/diseases-hcp/strep-throat.html. Accessed March 13, 2024.

SIGNS AND SYMPTOMS OF WHOOPING COUGH

Symptoms of whooping cough typically appear within 5–10 days after exposure to the bacteria that cause it. In some cases, symptoms may not manifest for up to three weeks.

Early Symptoms: Stage 1

Early symptoms can last for one to two weeks and usually include the following:

- runny or stuffed-up nose
- low-grade fever (less than 100.4 °F (38 °C))
- mild, occasional cough (babies do not do this)
- apnea (life-threatening pauses in breathing) and cyanosis (turning blue or purple) in babies and young children

In its early stages, whooping cough can resemble nothing more than the common cold. As a result, doctors often do not suspect or diagnose it until the more severe symptoms appear.

Later Symptoms: Stage 2

One to two weeks after the onset of symptoms, individuals with whooping cough may experience paroxysms—rapid, violent, and uncontrollable coughing fits. These fits typically persist for one to six weeks but can extend up to 10 weeks. As the illness progresses, coughing fits generally worsen and become more frequent. These fits can cause individuals to:

- make a high-pitched "whoop" sound when they are finally able to inhale at the end of a coughing fit
- vomit during or after coughing fits
- feel very tired after the fit, but usually seem well in between fits
- struggle to breathe

Babies May Struggle to Breathe, While Teens and Adults Usually Have Mild Symptoms

Many babies with whooping cough do not cough at all; instead, it may cause them to turn blue or struggle to breathe. The infection can resemble a common cold throughout the entire illness, not just at the beginning. Generally, the illness is milder in teens and adults who have been vaccinated against whooping cough compared to babies and children. In milder cases, the characteristic "whoop" sound may not be present. However, serious cases can occur in teens and adults, particularly those who were not vaccinated against whooping cough. These individuals may experience prolonged coughing fits that disrupt sleep and are described as the worst cough of their lives. Whooping cough can also lead to significant disruptions in daily life and serious complications.

Vaccinated People May Not Get as Sick

Whooping cough vaccines are effective but not flawless. The infection typically causes less severe illness in vaccinated individuals who still contract whooping cough. In vaccinated people who develop whooping cough:

- the cough usually would not last as many days
- coughing fits, whooping, and vomiting after coughing fits are less common
- apnea and cyanosis are less common (in vaccinated babies and children)

Recovery: Stage 3

Recovery from whooping cough can be gradual. The cough becomes less severe and less frequent as recovery progresses. Coughing fits may cease for a period but can recur if the individual contracts other respiratory infections. These fits can return many months after the onset of whooping cough.

HOW WHOOPING COUGH SPREADS

The bacteria that cause whooping cough spread easily from person to person through the air. When a person with whooping cough sneezes or coughs, they release small particles containing the bacteria. Others then inhale these bacteria. Transmission also occurs when people spend extended time together or share breathing space, such as when holding a newborn on the chest.

People Can Be Contagious for Weeks

People can spread the bacteria from the onset of the first symptoms and for at least two weeks after coughing begins. Early administration of antibiotics during the illness may reduce the contagious period.

People Can Spread the Disease Even If They Do Not Know They Have It

Some people have mild symptoms and may not realize they have whooping cough, but they can still transmit the bacteria to others. Many babies who contract whooping cough are infected by older siblings, parents, or caregivers who are unaware they have the infection.

COMPLICATIONS OF WHOOPING COUGH

Babies and Children

Whooping cough can cause serious and sometimes deadly complications in babies and young children who have not received all recommended vaccines. Approximately one-third of infants younger than one year old with whooping cough require hospital care. The younger the infant, the more likely they are to need hospitalization. Among infants under one year old hospitalized with whooping cough:

- 2 in 3 (68%) will have apnea (life-threatening pauses in breathing)
- 1 in 5 (22%) get pneumonia (lung infection)
- 1 in 50 (2%) will have convulsions (violent, uncontrolled shaking)
- 1 in 150 (0.6%) will have encephalopathy (disease of the brain)
- 1 in 100 (1%) will die

DIAGNOSIS OF WHOOPING COUGH

Doctors diagnose whooping cough by considering if you have been in contact with someone who has whooping cough and by performing a:

- history of typical signs and symptoms
- physical exam

- laboratory test of a mucus sample from the back of the throat
- blood test

TREATMENT FOR WHOOPING COUGH

Doctors typically treat whooping cough with antibiotics. Several antibiotics are available for treating whooping cough. It is crucial to initiate treatment early, ideally before coughing fits commence. Early treatment of whooping cough can:

- make the illness less serious
- help prevent the spreading of the bacteria that cause it to others

Starting treatment after three weeks of illness is unlikely to be beneficial, even though most people will still experience symptoms. By that point, your body has already cleared the bacteria, but the symptoms persist due to the damage already inflicted on your body.

Managing Symptoms at Home

Manage whooping cough symptoms and reduce the risk of spreading the bacteria to others.

- Take antibiotics exactly as prescribed by the doctor.
- Keep your home free from irritants, such as smoke, dust, and chemical fumes, as much as possible to reduce cough triggers.
- Use a clean, cool mist humidifier to help loosen mucus and soothe the cough.
- Wash hands often with soap and water for at least 20 seconds.
- Eat small meals every few hours to help prevent vomiting.
- Stay hydrated by consuming plenty of fluids, including water, juices, soups, and fruits, to prevent dehydration.
- Do not administer cough medicine unless recommended by your doctor; it typically does not

provide relief and is often not recommended for children under four years old.

Report signs of dehydration to your doctor immediately. Signs of dehydration include the following:

- dry, sticky mouth
- sleepiness or tiredness
- thirst
- decreased urination or fewer wet diapers
- few or no tears when crying
- muscle weakness
- headache
- dizziness or lightheadedness

GETTING TREATMENT IN A HOSPITAL

Whooping cough can sometimes be very serious and lead to complications, especially in babies. Individuals with severe illness or complications often require hospital care. Approximately one-third of infants younger than one year old who contract whooping cough need hospitalization. Hospital treatment for whooping cough typically focuses on the following:

- **Keeping breathing passages clear**. This may require suctioning (drawing out) mucus.
- **Monitoring breathing and giving oxygen, if needed.**
- **Preventing or treating dehydration**. People might need intravenous (IV, through the vein) fluids if they show signs of dehydration or have difficulty eating.

PREVENTION OF WHOOPING COUGH

Vaccines

The best way to prevent whooping cough is to get vaccinated. The Centers for Disease Control and Prevention (CDC) recommends whooping cough vaccination for everyone.

Preventive Antibiotics

Preventive antibiotics, also known as "postexposure antimicrobial prophylaxis" (PEP), are medications administered to individuals who have been exposed to harmful bacteria to prevent illness. Doctors and local health departments typically determine who should receive preventive antibiotics. For individuals exposed to whooping cough, the CDC recommends preventive antibiotics only if they:

- live with a person who has been diagnosed with whooping cough
- are at increased risk for serious disease (e.g., babies, people with certain medical conditions) or will have close contact with someone who is at increased risk for serious disease (e.g., women in their third trimester of pregnancy, people who work with or care for high-risk individuals)

If you have been exposed to the bacteria that cause whooping cough, discuss with your doctor whether you need preventive antibiotics. This is particularly important if there is a baby or pregnant woman in your household, or if you anticipate having contact with a baby or pregnant woman.

Good Hygiene

The CDC recommends practicing good hygiene to prevent the spread of the bacteria that cause whooping cough and other respiratory illnesses.

COVER YOUR COUGH OR SNEEZE

- Cover your mouth and nose with a tissue when you cough or sneeze.
- Throw away used tissues in the wastebasket right away.
- Cough or sneeze into your upper sleeve or elbow if you do not have a tissue. Avoid coughing into your hands as this can spread germs.

WASH YOUR HANDS OFTEN

- Wash your hands often with soap and water for at least 20 seconds.
- Use an alcohol-based hand sanitizer if soap and water are not available.

Temporary Immunity after Getting Sick

People who have had whooping cough develop some natural immunity (protection) against future infections. However, getting sick with whooping cough does not provide lifelong protection.

FIVE THINGS TO KNOW ABOUT WHOOPING COUGH

- Whooping cough can be very serious, especially for babies.
- Whooping cough can cause serious illness in people of all ages and can be life-threatening, especially in babies.
- About one-third of babies younger than one year old who contract whooping cough require hospital care, and 1 out of 100 babies hospitalized for treatment die.
- Whooping cough is very contagious.
    - The bacteria that cause whooping cough spread easily from person to person through coughing and sneezing.
    - Some people have mild symptoms and may not realize they have whooping cough, but they can still spread the bacteria to others, including babies.
- Severe coughing fits can last for weeks.
    - Pertussis is known as "whooping cough" because of the "whooping" sound people can make when gasping for air after coughing.
    - Whooping cough can cause rapid, violent, and uncontrolled coughing fits until all air is gone from the lungs. These coughing fits can go on for up to 10 weeks or more.
- Babies may not cough at all.
    - Babies may not cough at all. Instead, they may experience apnea (life-threatening pauses in breathing) or struggle to breathe.

    - Any time someone struggles to breathe, it is important to get them to a doctor immediately.
- Vaccines are the best protection against whooping cough.
    - The best way to protect yourself and your loved ones is to stay updated with recommended whooping cough vaccines.
    - Two vaccines in the United States help prevent whooping cough: diphtheria, tetanus, and pertussis (DTaP) and tetanus, diphtheria, and pertussis (Tdap) vaccines. Children younger than seven years old get DTaP vaccine, while older children, teens, and adults get Tdap vaccine.
- Women should get a Tdap vaccine during the third trimester of each pregnancy to help protect their baby early in life.[6]

Section 22.7 | **Childhood Asthma**

Asthma often begins during childhood when the immune system is still developing. Viral infections and exposure to allergens, such as cigarette smoke during infancy or early childhood, can increase a child's risk of developing asthma. Having a parent with asthma, particularly the mother, also raises a child's risk. Boys are more likely than girls to have asthma during childhood.

DIAGNOSING ASTHMA IN CHILDREN YOUNGER THAN SIX

It can be challenging to distinguish whether a child under the age of six has asthma or another condition affecting breathing because young children often cannot perform the most common test for diagnosing asthma, which is spirometry. Instead, your child's doctor will inquire about their medical history and symptoms. They may prescribe asthma medications for a few months to assess your child's response.

[6] "Whooping Cough (Pertussis)," Centers for Disease Control and Prevention (CDC), August 8, 2022. Available online. URL: www.cdc.gov/pertussis/index.html. Accessed March 13, 2024.

MANAGING ASTHMA IN CHILDREN

There is no cure for asthma in children. Your child's doctor will assist you in learning to control it by avoiding triggers, administering medication, and monitoring symptoms. Additionally, your child's doctor will collaborate with you to develop an asthma action plan. This plan will outline triggers to avoid and steps to take during an asthma attack. Be sure to provide a copy of your child's asthma action plan to school staff and other caregivers.

HOW TO TELL IF YOUR CHILD'S ASTHMA IS NOT WELL-CONTROLLED

If your young child's asthma is not well-controlled, you may notice increased nighttime coughing and decreased appetite. Your child may also appear more fatigued, irritable, or moody.

When to Call 911

For young children with asthma, call 911 if they:

- seem drowsy, confused, or troubled
- have a blue tint to the skin and lips
- have a fast heartbeat

If your child does not have the previously mentioned symptoms but is experiencing difficulty breathing or persistent coughing, contact your doctor immediately. It is important to follow your child's asthma action plan whenever possible.[7]

WHAT ARE THE TREATMENTS FOR ASTHMA IN CHILDREN?

If your child has asthma, you'll collaborate with their health-care provider to develop a treatment plan. This plan will include strategies to manage your child's asthma symptoms and prevent asthma attacks, such as:

- **Strategies to avoid triggers**. For example, if tobacco smoke is a trigger for your child, you should not allow anyone to smoke in your home or car.

[7] "Asthma in Children," National Heart, Lung, and Blood Institute (NHLBI), March 24, 2022. Available online. URL: www.nhlbi.nih.gov/health/asthma/children. Accessed March 13, 2024.

- **Short-term relief medicines.** This is also called "quick-relief medicines." They help prevent or relieve symptoms during an asthma attack. These include an inhaler that your child should have at all times, along with other medications that quickly open your child's airways.
- **Control medicines.** They work by reducing airway inflammation and preventing the narrowing of the airways. Not all children will require control medicines. Whether your child needs them depends on the severity of their asthma and the frequency of their symptoms.[8]

CONTROLLING CHILDHOOD ASTHMA

Asthma is a chronic lung disease affecting approximately 25 million people of all ages in the United States. Among them, an estimated 7 million are children, with about 3 million aged 5–11. Asthma inflames and narrows the airways, leading to symptoms such as coughing, wheezing, chest tightness, and shortness of breath.

For most individuals, managing asthma involves daily medication to prevent symptoms. Inhaled steroids are commonly used for long-term control, including in young children. An asthma flare-up, or attack, occurs when symptoms worsen or new symptoms arise. Prompt treatment of symptoms can help prevent severe flare-ups. Quick-acting medications like inhaled albuterol are used as needed to open the airways. Oral steroids such as prednisone may be necessary for short periods to manage acute asthma episodes. Severe flare-ups may require emergency care and can be life-threatening.

Many health-care providers recommend increasing the dose of inhaled steroids at the first signs of asthma symptoms such as coughing, wheezing, and shortness of breath. To evaluate this approach in children, Dr. Daniel J. Jackson, MD, an Associate Professor of Pediatrics at the University of Wisconsin, led a study funded by the National Institutes of Health (NIH), specifically the National Heart, Lung, and Blood Institute (NHLBI). The study aimed to determine whether a short-term increase in the dose of

---

[8] MedlinePlus, "Asthma in Children," National Institutes of Health (NIH), January 26, 2024. Available online. URL: https://medlineplus.gov/asthmainchildren.html. Accessed March 27, 2024.

inhaled steroids could prevent asthma flare-ups. The results of the study were published on March 8, 2018, in the *New England Journal of Medicine*. The researchers examined 254 children aged 5–11 with mild to moderate asthma from 2016 to 2017. These children were administered low-dose inhaled steroids (two puffs of fluticasone from an inhaler twice daily) over a span of 48 weeks. At the first signs of an asthma flare-up, half of the children utilized high-dose (5 times the standard dose) inhaled steroids twice daily for seven days, while the remaining 127 children adhered to low-dose inhaled steroids throughout each episode.

The team found that the increased dose made little difference in preventing severe flare-ups: 38 children in the high-dose group and 30 in the low-dose group required oral prednisone treatment for a flare-up at least once. Both groups showed similar numbers of asthma symptoms, time to the first severe flare-up, and use of quick-relief medicine (albuterol). Additionally, the study noted a slightly lower growth rate among children under eight years who received the high-dose steroid.

"These findings suggest that a short-term increase to high-dose inhaled steroids should not be routinely included in asthma treatment plans for children with mild-moderate asthma who are regularly using low-dose inhaled corticosteroids," Dr. Jackson says. "Low-dose inhaled steroids remain the cornerstone of daily treatment in affected children."[9]

ASTHMA IS THE MOST COMMON CHRONIC DISEASE OF CHILDHOOD

- In an average classroom of 30 kids, about 3 have asthma.
- About 4 in 10 children who wheeze when they get colds or respiratory infections will be diagnosed with asthma.

An estimated 5 million children in the United States have asthma. Among all U.S. children, asthma affects about:

- 11 percent of all children living in poverty

[9] News and Events, "Controlling Childhood Asthma," National Institutes of Health (NIH), March 13, 2018. Available online. URL: www.nih.gov/news-events/nih-research-matters/controlling-childhood-asthma. Accessed March 13, 2024.

- 11 percent of all boys ages 5–14
- 14 percent of all Black children

Each year, children with poorly managed asthma experience more than:

- 10 million missed school days
- 74,000 hospital stays
- 767,000 trips to the emergency room

Children with asthma may experience:

- coughing
- wheezing
- chest tightness
- shortness of breath

If your child has asthma, work with their health-care provider to:

- develop an asthma action plan
- identify and avoid triggers
- take medicines as prescribed,
- watch for any changes

Share the asthma action plan with your child's caretakers and school. With proper asthma management, your child can lead a full and active life.[10]

Section 22.8 | **COVID-19 in Children**

Coronavirus disease 2019 (COVID-19) is caused by a virus named severe acute respiratory syndrome coronavirus 2 (SARS-CoV-2). It is highly contagious and spreads rapidly (see Figure 22.1). Over 1 million people have died from COVID-19 in the United States. COVID-19 commonly presents with respiratory symptoms similar

[10] "Asthma in Kids," National Heart, Lung, and Blood Institute (NHLBI), April 18, 2022. Available online. URL: www.nhlbi.nih.gov/LMBBasthma/asthma-kids. Accessed April 17, 2024.

to those of a cold, flu, or pneumonia. However, it can also affect other parts of the body. While most people experience mild symptoms, some become severely ill. Additionally, individuals with minor or no symptoms may develop post-COVID conditions, also known as "Long COVID."[11]

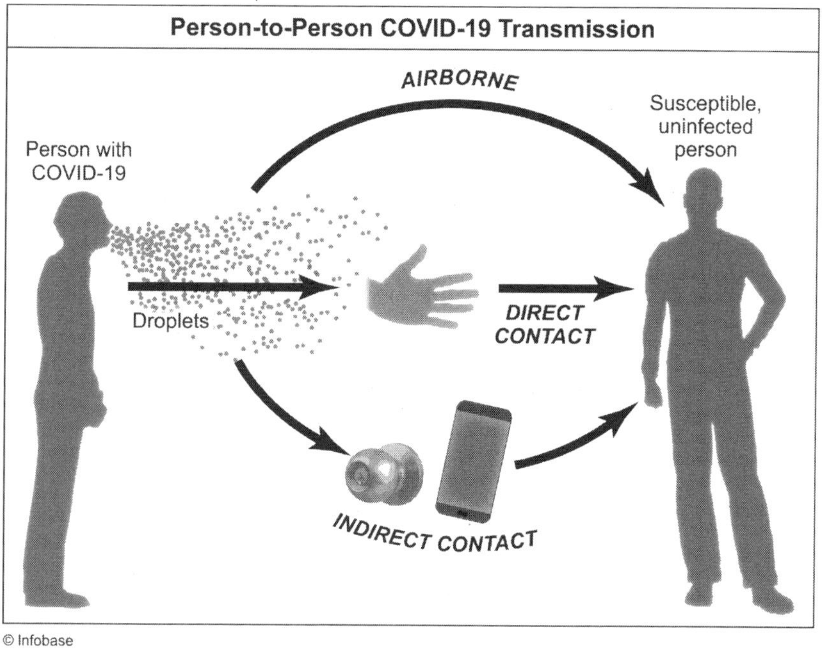

Figure 22.1. Transmission of COVID-19
Infobase

EPIDEMIOLOGY IN CHILDREN

Data from the Centers for Disease Control and Prevention (CDC) indicate that severe disease and fatalities from COVID-19 are less common in children compared to adults. However, knowledge about the pathogenesis and clinical presentation of SARS-CoV-2 infection in children remains limited compared to adults. While only a small percentage of children with COVID-19 need medical care, the rate of intensive care unit (ICU) admissions among

[11] "About COVID-19," Centers for Disease Control and Prevention (CDC), July 10, 2023. Available online. URL: www.cdc.gov/coronavirus/2019-ncov/your-health/about-covid-19.html. Accessed March 13, 2024.

hospitalized children is similar to that of hospitalized adults with COVID-19.

Children from certain racial and ethnic groups experience higher rates of COVID-19-related hospitalization, potentially due to barriers in accessing health care and economic and structural inequities. In the United States from 2020 to 2021, Black/African-American children with COVID-19 were twice as likely to be hospitalized and five times more likely to require ICU admission compared to white children.

A study conducted in the United States on children hospitalized with COVID-19 between April and September 2020 found an association between race/ethnicity and disease severity. Similarly, a recent study in the United Kingdom identified an independent association between admission to critical care and children hospitalized with COVID-19 who self-identified as Black. In England, research indicated that children identifying as Asian were more likely than those identifying as white to require hospitalization for COVID-19 and admission to an ICU. Additionally, the study noted significantly higher hospitalization rates among children identifying as Black, mixed race, or other ethnicities compared to those identifying as white.

CLINICAL FEATURES OF COVID-19

The signs and symptoms of SARS-CoV-2 infection in symptomatic children closely resemble those in adults. However, a higher proportion of children may be asymptomatic or experience only mild illness compared to adults. While the exact incidence of asymptomatic SARS-CoV-2 infection remains unclear, a small study indicated that 45 percent of children tested for surveillance during hospitalization for non-COVID-19 reasons had asymptomatic infection. Common signs and symptoms of COVID-19 in hospitalized children include fever, nausea/vomiting, cough, shortness of breath, and upper respiratory symptoms. These symptoms can overlap significantly with those of influenza and other respiratory and gastrointestinal viral infections. Critical illnesses such as respiratory failure, acute respiratory distress syndrome (ARDS), and, less frequently, shock, can occur in children with COVID-19.

RISK FACTORS FOR SEVERE COVID-19

Observational studies and meta-analyses indicate that children with certain comorbidities face an increased risk of severe COVID-19. These comorbidities include cardiac disease, neurologic disorders, prematurity (in young infants), diabetes, obesity (especially severe obesity), chronic lung disease, feeding tube dependence, and immunocompromised status. Demographic factors such as age (< 1 year and 10–14 years) and non-white race/ethnicity have also been linked to severe disease outcomes. However, many studies did not evaluate the relative severity of underlying medical conditions in children with severe COVID-19. Assessing the risk of severe disease is crucial for guiding treatment decisions, particularly regarding antiviral treatment, which may benefit nonhospitalized children with mild to moderate COVID-19 who are at high risk of severe illness, such as those with severe comorbidities.

COVID-19 Vaccination

Staying current with COVID-19 vaccinations remains the most effective measure to prevent severe illness from COVID-19. Vaccine effectiveness varies across age groups and time periods. From July 2022 to September 2023, during the dominance of Omicron subvariants in the United States, 86 percent of eligible children aged six months to under five years who were hospitalized or sought care in emergency departments for acute respiratory illness had not received any COVID-19 vaccines. Two or more doses of the COVID-19 vaccine showed 40 percent effectiveness in preventing emergency department visits or hospitalizations due to COVID-19 compared to unvaccinated children in the same age group. In a study involving U.S. children aged eight months to under five years hospitalized for COVID-19 from September 20, 2022, to May 31, 2023, only 4.5 percent had completed their primary COVID-19 vaccine series.

During the period when the Delta variant predominated in the United States, vaccine effectiveness against severe COVID-19 in adolescents aged 12–18 years exceeded 90 percent. However, when the Omicron variant became dominant, vaccine effectiveness against hospitalization for noncritical COVID-19 dropped to 20 percent in adolescents, while effectiveness against critical illness remained at 79 percent in this age group. In children aged 5–11 years, vaccine effectiveness against hospitalization varied more, with an estimated effectiveness of 68 percent after Omicron became the dominant variant in the United States.

A meta-analysis of COVID-19 vaccination in adolescents aged 12–17 years found a vaccine effectiveness of 88 percent against severe disease and 35 percent against non-severe COVID-19. In Italy, during the Omicron period, vaccine effectiveness was estimated at 38 percent in children aged 5–11 years. Similarly, a Canadian study indicated that the effectiveness of two doses of COVID-19 vaccine against symptomatic COVID-19 in children aged 5–11 years varied widely, declining over time after the last dose and particularly against Omicron subvariants that were antigenically distinct from the vaccine.

MORTALITY

Death from COVID-19 is rare among children. Risk factors associated with higher mortality include chronic conditions like neurological or cardiac diseases, as well as multiple comorbidities. In the United States, deaths related to COVID-19 have been more prevalent among children aged 10–20 years, particularly among young adults aged 18–20 years, and those identifying as Hispanic, Black, or American Indian/Alaskan Native.

A systematic review and meta-analysis indicated that neurologic or cardiac comorbidities conferred the highest risk of death among hospitalized children with COVID-19. Additionally, an individual patient data meta-analysis within the same study revealed that the risk of death from COVID-19 was higher in children with one chronic condition compared to those without comorbidities, with a substantial increase in risk as the number of comorbidities increased.

VERTICAL TRANSMISSION AND INFANTS BORN TO PEOPLE WITH SARS-COV-2 INFECTION

Systematic reviews and meta-analyses have indicated that confirmed vertical transmission of SARS-CoV-2 appears to be rare, but severe maternal COVID-19 has been linked to SARS-CoV-2 infection in babies. In two large combined cohorts of pregnant individuals from the United States and the United Kingdom, SARS-CoV-2 infection was reported in 1.8 and 2 percent of babies born to individuals with SARS-CoV-2 infection. A systematic review and meta-analysis of prospective observational studies from high-income countries estimated that the frequency of SARS-CoV-2 infection in infants born to individuals with SARS-CoV-2 infection was 2.3 percent.

Case reports have documented intrauterine fetal demise during the third trimester of pregnancy in individuals with mild COVID-19 caused by infection with the Delta variant. These individuals exhibited evidence of placental SARS-CoV-2 infection, placental malperfusion, and placental inflammation. One case report involved a person with asymptomatic SARS-CoV-2 infection and severe preeclampsia who underwent emergency cesarean delivery at 25 weeks of gestation. The neonate passed away on day four, with evidence of SARS-CoV-2 infection detected in placental tissues and in the infant's lungs and vascular endothelium during autopsy. Evidence of placental SARS-CoV-2 infection was also noted in five stillbirths and in a live-born neonate in Sweden.

A systematic review of neonatal SARS-CoV-2 infections indicated that 70 percent were attributed to postpartum transmission, while 30 percent resulted from vertical transmission from the infected birth parent. Two systematic reviews also reported that newborn infants who roomed in with an infected birth parent did not show an elevated risk of SARS-CoV-2 transmission compared to newborns who were isolated from the birth parent.

Detection of SARS-CoV-2 RNA in the breast milk of individuals with confirmed cases of COVID-19 is rare. There is no evidence of SARS-CoV-2 transmission through breast milk. Breast milk from people with SARS-CoV-2 infection can contain antibodies to SARS-CoV-2.

MULTISYSTEM INFLAMMATORY SYNDROME IN CHILDREN

A small subset of children and young adults with SARS-CoV-2 infection, including those with asymptomatic infection, may develop MIS-C. This syndrome is also called "Pediatric Inflammatory Multisystem Syndrome Temporally Associated with SARS-CoV-2" (PIMS-TS). Although the case definitions for these syndromes differ slightly, they are likely the same disease. The syndrome was first described in Europe, where previously healthy children with severe inflammation and features similar to Kawasaki disease were identified as having infection with SARS-CoV-2. Subsequently, children with MIS-C were identified in the United States and in many other locations outside of Europe.

Although risk factors for the development of MIS-C have not been established, an analysis of MIS-C cases in the United States found that ICU admission was more likely for patients aged 6–12 years than for younger children, and it was more likely for children who identified as non-Hispanic Black than for those who identified as non-Hispanic white. Unlike most children who present with severe COVID-19, the majority of children who present with MIS-C do not seem to have common underlying comorbidities other than obesity. Additionally, children whose deaths were related to MIS-C were less likely to have underlying medical conditions than children who died of COVID-19.

Several studies have suggested that COVID-19 vaccination protects against the development of MIS-C. Following the emergence of the Omicron variant, the incidence of MIS-C and its clinical severity have declined. This decline may be attributed to several factors. For instance, more children have now received COVID-19 vaccines and have had infections with SARS-CoV-2, which may provide some protection against MIS-C.

POST-COVID CONDITIONS

The persistent symptoms after COVID-19 that have been described in children are similar to those seen in adults. The terminology for these collective symptoms is evolving and includes long COVID, post–COVID-19 condition, and postacute sequelae of SARS-CoV-2 infection (PASC). The data on the incidence of post-COVID conditions in children are limited and somewhat conflicting, but the overall incidence appears to be lower in children than in adults.

Case definitions for post-COVID conditions vary between studies, making it challenging to determine the true incidence of these conditions. The incidence of post-COVID symptoms in children appears to increase with age. The most commonly reported symptoms include persistent fatigue, headache, shortness of breath, sleep disturbances, gastrointestinal (GI) symptoms, and an altered sense of smell. Additionally, cardiopulmonary injury, neurocognitive impairment, and new-onset diabetes may occur. However, some studies did not include control groups of children without SARS-CoV-2 infection, which complicates assessing the relative risk of these symptoms.[12]

[12] "Special Considerations in Children," National Institutes of Health (NIH), February 29, 2024. Available online. URL: www.covid19treatmentguidelines.nih.gov/management/clinical-management-of-children/special-considerations-in-children. Accessed March 13, 2024.

Chapter 23 | **Other Infections in Children**

Chapter Contents

Newborns with symptoms of conjunctivitis (pink eye) should see a doctor right away. Neonatal conjunctivitis is a red eye in a newborn caused by infection, irritation, or a blocked tear duct. When caused by an infection, neonatal conjunctivitis can be very serious.

SYMPTOMS AND CAUSES OF CONJUNCTIVITIS IN NEWBORNS

Newborns with conjunctivitis develop drainage from the eyes within a few days to several weeks after birth. Their eyelids become puffy, red, and tender. The cause of neonatal conjunctivitis is often difficult to determine because, in many instances, the symptoms do not vary by cause. Conjunctivitis in a newborn may be caused by a blocked tear duct, irritation produced by the topical antimicrobials given at birth, or infection with a virus or bacterium passed from the mother to her baby during childbirth. Even mothers without symptoms (asymptomatic) at the time of delivery can carry and pass bacteria or viruses to babies during birth. The most common types of neonatal conjunctivitis include the following:

- **Inclusion (chlamydial) conjunctivitis**. *Chlamydia trachomatis* can cause inclusion conjunctivitis and genital infections (chlamydia). A woman with untreated chlamydia can pass the bacteria to her baby during childbirth. Symptoms of inclusion conjunctivitis include redness of the eye(s), swelling of the eyelids, and discharge of pus. Symptoms are likely to appear 5–12 days after birth but can develop earlier if the amniotic sac is ruptured during delivery. Some newborns with chlamydial conjunctivitis can have the infection in other parts of their bodies. The bacteria can infect the lungs and nasopharynx (where the back of the nose connects to the mouth).
- **Gonococcal conjunctivitis**. *Neisseria gonorrhoeae* can cause gonococcal conjunctivitis, as well as the sexually transmitted infection (STI) called "gonorrhea." A woman with untreated gonorrhea can pass the bacteria

to her baby during childbirth. Symptoms usually include red eyes, thick pus in the eyes, and swelling of the eyelids. This type of conjunctivitis usually begins in the first two to five days of life. It can also progress to serious infections of the bloodstream (bacteremia) and the lining of the brain and spinal cord (meningitis) in newborns.

- **Chemical conjunctivitis**. When eye drops are given to newborns to help prevent a bacterial infection, the newborn's eye(s) may become irritated. This may be diagnosed as chemical conjunctivitis. Symptoms of chemical conjunctivitis usually include mildly red eye(s) and some swelling of the eyelids. Symptoms are likely to last for only 24–36 hours.
- **Other neonatal conjunctivitis**. Viruses and bacteria other than *Chlamydia trachomatis* and *Neisseria gonorrhoeae* can cause conjunctivitis. For example, bacteria that normally live in a woman's vagina and are not sexually transmitted can cause conjunctivitis. Additionally, the viruses that cause genital and oral herpes can cause neonatal conjunctivitis and severe eye damage. The mother may pass these viruses to her baby during childbirth. However, herpes conjunctivitis is less common than conjunctivitis caused by gonorrhea and chlamydia. Symptoms usually include red eye(s) and swollen eyelids with some pus.

PREVENTION AND TREATMENT OF CONJUNCTIVITIS IN NEWBORNS

To prevent neonatal conjunctivitis, most states have laws requiring providers to put drops or ointment in a newborn's eyes, typically within two to three hours of birth. In the past, hospitals used silver nitrate; now, hospitals mostly use antibiotic eye drops, typically erythromycin. During pregnancy and prior to giving birth, women with genital herpes should consult with their physician about ways to minimize the chances of spreading the infection to their newborn baby.

Doctors may treat neonatal conjunctivitis caused by a bacterial infection with antibiotics, depending on the severity of the infection and the bacteria that caused it. Some antibiotics are applied as eye drops or ointments (topical). Other antibiotics are given by mouth (orally), through a vein (intravenously), or as a shot (intramuscularly). Doctors may treat a newborn's conjunctivitis with a combination of topical and either oral, intravenous, or intramuscular antibiotics. Rinsing the newborn's infected eye with a saline solution will remove any debris that may develop in response to the infection.

If a blocked tear duct causes conjunctivitis, a gentle, warm massage between the eye and nasal area may help. If the blocked tear duct does not clear by one year of age, the newborn may require surgery. Treatments for the common causes of neonatal conjunctivitis are as follows:

- **Inclusion (chlamydial) conjunctivitis.** Doctors usually use oral antibiotics to treat inclusion conjunctivitis.
- **Gonococcal conjunctivitis.** Doctors give IV or IM antibiotics to treat gonococcal conjunctivitis. If untreated, the newborn could develop corneal ulcerations (open sores in the cornea) and blindness.
- **Chemical conjunctivitis.** Since this type of conjunctivitis is caused by chemical irritation, treatment is usually not required. The newborn will usually get better in 24–36 hours.
- **Other bacterial and viral conjunctivitis.** Doctors usually prescribe antibiotic drops or ointments to treat conjunctivitis caused by bacteria. For both bacterial and viral conjunctivitis, a warm compress to the eye may relieve swelling and irritation. Be sure to wash your hands before and after touching the infected eyes.[1]

[1] "Conjunctivitis (Pink Eye) in Newborns," Centers for Disease Control and Prevention (CDC), January 4, 2019. Available online. URL: www.cdc.gov/conjunctivitis/newborns.html. Accessed March 13, 2024.

Section 23.2 | Chronic Diarrhea

WHAT IS CHRONIC DIARRHEA IN CHILDREN?

Chronic diarrhea is characterized by passing loose, watery stools three or more times a day for at least four weeks. Children with chronic diarrhea may have loose, watery stools continually, or their diarrhea may come and go. Chronic diarrhea can affect children of any age. In contrast, diarrhea that lasts only a short time is called "acute diarrhea." Acute diarrhea, a common problem in children, usually lasts a few days and resolves on its own.

WHAT CAUSES CHRONIC DIARRHEA IN CHILDREN?

Infections of the Digestive Tract

Infections from harmful viruses, bacteria, or parasites can sometimes lead to chronic diarrhea. Children may become infected through contaminated water, beverages, or food, or through person-to-person contact. After an infection, some children have problems digesting carbohydrates such as lactose or proteins in foods such as milk, milk products, or soy. These problems can cause prolonged diarrhea, often lasting up to six weeks after an infection. Additionally, some bacterial and parasitic infections that cause diarrhea do not resolve quickly without treatment.

Celiac Disease

Celiac disease is a digestive disorder that damages the small intestine. The disease is triggered by eating foods containing gluten, a protein found naturally in wheat, barley, and rye. Gluten is common in foods such as bread, pasta, cookies, and cakes. Celiac disease can cause chronic diarrhea in children of any age.

Functional Gastrointestinal Disorders

In functional GI disorders, symptoms are caused by changes in how the digestive tract works. Children with a functional GI disorder have frequent symptoms, yet the digestive tract does not become damaged. Functional GI disorders are not diseases; they are groups of symptoms that occur together. Two functional GI disorders that cause chronic diarrhea in children are toddler's diarrhea and irritable bowel syndrome (IBS).

Toddler's Diarrhea

Toddler's diarrhea, also called "functional diarrhea" or "chronic nonspecific diarrhea of childhood," is a common cause of chronic diarrhea in toddlers (aged 1–3) and preschool-age children (aged 3–5). Children with toddler's diarrhea pass four or more watery or loose stools a day and do not have any other symptoms. They typically are growing well, gaining weight, and are healthy. Toddler's diarrhea develops between the ages of three months and three years and usually resolves on its own by the time children begin grade school. Researchers think that drinking too many sugar-sweetened beverages, especially those high in high-fructose corn syrup and sorbitol, may cause toddler's diarrhea.

Irritable Bowel Syndrome

The most common symptoms of IBS are abdominal pain, discomfort, or cramping, along with diarrhea, constipation, or both. The pain or discomfort of IBS typically improves with the passage of stool or gas. IBS does not cause symptoms such as weight loss, vomiting, or blood in the stool. IBS is a common cause of chronic diarrhea in grade school-age children and adolescents. Doctors rarely diagnose IBS in younger children because younger children are not able to report symptoms of IBS, such as abdominal pain or discomfort.

WHAT ARE THE SYMPTOMS OF CHRONIC DIARRHEA IN CHILDREN?

The main symptom of chronic diarrhea in children is passing loose, watery stools three or more times a day for at least four weeks. Depending on the cause, children with chronic diarrhea may also have one or more of the following symptoms:

- bloody stools
- chills
- fever

- loss of control of bowel movements
- nausea or vomiting
- pain or cramping in the abdomen

HOW DO DOCTORS FIND THE CAUSE OF CHRONIC DIARRHEA IN CHILDREN?

To find the cause of a child's chronic diarrhea, doctors may use information from the child's medical and family history, a physical exam, and tests.

Medical and Family History

Your child's doctor will ask you for information about your child's symptoms, such as:

- how long your child has had diarrhea
- how much stool your child passes
- how often your child has diarrhea
- how your child's stool looks, such as color and consistency
- whether your child has other symptoms along with diarrhea

The doctor will ask about the foods your child eats and the beverages he or she drinks. The doctor may recommend keeping a diary of what your child eats and drinks, as well as his or her bowel habits. Your child's doctor may also inquire about family medical history, as some conditions that cause chronic diarrhea, such as Crohn's disease and UC, run in families.

Physical Exam

During a physical exam, a doctor typically:

- checks blood pressure and pulse
- checks for symptoms of dehydration and malabsorption
- listens to sounds in your child's abdomen using a stethoscope
- taps on your child's abdomen to check for pain or tenderness

WHAT TESTS DO DOCTORS USE TO FIND THE CAUSE OF CHRONIC DIARRHEA IN CHILDREN?

Doctors may use the following tests to help find the cause of a child's chronic diarrhea:

Stool Test

Stool tests can show the presence of blood and signs of infection, food allergies, and digestive tract problems, such as malabsorption of certain sugars, proteins, or nutrients. A health-care professional will give you a container for catching and storing a sample of your child's stool, along with instructions on where to send or take the sample for testing. A doctor may also perform a digital rectal exam to check for blood in your child's stool.

Blood Tests

A health-care professional may take a sample of your child's blood to test for signs of certain diseases or disorders that can cause chronic diarrhea, such as infections or celiac disease.

Hydrogen Breath Tests

This test measures the amount of hydrogen in a child's breath. Normally, little hydrogen is found in a child's breath. However, bacteria break down sugars—such as lactose, fructose, and sucrose—that are not digested by the small intestine and produce high levels of hydrogen. By measuring the amount of hydrogen in a child's breath, a doctor can diagnose:

- lactose intolerance
- fructose intolerance
- sucrose intolerance
- small intestinal bacterial overgrowth (SIBO)

For a lactose intolerance test, your child will drink a beverage that contains a known amount of lactose. For a fructose intolerance test, your child will drink a beverage that contains a known amount of fructose. For a sucrose intolerance test, your child will drink a beverage that contains a known amount of sucrose. For an

SIBO test, your child will drink a beverage that contains a known amount of sugar. Your child will then breathe into a balloon-type container that measures hydrogen. If the hydrogen level is high, your doctor will diagnose one of these disorders.

Fasting Tests

To determine if a food allergy or intolerance is causing your child's chronic diarrhea, the doctor may recommend that your child avoid foods containing lactose, carbohydrates, wheat, or other ingredients to see if a change in diet reduces or stops the diarrhea.

Endoscopy

Your doctor may use endoscopy to look inside your child's body to help find the cause of his or her chronic diarrhea. Endoscopic procedures include the following:

- colonoscopy
- flexible sigmoidoscopy
- upper GI endoscopy

HOW DO DOCTORS TREAT CHRONIC DIARRHEA IN CHILDREN?

How doctors treat chronic diarrhea in children depends on the cause. By treating the cause, doctors may be able to reduce or stop chronic diarrhea.

Infections of the Digestive Tract

Your child's doctor may prescribe antibiotics to treat bacterial infections and medicines that target parasites to treat parasitic infections. If your child has long-lasting problems digesting certain carbohydrates or proteins after an infection, a doctor may recommend changes in the foods your child eats. Additionally, for treating your child's SIBO, the doctor may prescribe antibiotics and recommend dietary changes.

Functional Gastrointestinal Disorders

TODDLER'S DIARRHEA

For toddler's diarrhea, treatment is usually not needed. Most children outgrow toddler's diarrhea by the time they start school, around age five. In many cases, reducing sugar-sweetened beverages and increasing the amount of fiber and fat in the diet may improve symptoms of toddler's diarrhea.

IRRITABLE BOWEL SYNDROME

A doctor may treat your child's IBS with changes in what your child eats and medicines.

Food Allergies and Intolerances

FOOD ALLERGIES

If your child has a food allergy, the doctor will recommend avoiding foods that trigger the allergy. Keeping a diary of what your child eats and drinks, as well as his or her bowel habits, will help the doctor identify the foods that trigger the allergy.

CELIAC DISEASE

If your child has celiac disease, the doctor will recommend avoiding all foods and products that contain gluten.

LACTOSE INTOLERANCE

If your child is lactose intolerant, the doctor will recommend reducing or avoiding foods and beverages that contain milk or milk products. Most children with lactose intolerance can tolerate some amount of lactose in their diet. The amount of change needed depends on how much lactose a child can consume without symptoms. The doctor may recommend dietary supplements that contain lactase, the enzyme that helps digest lactose. Additionally, the doctor may recommend calcium supplements.

FRUCTOSE INTOLERANCE

If your child is fructose intolerant, the doctor will recommend reducing or avoiding foods and beverages that contain fructose.

SUCROSE INTOLERANCE

If your child is sucrose intolerant, the doctor will recommend reducing or avoiding foods and beverages that contain sucrose.

Inflammatory Bowel Disease

A doctor may use medicines, surgery, and changes in what your child eats to treat inflammatory bowel disease (IBD), such as Crohn's disease and UC.

WHAT SHOULD A CHILD WITH CHRONIC DIARRHEA EAT?

A child with chronic diarrhea should eat foods that may improve symptoms and ensure good nutrition for normal growth and development. Children whose chronic diarrhea was caused by an infection of the digestive tract should eat the foods they normally eat. If your child has long-lasting problems digesting certain carbohydrates or proteins after an infection, talk with your child's doctor about what foods your child should eat. Increasing the amount of fat and fiber in your child's diet may improve symptoms of toddler's diarrhea.

WHAT SHOULD A CHILD WITH CHRONIC DIARRHEA AVOID EATING?

What foods your child should avoid eating depends on the cause of chronic diarrhea. In general, your child should avoid foods that make symptoms worse. To find out if certain foods trigger your child's symptoms, keep a diary and track:

- what your child eats each day
- what symptoms your child has
- when the symptoms occur
- what foods make the symptoms worse

Take your notes to your child's doctor and discuss which foods seem to make your child's symptoms worse. Your child may need to avoid these foods or eat less of them.[2]

Section 23.3 | **Ear Infection**

WHAT IS AN EAR INFECTION?

There are different types of ear infections. Middle ear infection (acute otitis media (AOM)) is an infection in the middle ear. Another condition that affects the middle ear is called "otitis media" (OM) with effusion. This condition occurs when fluid builds up in the middle ear without causing an infection. OM with effusion does not cause fever, ear pain, or pus build-up in the middle ear. Swimmer's ear is an infection in the outer ear canal. Swimmer's ear is different from a middle ear infection.

CAUSES OF EAR INFECTION

Bacteria or viruses can cause a middle ear infection:

- bacteria, such as *Streptococcus pneumoniae* and *Haemophilus influenzae* (nontypeable) are the two most common bacteria causing middle ear infection
- viruses, such as those that cause colds, can cause middle ear infection

SYMPTOMS OF EAR INFECTION

Common symptoms of middle ear infection in children can include the following:

- ear pain
- fever

[2] "Chronic Diarrhea in Children," National Institute of Diabetes and Digestive and Kidney Diseases (NIDDK), February 21, 2017. Available online. URL: www.niddk.nih.gov/health-information/digestive-diseases/chronic-diarrhea-children. Accessed March 13, 2024.

- fussiness or irritability
- rubbing or tugging at an ear
- difficulty sleeping

WHEN TO SEEK MEDICAL CARE

See a doctor if your child has:

- a fever of 102.2 °F (39 °C) or higher
- pus, discharge, or fluid coming from the ear
- worsening symptoms
- symptoms of a middle ear infection that lasts for more than two to three days
- hearing loss

This list is not all-inclusive. Please see a doctor for any symptom that is severe or concerning.

TREATMENT OF EAR INFECTION

A doctor can diagnose a middle ear infection by asking about symptoms and examining your child. The doctor will look inside your child's ear to examine the eardrum and check for pus in the middle ear. The body's immune system can often fight off middle ear infections on its own, so antibiotics are sometimes not needed. However, severe middle ear infections or infections that last longer than two to three days require antibiotics right away. For mild middle ear infections, your doctor might recommend watchful waiting or delayed antibiotic prescribing.

- **Watchful waiting**. Your child's doctor may suggest observing your child for two to three days to see if antibiotics are needed. This gives the immune system time to fight off the infection. If your child's symptoms do not improve, the doctor may then prescribe an antibiotic.
- **Delayed prescribing**. Your child's doctor may prescribe an antibiotic but recommend waiting two to three days before filling the prescription. Your child may recover on their own and may not need the antibiotic.

HOW TO FEEL BETTER

The following are some ways to feel better, even if antibiotics are needed for an ear infection:

- rest
- extra water or other fluids
- over-the-counter (OTC) medicines to relieve pain or fever
- ask your doctor or pharmacist about OTC medicines that can help you feel better
- always use OTC medicines as directed

OVER-THE-COUNTER MEDICINE AND CHILDREN

Carefully read and follow the instructions on OTC medicine product labels before giving medicines to children. Some OTC medicines are not recommended for children of certain ages.

- Pain relievers:
  - **Children younger than six months**. Only give acetaminophen.
  - **For children six months or older**. It is ok to give acetaminophen or ibuprofen.
  - **Never give aspirin to children because it can cause Reye syndrome**. Reye syndrome is a very serious but rare illness that can harm the liver and brain.
- Cough and cold medicines:
  - **Children younger than four years old**. Do not use OTC cough and cold medicines in young children unless a doctor advises you. Cough and cold medicines can result in serious and sometimes life-threatening side effects in young children.
  - **Children years or older**. Discuss with your child's doctor if OTC cough and cold medicines are safe to give to your child.

Ask your doctor or pharmacist about the right dosage of OTC medicines for your child's age and size. Additionally, inform your child's doctor and pharmacist about all prescription and OTC medicines your child takes.

PREVENTION OF EAR INFECTION

You can help prevent ear infections by doing your best to stay healthy and keep others healthy, including the following:

- Receive recommended vaccines, such as flu vaccine and pneumococcal vaccine. The pneumococcal vaccine protects against a common cause of middle ear infections, *Streptococcus pneumoniae*.
- Clean your hands.
- Breastfeed exclusively until your baby is six months old, and continue breastfeeding for at least 12 months.
- Do not smoke and avoid exposure to secondhand smoke.
- Dry your ears thoroughly after swimming.[3]

Section 23.4 | **Sinus Infection**

If you have a stuffy nose that just is not getting better, you might have a sinus infection, also called "sinusitis."

CAUSES OF SINUS INFECTION

Sinus infections occur when fluid builds up in the air-filled pockets in the face (sinuses), allowing germs to grow. While viruses cause most sinus infections, bacteria can also be responsible for some sinus infections.

RISK FACTORS OF SINUS INFECTION

Several factors can increase your risk of getting a sinus infection:

- a previous cold
- seasonal allergies

---

[3] "Ear Infection," Centers for Disease Control and Prevention (CDC), July 1, 2021. Available online. URL: www.cdc.gov/antibiotic-use/ear-infection.html. Accessed March 13, 2024.

- smoking and exposure to secondhand smoke
- structural problems within the sinuses; for example, growths on the lining of the nose or sinuses, known as "nasal polyps"
- a weak immune system or taking drugs that weaken the immune system

SYMPTOMS OF SINUS INFECTION

Common symptoms of sinus infections include the following:

- runny nose
- stuffy nose
- facial pain or pressure
- headache
- mucus dripping down the throat (postnasal drip)
- sore throat
- cough
- bad breath

WHEN TO SEEK MEDICAL CARE

See a doctor if you have:

- severe symptoms, such as severe headaches or facial pain
- symptoms that get worse after improving
- symptoms lasting more than 10 days without getting better
- fever longer than three to four days
- you should also seek medical care if you have had multiple sinus infections in the past year

This list is not all-inclusive. Please see a doctor for any symptom that is severe or concerning.

TREATMENT OF SINUS INFECTION

Your doctor will determine if you have a sinus infection by asking about symptoms and examining you. Antibiotics are unnecessary for many sinus infections, as most get better independently without them. When antibiotics are not needed, they will not help you, and their side effects could cause harm. Side effects can range from mild reactions, such as a rash, to serious health problems, including severe allergic reactions, antibiotic-resistant infections, and *Clostridioides difficile* (*C. diff*) infection. *C. diff* causes diarrhea that can lead to severe colon damage and death. However, in some cases, you may need antibiotics. Talk to your doctor about the best treatment for your illness. Your doctor might recommend watchful waiting or delayed antibiotic prescribing for some sinus infections.

- **Watchful waiting**. Your doctor may suggest observing your symptoms for two to three days to see if antibiotics are needed. This gives the immune system time to fight off the infection. If your symptoms do not improve, the doctor may then prescribe an antibiotic.
- **Delayed prescribing**. Your doctor may prescribe an antibiotic but recommend waiting two to three days before filling the prescription. You may recover on your own and may not need the antibiotic.

HOW TO FEEL BETTER

The following are some ways to help relieve sinus pain and pressure:

- Put a warm compress over the nose and forehead to help relieve sinus pressure.
- Use a decongestant or saline nasal spray.
- Breathe in steam from a bowl of hot water or shower.

Ask your doctor or pharmacist about over-the-counter (OTC) medicines that can help you feel better. Always use OTC medicines as directed.

OVER-THE-COUNTER MEDICINE AND CHILDREN

Carefully read and follow instructions on OTC medicine product labels before giving medicines to children. Some OTC medicines are not recommended for children of certain ages.

- Pain relievers:
    - **Children younger than six months**. Only give acetaminophen.

    - **Children six months or older**. It is ok to give acetaminophen or ibuprofen.
    - **Never give aspirin to children because it can cause Reye syndrome**. Reye syndrome is a very serious but rare illness that can harm the liver and brain.
- Cough and cold medicines:
    - **Children younger than four years old**. Do not use OTC cough and cold medicines in young children unless a doctor specifically tells you to. Cough and cold medicines can result in serious and sometimes life-threatening side effects in young children.
    - **Children four years or older**. Discuss with your child's doctor if OTC cough and cold medicines are safe to give to your child.

Ask your doctor or pharmacist about the right dosage of OTC medicines for your child's age and size. Additionally, inform your child's doctor and pharmacist about all prescription and OTC medicines your child is taking.[4]

Section 23.5 | **Group B Strep**

- Group B *Streptococcus* (group B strep; GBS) bacteria cause GBS disease.
- GBS disease includes many types of infections—some can be life-threatening.
- Anyone can get GBS disease, but it is most common in newborns.
- Pregnant women should get tested for GBS bacteria and get antibiotics during labor, if needed.

[4] "Sinus Infection (Sinusitis)," Centers for Disease Control and Prevention (CDC), August 27, 2019. Available online. URL: www.cdc.gov/antibiotic-use/sinus-infection.html. Accessed March 13, 2024.

WHAT IS GROUP B STREP DISEASE

Group B strep disease is a name for any infection caused by GBS bacteria. These bacteria that commonly live in people's gastrointestinal and genital tracts.

- **Gastrointestinal tract**. The part of the body that digests food and includes the stomach and intestines.
- **Genital tract**. The part of the body involved in reproduction and includes the vagina in women.

Most of the time, the bacteria are not harmful and do not make people feel sick (have any symptoms).

TYPES OF GROUP B STREP INFECTIONS

Group B strep bacteria can cause many types of infections. Some of these infections can be life-threatening.

Infections include:

- bacteremia (bloodstream infection)
- sepsis (the body's extreme response to an infection)
- bone and joint infections
- urinary tract (bladder) infections
- meningitis (infection of the lining of the brain and spinal cord)
- pneumonia (lung infection)
- skin and soft tissue infections

Most Common Infections

NEWBORNS

Group B strep bacteria most commonly cause bacteremia, sepsis, pneumonia, and meningitis.

ADULTS

Bloodstream infections, pneumonia, and skin and bone infections are the most common GBS infections among nonpregnant adults. It Is very uncommon for GBS bacteria to cause meningitis in adults.

SYMPTOMS

Symptoms of GBS disease depend on the part of the body that is infected.

Newborns

Most newborns who get GBS disease in the first week of life show symptoms on the day of birth. Babies who develop the disease later can appear healthy at birth and during their first week of life.

GBS disease symptoms can seem like other health problems in newborns and babies. Symptoms include:

- fever
- difficulty feeding
- irritability or lethargy (limpness or baby is hard to wake up)
- difficulty breathing
- bluish color to skin

Pregnant Women Who Test Positive

About one in four women test positive for GBS bacteria during routine screening toward the end of their pregnancy.

No symptoms: These women usually do not feel sick or have any symptoms.

WHO IS AT RISK

Anyone can get GBS disease, but some people are at greater risk than others. Being a certain age or having certain medical conditions can put you at increased risk for GBS disease.

HOW IT SPREADS

GBS bacteria come and go naturally in people's bodies. How people spread GBS bacteria to others is generally unknown.

From Mothers to Babies

Pregnant women can pass the bacteria to their babies during delivery. Most babies who get GBS disease in the first week of life are exposed to the bacteria this way. It can be hard to determine how babies who develop GBS disease later acquired the bacteria. The bacteria may have come from the mother during birth or from another source.

PREVENTION

There are currently no vaccines to prevent GBS disease, but they are under development. Unfortunately, experts have not identified effective ways to prevent GBS disease in people older than one week.

In Newborns

Health-care providers can take steps to help prevent GBS disease during the first week of a newborn's life.

SCREENING AND DIAGNOSIS

Screening

All pregnant women should get screened for GBS bacteria.

Diagnosing GBS Disease

After seeing someone who is sick, health-care providers may take samples depending on the type of infection they suspect:

- blood
- spinal fluid
- urine

Health-care providers may also order a chest x-ray to help determine if someone has GBS disease.

TREATMENT AND RECOVERY

Doctors usually treat GBS disease with antibiotics. Sometimes, people with soft tissue and bone infections may need additional treatment, such as surgery. The treatment will depend on the type of infection caused by the GBS bacteria.

It is important to start treatment as soon as possible.[5]

Section 23.6 | **Chickenpox**

Chickenpox is a highly contagious disease caused by the varicella-zoster virus (VZV). It can cause an itchy, blister-like rash, among other symptoms. The rash first appears on the chest, back, and face and then spreads over the entire body. Chickenpox can be serious, especially during pregnancy, in babies, adolescents, adults, and people with weakened immune systems (lowered ability to fight germs and sickness). The best way to prevent chickenpox is to get the chickenpox vaccine.

SIGNS AND SYMPTOMS OF CHICKENPOX

Anyone who has not had chickenpox or gotten the chickenpox vaccine can get the disease. Chickenpox illness usually lasts about four to seven days. The classic symptom of chickenpox is a rash that turns into itchy, fluid-filled blisters that eventually turn into scabs. The rash may first appear on the chest, back, and face, and then spread over the entire body, including inside the mouth, eyelids, or genital area. It usually takes about one week for all of the blisters to become scabs. Other typical symptoms that may begin to appear one to two days before the rash include:

- fever
- tiredness
- loss of appetite
- headache

[5] "About Group B Strep Disease," Centers for Disease Control and Prevention (CDC), January 3, 2024. Available online. URL: www.cdc.gov/group-b-strep/about/index.html. Accessed July 1, 2024.

CHICKENPOX IN VACCINATED PEOPLE (BREAKTHROUGH CHICKENPOX)

Some people who have been vaccinated against chickenpox can still get the disease. However, they usually have milder symptoms with fewer or no blisters (or just red spots), a mild or no fever, and are sick for a shorter period of time than those who are not vaccinated. However, some vaccinated people who get chickenpox may still experience a disease similar to that of unvaccinated individuals.

COMPLICATIONS OF CHICKENPOX

Complications from chickenpox can occur, but they are not common in healthy people who get the disease. People who may get a serious case of chickenpox and are at high risk for complications include the following:

- infants
- adolescents
- adults
- people who are pregnant
- people with bodies that have a lowered ability to fight germs and sickness (weakened immune systems) because of illness or medications

Serious complications from chickenpox include the following:

- bacterial infections of the skin and soft tissues in children, including Group A streptococcal infections
- infection of the lungs (pneumonia)
- infection or swelling of the brain (encephalitis, cerebellar ataxia)
- bleeding problems (hemorrhagic complications)
- bloodstream infections (sepsis)
- dehydration

Some people with serious complications from chickenpox can become so sick that they need to be hospitalized. Chickenpox can also cause death. Deaths are very rare now due to the vaccine program. However, some deaths from chickenpox continue to occur in healthy, unvaccinated children and adults. In the past, many healthy adults who died from chickenpox contracted the disease from their unvaccinated children.

TRANSMISSION OF CHICKENPOX

Chickenpox is a highly contagious disease caused by the VZV. The virus spreads easily from people with chickenpox to others who have never had the disease or have never been vaccinated. If one person has it, up to 90 percent of the people close to that person who are not immune will also become infected. The virus spreads mainly through close contact with someone who has chickenpox. A person with chickenpox is considered contagious from one to two days before the rash appears until all the chickenpox lesions have crusted (scabbed). Vaccinated people who get chickenpox may develop lesions that do not crust. These people are considered contagious until no new lesions have appeared for 24 hours.

The VZV also causes shingles. After chickenpox, the virus remains dormant in the body. People get shingles when VZV reactivates in their bodies after they have already had chickenpox. People with shingles can spread VZV to those who have never had chickenpox or never received the chickenpox vaccine. This can happen through direct contact with fluid from shingles rash blisters or through breathing in virus particles that come from the blisters. If they get infected, they will develop chickenpox, not shingles. It takes about two weeks (from 10 to 21 days) for someone to develop chickenpox after exposure to a person with chickenpox or shingles. If a vaccinated person gets the disease, they can still spread it to others. For most people, getting chickenpox once provides immunity for life. It is possible to get chickenpox more than once, but this is uncommon.

PEOPLE AT RISK FOR SEVERE CHICKENPOX

Some people who get chickenpox may have more severe symptoms and may be at higher risk for complications.

TREATMENTS AT HOME FOR PEOPLE WITH CHICKENPOX

There are several things you can do at home to help relieve chickenpox symptoms and prevent skin infections. Calamine lotion and a cool bath with added baking soda, uncooked oatmeal, or colloidal oatmeal may help relieve some of the itching. Try to keep fingernails trimmed short and minimize scratching to prevent the virus from spreading to others and to help prevent skin infections. If you accidentally scratch a blister, wash your hands with soap and water for at least 20 seconds.

TREATMENTS PRESCRIBED BY YOUR HEALTH-CARE PROVIDER FOR PEOPLE WITH CHICKENPOX

Your health-care provider can advise you on treatment options. Antiviral medications are recommended for people with chickenpox that are more likely to develop serious illness, including:

- otherwise, healthy people older than 12 years of age
- people with chronic skin or lung disease
- people receiving long-term salicylate therapy or steroid therapy
- people who are pregnant
- people with a weakened immune system

There are antiviral medications licensed for the treatment of chickenpox. The medication works best if it is given as early as possible, preferably within the first 24 hours after the rash starts.

PREVENTION OF CHICKENPOX

The best way to prevent chickenpox is to get the chickenpox vaccine. Everyone—including children, adolescents, and adults—should get two doses of the chickenpox vaccine if they have never had chickenpox or were never vaccinated. The chickenpox vaccine is very safe and effective at preventing the disease. Most people who get the vaccine will not get chickenpox. If a vaccinated person does get chickenpox, the symptoms are usually milder, with fewer or no blisters (they may have just red spots) and low or no fever. The chickenpox vaccine prevents almost all cases of severe illness.

Since the chickenpox vaccination program began in the United States, there has been a decrease of over 97 percent in chickenpox cases. Hospitalizations and deaths have become rare.[6]

Section 23.7 | **Hand-Foot-and-Mouth Disease**

Hand-foot-and-mouth disease (HFMD) is common in children under five years old, but anyone can get it. The illness is usually not serious, but it is very contagious. It can spread quickly at schools and daycare centers. HFMD is often confused with foot-and-mouth disease (also called "hoof-and-mouth disease"), which affects cows, sheep, goats, and pigs. Humans do not get the animal disease, and animals do not get the human disease. HFMD spreads easily through:

- person-to-person contact
- droplets made when a person who is sick with HFMD sneezes, coughs, or talks
- contact with contaminated surfaces and objects

IS HAND-FOOT-AND-MOUTH DISEASE CONTAGIOUS?

Yes, HFMD is caused by viruses. A person infected with one of these viruses is contagious, meaning they can pass the virus to other people. If someone is sick with HFMD, the virus can be found in their:

- nose and throat secretions, such as saliva, drool, or nasal mucus
- fluid from blisters
- feces (poop)

People with HFMD are usually most contagious during the first week that they are sick. However, they can still sometimes spread

[6] "About Chickenpox," Centers for Disease Control and Prevention (CDC), October 18, 2022. Available online. URL: www.cdc.gov/chickenpox/about/index.html. Accessed March 14, 2024.

the virus to others for days or weeks after symptoms go away, or even if they have no symptoms at all.

IS HAND-FOOT-AND-MOUTH DISEASE COMMON?

Yes, HFMD is common and, in the United States, occurs mostly in the summer and fall, but you can get it any time of year.

WHAT VIRUSES CAUSE HAND-FOOT-AND-MOUTH DISEASE?

Hand-foot-and-mouth disease is caused by viruses that belong to the enterovirus family:

- **Coxsackievirus A16 is typically the most common cause of HFMD in the United States.** Other coxsackieviruses can also cause the illness.
- **Coxsackievirus A6 can also cause HFMD.** The symptoms may be more severe.
- **Enterovirus 71 (EV-A71) has been associated with cases and outbreaks in East and Southeast Asia.** Although rare, EV-A71 has been associated with more severe diseases such as encephalitis (swelling of the brain).

SYMPTOMS OF HAND-FOOT-AND-MOUTH DISEASE

Fever and Flu-Like Symptoms

Children often get a fever and other flu-like symptoms three to five days after they catch the virus. These can include:

- fever
- eating or drinking less
- sore throat
- feeling unwell

Mouth Sores

Your child can get painful mouth sores. These sores usually start as small red spots, often on the tongue and insides of the mouth, that blister and can become painful. Signs that swallowing might be painful for your child:

- not eating or drinking
- drooling more than usual
- only wanting to drink cold fluids

Skin Rash

Your child can get a skin rash on the palms of the hands and soles of the feet. It can also show up on the buttocks, legs, and arms. The rash is usually not itchy and looks like flat or slightly raised red spots, sometimes with blisters that have an area of redness at their base. Fluid in the blisters can contain the virus that causes HFMD. Keep blisters clean and avoid touching them.

HOW TO TREAT HAND-FOOT-AND-MOUTH-DISEASE?

Most people with HFMD get better on their own in 7–10 days. There is no specific medical treatment for HFMD, but you can take steps to relieve symptoms and prevent dehydration while you or your child are sick. Take over-the-counter (OTC) medications to relieve fever and pain caused by mouth sores, such as acetaminophen or ibuprofen. Never give aspirin to children. Ensure you drink enough liquids. Mouth sores can make it painful to swallow, so your child may not want to drink much. Make sure they drink enough to stay hydrated.

WHEN TO SEE A HEALTH-CARE PROVIDER

- Your child is not able to drink normally, and you are worried they might be getting dehydrated.
- Your child's fever lasts longer than three days.
- Your child has a weakened immune system.
- Symptoms are severe.
- Your child is very young, especially younger than six months.

PREVENTING HAND-FOOT-AND-MOUTH DISEASE

Hand-foot-and-mouth disease is very contagious. You can help prevent catching or spreading HFMD by following simple steps below.

Wash Your Hands

Wash your hands often with soap and water for at least 20 seconds. If soap and water are not available, use an alcohol-based hand sanitizer. Always wash your hands:

- after changing diapers
- after using the toilet
- after blowing your nose, coughing, or sneezing
- before and after caring for someone who is sick

Help children wash their hands. Teach them how to wash their hands and make sure they wash them often. Help them keep blisters clean and avoid touching them.

Avoid Close Contact with People Who Are Sick

Avoid touching someone who has HFMD, such as hugging or kissing them.

CAN YOUR CHILD RETURN TO SCHOOL IF THEY ARE SICK?

Because HFMD is normally mild, children can continue to go to childcare and schools as long as they:

- have no fever
- have no uncontrolled drooling with mouth sores
- feel well enough to participate in classroom activities

Talk with your child's health-care provider if you are still unsure when it is okay for them to return. In some cases, the local health department may require children with HFMD to stay home to control an outbreak.

Avoid Touching Your Eyes, Nose, and Mouth

You can get infected with HFMD if you have the virus on your hands and then touch your eyes, nose, or mouth. To reduce your chance of getting sick, avoid touching your eyes, nose, and mouth with unwashed hands.

Clean and Disinfect

Clean and disinfect frequently touched surfaces and shared items, such as toys and doorknobs.[7]

Section 23.8 | Jaundice and Kernicterus

WHAT ARE JAUNDICE AND KERNICTERUS?

Jaundice is the yellow color seen in the skin of many newborns. Jaundice occurs when a chemical called "bilirubin" builds up in the baby's blood. During pregnancy, the mother's liver removes bilirubin for the baby, but after birth, the baby's liver must remove the bilirubin. In some babies, the liver might not be developed enough to efficiently eliminate bilirubin. When too much bilirubin builds up in a new baby's body, the skin and whites of the eyes might look yellow. This yellow coloring is called "jaundice." When severe jaundice goes untreated for too long, it can cause a condition called "kernicterus." Kernicterus is a type of brain damage that can result from high levels of bilirubin in a baby's blood. It can cause athetoid cerebral palsy (CP) and hearing loss. Kernicterus also causes problems with vision and teeth and can sometimes lead to intellectual disabilities. Early detection and management of jaundice can prevent kernicterus.

SIGNS AND SYMPTOMS OF JAUNDICE

Jaundice usually appears first on the face and then moves to the chest, belly, arms, and legs as bilirubin levels increase. The whites of the eyes can also look yellow. Jaundice can be harder to see in babies with darker skin. The baby's doctor or nurse can test how

[7] "Hand, Foot, and Mouth Disease (HFMD)," Centers for Disease Control and Prevention (CDC), May 11, 2023. Available online. URL: www.cdc.gov/hand-foot-mouth/index.html. Accessed March 14, 2024.

much bilirubin is in the baby's blood. See your baby's doctor the same day if your baby:

- is very yellow or orange (skin color changes start from the head and spread to the toes)
- is hard to wake up or will not sleep at all
- is not breastfeeding or sucking from a bottle well
- is very fussy
- does not have enough wet or dirty diapers (at least four to six thoroughly wet diapers in 24 hours and three to three stools per day by the fourth day)

Get emergency medical help if your baby:

- is crying inconsolably or with a high pitch
- is arched like a bow (the head or neck and heels are bent backward and the body forward)
- has a stiff, limp, or floppy body
- has strange eye movements

RISK FACTORS OF JAUNDICE

About 60 percent of all babies have jaundice. Some babies are more likely to have severe jaundice and higher bilirubin levels than others. Babies with any of the following risk factors need close monitoring and early jaundice management.

Preterm Babies

Babies born before 37 weeks, or 8.5 months, of pregnancy might have jaundice because their liver is not fully developed. The young liver might not be able to get rid of so much bilirubin.

Babies with Darker Skin Color

Jaundice may be missed or not recognized in a baby with a darker skin color. Checking the gums and inner lips may detect jaundice. If there is any doubt, a bilirubin test should be done.

East Asian or Mediterranean Descent

A baby born to an East Asian or Mediterranean family is at a higher risk of becoming jaundiced. Also, some families inherit conditions (such as G6PD deficiency), and their babies are more likely to get jaundice.

Feeding Difficulties

A baby who does not eat, wet, or stool well in the first few days of life is more likely to develop jaundice.

Sibling with Jaundice

A baby with a sister or brother who has jaundice is more likely to develop jaundice.

Bruising

A baby with bruises at birth is more likely to get jaundice. A bruise forms when blood leaks out of a blood vessel and causes the skin to look black and blue. The healing of large bruises can cause high bilirubin levels and your baby might get jaundice.

Blood Type

Women with an O blood type or Rh-negative blood factor might have babies with higher bilirubin levels. A mother with Rh incompatibility should be given Rhogam.

DIAGNOSIS OF JAUNDICE

At a minimum, babies should be checked for jaundice every 8–12 hours in the first 48 hours of life. It is important for your baby to be seen by a nurse or doctor when the baby is between three and five days old because this is usually when a baby's bilirubin level is highest. If your baby is discharged before 72 hours of age, your baby should be seen within two days of discharge. The timing of this visit may vary depending on your baby's age when released from the hospital and other factors.

A doctor or nurse may check the baby's bilirubin using a light meter placed on the baby's head. This results in a transcutaneous bilirubin (TcB) level. If it is high, a blood test will likely be ordered. The best way to accurately measure bilirubin is with a small blood sample from the baby's heel, resulting in a total serum bilirubin (TSB) level. If the level is high, based on the baby's age in hours and other risk factors, treatment will likely follow. Repeat blood samples will also likely be taken to ensure that the TSB decreases with the prescribed treatment.

TREATMENT FOR JAUNDICE

No baby should develop brain damage from untreated jaundice. When being treated for high bilirubin levels, the baby will be undressed and placed under special lights. These lights will not harm the baby and can be used in the hospital or at home. The baby's milk intake may also need to be increased. In some cases, if the baby has very high bilirubin levels, the doctor will perform a blood exchange transfusion. Jaundice is generally treated before brain damage becomes a concern. Putting the baby in sunlight is not recommended as a safe way to treat jaundice.

IF YOU ARE CONCERNED

If you think your baby has jaundice, you should call and visit your baby's doctor right away. Ask your baby's doctor or nurse about a jaundice bilirubin test. If your baby does have jaundice, it is important to take it seriously and stick to the follow-up plan for appointments and recommended care. Ensure your baby is getting enough to eat. The process of removing waste also removes bilirubin from your baby's blood. If you are breastfeeding, you should nurse the baby at least 8–12 times a day for the first few days. This will help you produce enough milk and will help keep the baby's bilirubin level down. Support and advice for breastfeeding mothers can increase the chances of successful breastfeeding. If you are having trouble breastfeeding, ask your doctor, nurse, or lactation coach for help.[8]

---

[8] National Center on Birth Defects and Developmental Disabilities (NCBDDD), "What Are Jaundice and Kernicterus?" Centers for Disease Control and Prevention (CDC), December 8, 2020. Available online. URL: https://archive.cdc.gov/#/details?url=https://www.cdc.gov/ncbddd/jaundice/facts.html. Accessed March 14, 2024.

Section 23.9 | **Rubella**

Rubella is a contagious disease caused by a virus. It is also called "German measles," but it is caused by a different virus than measles. Rubella was eliminated from the United States in 2004. Rubella elimination is defined as the absence of continuous disease transmission for 12 months or more in a specific geographic area. Rubella is no longer endemic (constantly present) in the United States. However, rubella remains a problem in other parts of the world and can still be brought into the United States by people who get infected in other countries.

Before the rubella vaccination program started in 1969, rubella was a common and widespread infection in the United States. During the last major rubella epidemic in the United States from 1964 to 1965, an estimated 12.5 million people got rubella, 11,000 pregnant women lost their babies, 2,100 newborns died, and 20,000 babies were born with congenital rubella syndrome (CRS). Once the vaccine became widely used, the number of people infected with rubella in the United States dropped dramatically. Fewer than 10 people in the United States are reported as having rubella each year. Since 2012, all rubella cases had evidence that they were infected when they were living or traveling outside the United States. To maintain rubella elimination, it is important that children and women of childbearing age are vaccinated against rubella.

SIGNS AND SYMPTOMS OF RUBELLA

In children, rubella is usually mild, with few noticeable symptoms. For children who do have symptoms, a red rash is typically the first sign. The rash generally first appears on the face and then spreads to the rest of the body, lasting about three days. Other symptoms that may occur one to five days before the rash appears include:

- a low-grade fever
- headache
- mild pink eye (redness or swelling of the white of the eye)

- general discomfort
- swollen and enlarged lymph nodes
- cough
- runny nose

Most adults who get rubella usually have a mild illness, with low-grade fever, sore throat, and a rash that starts on the face and spreads to the rest of the body. Some adults may also experience a headache, pink eye, and general discomfort before the rash appears. About 25–50 percent of people infected with rubella will not experience any symptoms.

COMPLICATIONS OF RUBELLA

Up to 70 percent of women who get rubella may experience arthritis; this is rare in children and men. In rare cases, rubella can cause serious problems, including brain infections and bleeding issues. The most serious complication of rubella infection is the harm it can cause a pregnant woman's developing baby. If an unvaccinated pregnant woman gets infected with the rubella virus, she can have a miscarriage, or her baby can die shortly after birth. Additionally, she can pass the virus to her developing baby, who can develop serious birth defects such as:

- heart problems
- loss of hearing and eyesight
- intellectual disability
- liver or spleen damage

Serious birth defects are more common if a woman is infected early in her pregnancy, especially in the first trimester.

TRANSMISSION OF RUBELLA

Rubella spreads when an infected person coughs or sneezes. If a woman is infected with rubella while she is pregnant, she can pass it to her developing baby, causing serious harm. A person with rubella may spread the disease to others up to one week before the rash appears and remain contagious up to seven days after.

However, 25–50 percent of people infected with rubella do not develop a rash or have any symptoms, but they can still spread it to others. People infected with rubella should inform friends, family, and coworkers, especially pregnant women, if they have rubella. If your child has rubella, it is important to inform your child's school or daycare provider.

TREATMENT FOR RUBELLA

There is no specific medicine to treat rubella or expedite recovery. Symptoms are typically mild; for those with more severe symptoms, rest and fever-reducing medications like acetaminophen can help manage discomfort. If you have concerns about your symptoms or your child's, contact your doctor for guidance.[9]

Section 23.10 | **Parasitic Infections**

PARASITIC INFECTIONS IN CHILDREN

Parasitic infections or infestations can affect children of all ages. Infants, toddlers, and young children in day care settings are susceptible to giardiasis, a parasitic disease that causes diarrhea and spreads through contaminated feces. Pinworm infection (enterobiasis) is common among preschool and young school-age children. Additionally, both preschool and school-age children can contract head lice (pediculosis) or scabies, which spread through close person-to-person contact, often occurring during childhood play.

Children of all ages are susceptible to parasitic diseases such as giardiasis and cryptosporidiosis, which can result from swallowing contaminated water during activities like swimming or playing in contaminated recreational water sources such as pools, fountains, lakes, and rivers. Pets and other animals can also serve as sources of parasites that can affect children. Toxoplasmosis spreads through

[9] "About Rubella," Centers for Disease Control and Prevention (CDC), December 31, 2020. Available online. URL: www.cdc.gov/rubella/about/index.html. Accessed March 14, 2024.

ingestion of soil or litter-box contents contaminated with infectious cat feces. Additionally, children can acquire this infection if their mother was infected during pregnancy.

PARASITIC DISEASES IN THE UNITED STATES

Several parasitic diseases occur occasionally in the United States and more frequently in developing countries, but their prevalence has not been well studied. These diseases include strongyloidiasis, caused by a worm infection that poses particular danger to children with impaired immune systems. It is acquired when larvae (immature worms) in soil contaminated with infected human feces come into contact with and penetrate the skin. Other diseases in this category include visceral toxocariasis, which spreads when children ingest soil contaminated with dog or cat feces containing the eggs of roundworms from cats or dogs, and cutaneous larva migrans, transmitted when children walk barefoot on soil contaminated with hookworm larvae from cats or dogs that penetrate their skin.

Other parasitic diseases are rare among children in the United States but are widespread and account for a significant disease burden among children in developing countries. The most significant of these is malaria. Children in malaria-endemic countries face a high risk of severe outcomes from malaria infection. The majority of global malaria deaths occur in African children under five years of age. Children from the United States also face a high risk of malaria infection when traveling to malaria-endemic countries. They should ensure to take antimalarial drugs before, during, and after the trip, use repellent, sleep under an insecticide-treated bed net or in an air-conditioned room, and wear protective clothing.

SOIL-TRANSMITTED HELMINTH DISEASE

Soil-transmitted helminth (STH) diseases (where "helminth" refers to parasitic worms) are of significant importance in developing countries. They are caused by infection with roundworm, hookworm, or whipworm and can manifest as diarrhea, abdominal pain, intestinal obstruction, anemia, and stunted growth and cognitive development. Children typically acquire these infections by ingesting roundworm and whipworm eggs that have matured in soil contaminated by human feces, or by walking barefoot on contaminated soil where human hookworm eggs have hatched, releasing larvae that penetrate the skin. Schistosomiasis, another major parasitic disease among children in certain developing countries, can also result in impaired growth and development and may lead to severe health complications later in life.

Onchocerciasis (river blindness) is caused by a helminth that spends part of its life cycle in certain types of snails and penetrates the skin of individuals when they stand or swim in water inhabited by these snails. The helminth responsible for lymphatic filariasis is transmitted to children through mosquito bites. Although damage to the lymphatic system in children is usually asymptomatic, it can become symptomatic by puberty, leading to swollen arms and legs, as well as an enlarged, fluid-filled scrotum in adulthood. These diseases (STHs, onchocerciasis, schistosomiasis, and lymphatic filariasis) are categorized as neglected tropical diseases (NTDs) because they disproportionately affect impoverished populations.

PREVENTION OF PARASITIC INFECTIONS

One of the most crucial ways to prevent these parasitic diseases is by teaching children the importance of thorough handwashing with soap and running warm water, especially after using the toilet and before eating. In many developing countries, it is also essential to ensure proper disposal of feces, avoid walking barefoot outdoors, sleep under an insecticide-treated bed net, and minimize exposure to water potentially contaminated with the parasite that causes schistosomiasis. Periodic mass drug administrations for soil-transmitted helminth infections, schistosomiasis, onchocerciasis, and lymphatic filariasis can significantly reduce these infections and the associated diseases, potentially leading to the elimination of onchocerciasis and lymphatic filariasis. During mass drug administrations, all members of selected at-risk age groups receive treatment.[10]

[10] "Parasites," Centers for Disease Control and Prevention (CDC), October 21, 2020. Available online. URL: www.cdc.gov/parasites/children.html. Accessed March 14, 2024.

Chapter 24 | Growth Plate Injuries

The growth plate is the area of tissue near the ends of long bones in children and teens that determines the future length and shape of mature bones. Each long bone typically has at least two growth plates, one at each end, which are longer than they are wide. Examples include the femur (thigh bone), radius and ulna (forearm), and the metacarpal bones (hands and fingers). As a child's growth nears completion, usually during adolescence, the growth plates close and are replaced by solid bone.

These growth plates are relatively weak compared to nearby ligaments and tendons, making them vulnerable to injury. Growth plate fractures can occur due to a single traumatic event like a fall or automobile accident, or from chronic stress and overuse. Prompt treatment is often necessary to prevent complications in bone growth for children and teens with growth plate injuries. Fortunately, with proper care, most growth plate fractures heal completely without lasting effects.

WHO GETS GROWTH PLATE INJURIES?

Because the growth plate is the last area of bone to harden during growth, children and teens are particularly vulnerable to growth plate fractures or injuries. A comparable injury in an adult can result in a sprain. The following factors may increase the chance that your child or teen may injure or fracture their growth plate:

- **Sex.** Growth plate fractures occur more frequently in boys than in girls. Girls typically mature earlier than boys, leading to earlier completion of bone growth and replacement of the growth plate with stronger, solid bone.

- **Competitive sports**. Growth plate injuries often occur in children and teens who participate in competitive sports or activities that heighten the risk of falling or being hit, such as:
  - football
  - basketball
  - gymnastics
  - biking
  - sledding
  - skiing
  - skateboarding
- **Repetitive use**. Specializing in one sport and overusing certain limbs or areas of the body before puberty finishes can contribute to growth plate injuries.

TYPES OF GROWTH PLATE INJURIES

Doctors use a classification system called the "Salter-Harris" to categorize most growth plate injuries and fractures into five types. Understanding the anatomy of long bones can aid in comprehending the various types of growth plate injuries. Long bones have four major areas:

- **Epiphysis**. The end of the bone near the joint.
- **Physis**. The growth plate.
- **Metaphysis**. The area between the growth plate and the shaft.
- **Diaphysis**. The shaft of the long bone between growth plates above and below.

The Salter-Harris types are as follows:

- **Type I**. This happens when the fracture passes through the physis but does not involve the area of bone around the growth plate.
- **Type II**. This happens when the fracture runs through the physis and the metaphysis. It is the most common type of growth plate fracture.

- **Type III**. This happens when fractures run through the epiphysis and growth plate. It leads to a separation of epiphysis and physis from the metaphysics.
- **Type IV**. This happens when fractures run through the physis, metaphysis, and epiphysis.
- **Type V**. A compression fracture through the physis that happens when the end of the bone is crushed, and the physis is compressed. This type of fracture is rare.

Sometimes doctors use the Peterson classification to describe growth plate injuries, which includes a type VI. Type VI injuries occur when a portion of the epiphysis, physis, and metaphysis are missing, typically due to severe traumatic injuries involving open wounds or compound fractures.

CAUSES OF GROWTH PLATE INJURIES

Growth plate injuries can occur for various reasons. A sudden accident, such as trauma from a blow or fall, can lead to growth plate injuries in children. Additionally, participation in competitive sports or recreational activities can also result in these injuries. Furthermore, overuse of a specific part of the body can cause growth plate injuries, particularly in young children who specialize in a sport or activity and undergo extensive training. This may be seen in:

- gymnasts who practice for hours
- long-distance runners
- baseball pitchers

Although most growth plate injuries occur during play or athletic activity, growth plates are also susceptible to medical disorders that can disrupt their normal growth and development.

SYMPTOMS OF GROWTH PLATE INJURIES

Symptoms of a growth plate injury include the following:

- persistent pain and tenderness after a sudden or overuse injury
- deformity, warmth, or swelling at the end of a bone

- changes in how your child bends their limb
- inability to move, put pressure on, or bear weight on a limb because of pain

You may notice that your child self-limits the amount of time playing after a prior injury.

DIAGNOSIS OF GROWTH PLATE INJURIES

Doctors diagnose growth plate injuries by:

- asking about the pain and injury, including when the pain started and how the injury happened
- examining your child, which may include checking the injured area for tenderness, swelling, and deformity
- ordering x-rays

Because growth plates have not yet hardened into solid bone, neither the structures themselves nor injuries to them appear on x-rays. Instead, growth plates appear as gaps between the shaft of a long bone (metaphysis) and the end of the bone (epiphysis). Therefore, a growth plate injury may not be visible on an x-ray. Other tests doctors may use to diagnose your child's growth plate injury include the following:

- magnetic resonance imaging (MRI)
- computed tomography (CT)
- ultrasound

Because these tests allow doctors to visualize the growth plate and other soft tissue areas, they can effectively identify and classify growth plate injuries.

TREATMENT OF GROWTH PLATE INJURIES

Treatment for growth plate injuries depends on the type of injury. Treatment should start as soon as possible after injury and generally involves one or more of the following treatments.

Reduction of Fracture and Immobilization

The doctor immobilizes the injured limb in a cast or splint once normal alignment of the broken bones is established, preventing movement to allow the bone to rest and heal. To aid healing, it's important for your child or teen to avoid activities that exert pressure on the injured area. If the injuries result in displaced ends of the bones, the doctor typically performs a procedure called "reduction of fractures" to realign the bones or joints into their correct positions. Depending on the type of growth plate fracture your child has, doctors can set bones by:

- **Closed reduction**. When the doctor aligns and sets the bone using their hands.
- **Open reduction**. Some growth plate injuries require surgery to align and set the bones. This procedure typically involves the use of smooth metal pins to stabilize the bones without prematurely fusing the injured growth plates.
  - After surgery, the doctor often uses a cast to immobilize the injured area. The cast is left in place until the injury heals.
  - The need for surgery depends on the location and extent of the injury, its effect on nearby nerves and blood vessels, and the child's age.

If the injury is severe or treatment is delayed, a growth plate fracture can disrupt the normal growth of the bone. This may result in the bone being crooked or slightly longer or shorter than expected. To prevent complications with bone growth, healthcare providers typically recommend follow-up appointments to monitor bone development for any changes. With prompt treatment, most children and teens recover without additional growth issues. The timeline for returning to regular activities and sports depends on their recovery progress and the nature of the activity involved.

Strengthening and Range-of-Motion Exercises

After the injury has healed, your child's doctor may suggest exercises to strengthen the muscles supporting the injured bone area. Strengthening exercises can enhance your child's ability to move the joint correctly. A physical therapist can collaborate with your child to create an individualized exercise regimen.

WHO TREATS GROWTH PLATE INJURIES?

The following health-care providers may help diagnose and treat growth plate injuries:

- **Pediatric orthopedists**. Treat and perform surgery for bone and joint diseases in children and teens.
- **Occupational therapists**. Teach ways to protect joints and perform activities of daily living.
- **Pediatricians**. Diagnose and treat children.
- **Physical therapists**. Specialize in movement and strengthening muscles.
- **Sports medicine physicians**. Treat musculoskeletal injuries from participation in sports.[1]

[1] "Growth Plate Injuries," National Institute of Arthritis and Musculoskeletal and Skin Diseases (NIAMS), December 1, 2023. Available online. URL: www.niams.nih.gov/health-topics/growth-plate-injuries. Accessed March 14, 2024.

Chapter 25 | **Common Medical Problems in Children**

Chapter Contents

Section 25.1 | **Childhood Overweight and Obesity**

Childhood obesity is a significant health issue in the United States, affecting one in five children and adolescents. While certain groups of children are more affected than others, all children are susceptible to gaining weight that exceeds healthy levels.

Obesity is a complex issue influenced by various factors, including behavior, genetics, and certain medications. However, societal and community factors also play significant roles:

- Childcare and school environments, neighborhood design, access to healthy, affordable foods and beverages, and access to safe and convenient places for physical activity affect our ability to make healthy choices.
- Every child deserves a healthy start in life.

PREVALENCE OF CHILDHOOD OBESITY IN THE UNITED STATES

Childhood obesity remains a serious problem in the United States, placing children and adolescents at risk for poor health. The prevalence of obesity among children and adolescents remains unacceptably high. For children and adolescents aged 2–19 years in 2017–2020:

- The prevalence of obesity was 19.7 percent and affected about 14.7 million children and adolescents.
- Obesity prevalence was 12.7 percent among 2–5-year-olds, 20.7 percent among 6–11-year-olds, and 22.2 percent among 12–19-year-olds. Childhood obesity is also more common among certain populations.
- Obesity prevalence was 26.2 percent among Hispanic children, 24.8 percent among non-Hispanic Black children, 16.6 percent among non-Hispanic white children, and 9.0 percent among non-Hispanic Asian children.

- Obesity-related conditions include high blood pressure (HBP), high cholesterol, type 2 diabetes, breathing problems such as asthma and sleep apnea, and joint problems.

Note: *Obesity is defined as a body mass index (BMI) at or above the 95th percentile of the Centers for Disease Control and Prevention (CDC) sex-specific BMI-for-age growth charts.*

BODY MASS INDEX AND BODY MASS INDEX CATEGORIES FOR CHILDREN AND TEENS

Body mass index (BMI) is an anthropometric measure of weight and height calculated by dividing a person's weight (in kilograms) by the square of their height (in meters). Because children and teens are still growing, the ranges for height, weight, and BMI vary by age and sex. Therefore, BMI values must be interpreted relative to other children of the same age and sex.

The Centers for Disease Control and Prevention (CDC) growth charts display sex-specific BMI-for-age percentile curves, which can be used to monitor the growth of children and teens aged 2–19 years. BMI categories for children and teens are defined based on sex- and age-specific BMI percentiles, while BMI categories for adults are based solely on BMI values. Table 25.1 illustrates the BMI categories for children and teens along with their corresponding sex- and age-specific BMI percentiles.

Table 25.1. Child Body Mass Index Categories and Percentiles

Body Mass Index Category	Body Mass Index Range
Underweight	Less than the 5th percentile
Healthy weight	5th percentile to less than the 85th percentile
Overweight	85th percentile to less than the 95th percentile
Obesity	95th percentile or greater
Severe obesity	120 percent of the 95th percentile or greater or 35 kg/m^2 or greater

For example, a 10-year-old boy who is 54.5 inches tall (at the 50th percentile for height) and weighs 96 pounds would have a BMI of 22.5 kg/m^2. This BMI places him at the 96th percentile for his age and sex, categorizing him in the obesity category. This indicates that the boy's BMI exceeds that of 96 percent of 10-year-old boys in the reference population. An expanded definition of severe obesity is used by the American Academy of Pediatrics (AAP):

- **Class 2 obesity**. BMI ≥120 percent to < 140 percent of the 95th percentile or BMI ≥35 to < 40 kg/m^2.
- **Class 3 obesity**. BMI ≥140 percent of the 95th percentile or BMI ≥40 kg/m^2.

For example, a 15-year-old girl who is 63.7 inches tall (at the 50th percentile for height) and weighs 210 pounds would have a BMI of 36.4 kg/m^2. This BMI places her at the 99th percentile for her age and sex. Her BMI is 129 percent of the 95th percentile, which classifies her as having class 2 obesity based on the expanded definition of severe obesity.

Having a high BMI-for-age percentile is associated with clinical risk factors for cardiovascular disease, such as high cholesterol, HBP, and other chronic conditions. In 2023, the AAP released the Clinical Practice Guideline for the Evaluation and Treatment of Children and Adolescents with Obesity to guide pediatric health-care providers on the standard of care for youth with overweight and obesity and associated comorbidities.

CAUSES OF OBESITY

Obesity is a complex disease characterized by an individual's weight exceeding healthy levels for their height. It affects both children and adults alike. Multiple factors contribute to excess weight gain, including eating habits, physical activity levels, and sleep patterns. Social determinants of health, genetics, and certain medications also influence obesity.

Food, Activity, and Sleep

Eating and physical activity patterns, inadequate sleep, and various other factors contribute to excess weight gain.

Social Determinants of Health

The conditions in which we live, learn, work, and play are referred to as "social determinants of health" (SDOH). Making healthy food choices and engaging in adequate physical activity can be challenging if these conditions do not support health. Disparities in SDOH influence chronic disease outcomes and risks, including obesity, across racial, ethnic, and socioeconomic groups, as well as in different geographical locations and among individuals with varying physical abilities. Settings such as childcare centers, schools, and communities influence eating habits and physical activity through the availability of foods and beverages and the opportunities for physical activity they provide. Other community factors influencing obesity include the affordability of healthy food choices, social and peer support, marketing strategies, and policies influencing community design.

Genetics

Genetic changes in human populations evolve too slowly to account for the obesity epidemic. However, variants in several genes can contribute to obesity by increasing hunger and food intake. In rare cases, a specific variant of a single gene (known as "monogenic obesity") can lead to a distinct pattern of inherited obesity within a family.

Illnesses and Medications

Certain illnesses, such as Cushing disease, can contribute to obesity or weight gain. Additionally, drugs such as steroids and certain antidepressants may induce weight gain. Ongoing research explores the consequences of other factors, including chemical exposures and the role of the microbiome, in relation to obesity.

What Can Be Done?

EATING PATTERNS

Healthy eating adheres to the 2020–2025 *Dietary Guidelines for Americans*, focusing on consuming a variety of vegetables and fruits, whole grains, lean protein foods, and low-fat or fat-free dairy products. It also involves limiting foods and beverages high in added sugars, solid fats, or sodium. Managers of worksites and public facilities can enhance the nutritional quality of food and beverages offered in those environments.

PHYSICAL ACTIVITY

The *Physical Activity Guidelines for Americans* recommend that children aged three through five should engage in physical activity throughout the day. Children aged 6–17 require at least 60 minutes of moderate to vigorous physical activity daily. Adults should aim for 150 minutes of moderate-intensity physical activity per week. The communities can facilitate physical activity by designing or adapting environments to encourage walking or biking for everyday trips.

SLEEP

Newborns typically require 14–17 hours of sleep per day. This amount decreases with age; teenagers generally need 8–10 hours of sleep per day, while adults should aim for seven or more hours of sleep per day.

SOCIAL DETERMINANTS OF HEALTH

State early care and education systems can implement standards that address nutrition, infant feeding, physical activity, and screen time. By collaborating with communities, programs, initiatives, and public health practitioners, they can collectively work to eliminate barriers to health and promote overall well-being.

CONSEQUENCES OF OBESITY

Individuals with obesity face an elevated risk of numerous serious diseases and health conditions compared to those with a healthy weight. Moreover, obesity and its associated health issues impose a substantial economic burden on the U.S. health-care system. Obesity also affects military readiness.

Health Conditions

Obesity in children and adults increases the risk for the following health conditions.

- high blood pressure and high cholesterol, which are risk factors for heart disease
- type 2 diabetes
- breathing problems, such as asthma and sleep apnea
- joint problems, such as osteoarthritis and musculoskeletal discomfort
- gallstones and gallbladder disease

Childhood obesity is also associated with:

- psychological problems such as anxiety and depression
- low self-esteem and lower self-reported quality of life
- social problems such as bullying and stigma
- obesity as adults
- adults with obesity have higher risks for stroke, many types of cancer, premature death, and mental illness such as clinical depression and anxiety

Economic Effect

Annual obesity-related medical care costs in the United States, in 2019 dollars, were estimated to be nearly $173 billion. Annual nationwide productivity costs of obesity-related absenteeism range from $3.38 billion ($79 per individual with obesity) to $6.38 billion ($132 per individual with obesity).

Direct medical costs encompass preventive, diagnostic, and treatment services. Indirect costs are associated with illness and death, encompassing lost productivity. Productivity measures include absenteeism due to obesity-related health issues, reduced productivity while at work, and premature death and disability.

Military Readiness

Just over one in three young adults aged 17–24 are too heavy to serve in the United States military. Among those who meet weight requirements, only three in four report physical activity levels sufficient to prepare them for challenges in basic training. As a result, only two in five young adults meet both weight eligibility and adequate physical activity criteria for military service.

Additionally, in 2020, 19 percent of active-duty service members had obesity, up from 16 percent in 2015. These individuals are less likely to be medically ready for deployment. Between 2008 and 2017, active-duty soldiers experienced over 3.6 million musculoskeletal injuries. One study revealed that active-duty soldiers with obesity were 33 percent more likely to sustain such injuries.[1]

Section 25.2 | **Diabetes in Children**

WHAT IS DIABETES TYPE 1?

Diabetes refers to elevated blood glucose or blood sugar levels. In type 1 diabetes, the pancreas does not produce insulin, a hormone essential for transporting glucose into cells to provide energy. Without insulin, excess glucose remains in the bloodstream. Prolonged high blood glucose levels can lead to severe complications affecting the heart, eyes, kidneys, nerves, gums, and teeth.

Type 1 diabetes happens most often in children and young adults but can appear at any age. Symptoms may include the following:

- being very thirsty
- urinating often
- feeling very hungry or tired
- losing weight without trying
- having sores that heal slowly
- having dry, itchy skin
- losing the feeling in your feet or having tingling in your feet
- having blurry eyesight

[1] "Childhood Overweight and Obesity," Centers for Disease Control and Prevention (CDC), April 1, 2022. Available online. URL: www.cdc.gov/obesity/childhood/index.html. Accessed March 14, 2024.

A blood test can diagnose diabetes. If diagnosed, you will likely require lifelong insulin therapy. The A1C blood test assesses how effectively you are managing your diabetes.[2]

WHAT CAUSES TYPE 1 DIABETES?

Type 1 diabetes is believed to result from an autoimmune reaction where the body mistakenly attacks itself. This autoimmune response targets and destroys the insulin-producing beta cells in the pancreas. This process can occur over months or years before symptoms become evident.

Some individuals inherit certain genes that increase their susceptibility to developing type 1 diabetes. However, not everyone with these genes will necessarily develop the condition. Environmental triggers, such as viral infections, are also believed to contribute to the onset of type 1 diabetes. It's important to note that diet and lifestyle habits do not cause type 1 diabetes.

SYMPTOMS AND RISK FACTORS OF TYPE 1 DIABETES

Symptoms of type 1 diabetes may take months or years to manifest. They can develop within a few weeks or months, and once present, they can be severe. Some symptoms overlap with those of other health conditions. It's crucial not to self-diagnose. If you suspect type 1 diabetes, consult your doctor for a blood sugar test. Untreated diabetes can lead to serious—even fatal—health complications. While risk factors for type 1 diabetes are not as well-defined as for prediabetes and type 2 diabetes, family history is known to play a role.

TESTING FOR TYPE 1 DIABETES

A simple blood test can determine if you have diabetes. If you were tested at a health fair or pharmacy, follow up at a clinic or doctor's office to ensure accurate results. If type 1 diabetes is suspected,

[2] MedlinePlus, "Diabetes Type 1," National Institutes of Health (NIH), June 29, 2020. Available online. URL: medlineplus.gov/diabetestype1.html. Accessed March 28, 2024.

your blood may also be tested for autoantibodies, which indicate autoimmune activity typically associated with type 1 but not type 2 diabetes. Urine testing for ketones may also be recommended, as ketones are produced when the body metabolizes fat for energy—a characteristic more commonly seen in type 1 diabetes than type 2.

WAYS TO HELP MANAGE YOUR CHILD'S TYPE 1 DIABETES

Learn Everything You Can

Treatment options, managing blood sugar fluctuations, carbohydrate counting, ketones, handling illness, and strategies for managing diabetes at school are essential topics to explore. Consider reading books, participating in support groups and online forums, and consulting your child's health-care team and other parents for guidance. Important things to know will include the following items:

- when your child needs to take insulin, what types of insulin, and in what combination
- what device will they use to take insulin, and how to use it
- how and when to check for high and low blood sugar and ketones
- what items to have on hand, including glucagon, gels, snacks, and drinks for low blood sugar
- signs of low blood sugar (They are different for every child.)
- how to make a diabetes management plan for school
- when to contact your health-care team
- where to go for help and support[3]

WHAT IS TYPE 2 DIABETES?

Healthy eating is essential for managing diabetes. Approximately 38 million Americans have diabetes (about 1 in 10), with approximately 90–95 percent of them having type 2 diabetes. While type

[3] "Three Ways to Help Manage Your Child's Type 1 Diabetes," Centers for Disease Control and Prevention (CDC), June 20, 2022. Available online. URL: www.cdc.gov/diabetes/library/features/parents-type1.html. Accessed March 28, 2024.

2 diabetes typically develops in individuals over age 45, an increasing number of children, teens, and young adults are also being diagnosed.

WHAT CAUSES TYPE 2 DIABETES?

Insulin, a hormone produced by the pancreas, functions like a key, enabling blood sugar to enter cells for energy use in the body. In type 2 diabetes, cells do not respond properly to insulin, a condition known as "insulin resistance." To compensate, the pancreas increases insulin production in an effort to elicit a response from cells. Over time, the pancreas becomes unable to maintain this increased production, leading to elevated blood sugar levels and paving the way for prediabetes and type 2 diabetes. Elevated blood sugar levels can damage the body and contribute to serious health issues such as heart disease, vision impairment, and kidney disease.

SYMPTOMS AND RISK FACTORS OF TYPE 2 DIABETES

Symptoms of type 2 diabetes typically develop gradually over several years and may persist unnoticed; in some cases, symptoms may not be apparent at all. Due to their subtle nature, it is crucial to be aware of the risk factors and to undergo blood sugar testing by a doctor if any of these factors are present.

TESTING FOR TYPE 2 DIABETES

A straightforward blood test can determine if you have diabetes. If you've had your blood sugar tested at a health fair or pharmacy, it's advisable to follow up at a clinic or doctor's office to ensure the accuracy of the results.[4]

PREVENTING TYPE 2 DIABETES

There is a rising issue of type 2 diabetes among young people. However, parents can play a crucial role in reversing this trend

[4] "Type 2 Diabetes," Centers for Disease Control and Prevention (CDC), April 18, 2023. Available online. URL: www.cdc.gov/diabetes/basics/type2.html. Accessed March 14, 2024.

through healthy changes beneficial for the entire family. Type 2 diabetes was once known as "adult-onset diabetes" because it rarely affected young children and teens. Now, approximately one-third of American youth are overweight, a factor closely linked to the growing number of children diagnosed with type 2 diabetes, some as young as 10 years old.

Weight Matters

People who are overweight, particularly those with excess belly fat, are at higher risk of developing insulin resistance, including children. Insulin resistance is a significant risk factor for type 2 diabetes. Insulin, a hormone produced by the pancreas, functions like a key to facilitate the entry of blood sugar into cells for energy use. Due to genetic predisposition (inherited traits) or lifestyle factors (such as overeating and physical inactivity), cells may become less responsive to insulin. This prompts the pancreas to produce more insulin in an attempt to stimulate cells to absorb and utilize blood sugar.

As long as sufficient insulin is produced, blood sugar levels remain within normal range. This can persist for several years, but eventually, the pancreas becomes unable to maintain this level of insulin production. Blood sugar levels begin to rise, initially after meals and eventually throughout the day. This progression sets the stage for the development of type 2 diabetes.

Insulin resistance typically does not present with symptoms, though some children may develop patches of thickened, dark, velvety skin known as "acanthosis nigricans," often found in body creases and folds such as the back of the neck or armpits. They may also have other conditions related to insulin resistance, including:

- high blood pressure (HBP)
- high cholesterol
- polycystic ovary syndrome (PCOS)

Activity Matters

Physical activity reduces the risk of type 2 diabetes by enhancing the body's insulin utilization, thereby decreasing insulin resistance.

Additionally, physical activity improves overall health by helping control blood pressure and boosting mental health.

Age Matters

Children who develop type 2 diabetes are typically diagnosed during their early teens. Hormones present during puberty can make it more challenging for the body to effectively use insulin, particularly affecting girls more than boys in developing type 2 diabetes. This underscores the importance of guiding children to take proactive steps toward managing their health from a young age.

More Risk Factors

These factors also increase kids' risk for type 2 diabetes:

- having a family member with type 2 diabetes
- being born to a mom with gestational diabetes (diabetes while pregnant)
- being African American, Hispanic/Latino, Native American/Alaska Native, Asian American, or Pacific Islander
- having one or more conditions related to insulin resistance

If your child is overweight and exhibits any two of the previously listed risk factors, it's important to consult with your doctor about testing their blood sugar. Testing usually starts at 10 years old or when puberty begins, whichever comes first, and is repeated every three years.[5]

[5] "Prevent Type 2 Diabetes in Kids," Centers for Disease Control and Prevention (CDC), December 30, 2022. Available online. URL: www.cdc.gov/diabetes/prevent-type-2/type-2-kids.html. Accessed March 14, 2024.

Section 25.3 | **Epilepsy and Febrile Seizures**

WHAT IS EPILEPSY?

Epilepsy is a disorder of the brain that causes seizures. These seizures are not caused by a temporary underlying medical condition such as a high fever. Epilepsy can affect people in very different ways because there are many causes and different kinds of seizures. Some people may have multiple types of seizures or other medical conditions in addition to epilepsy. These factors play a major role in determining the severity of the person's condition and its effect on their life. How a seizure looks depends on the type of seizure a person is experiencing. Some seizures can look like staring spells, while others can cause a person to collapse, shake, and become unaware of what is happening around them. Epilepsy can be caused by different conditions that affect a person's brain, and many times the cause is unknown. Some causes include the following:

- stroke
- brain tumor
- traumatic brain injury (TBI) or head injury
- central nervous system (CNS) infection

A person with epilepsy is not contagious and cannot give epilepsy to another person.[6]

WHAT ARE FEBRILE SEIZURES?

Febrile seizures are convulsions that occur in young children. They are triggered by fever, typically above 101 °F (38.3 °C). Seizures may happen during illnesses such as a cold, the flu, or an ear infection. In some cases, a child may not have a fever at the time of the seizure but will develop one a few hours later. Having a febrile seizure does not mean a child has epilepsy. Epilepsy involves repeated

[6] "Epilepsy Fast Facts," Centers for Disease Control and Prevention (CDC), September 30, 2020. Available online. URL: www.cdc.gov/epilepsy/about/fast-facts.htm. Accessed March 14, 2024.

seizures that are not triggered by fever. Symptoms may include the following:

- loss of consciousness or passing out
- uncontrollable shaking
- eye-rolling
- rigid (stiff) limbs

Less commonly, a child can become rigid or have twitches in only part of the body. Most febrile seizures last a minute or two, though some may last only a few seconds, and others may last for more than 15 minutes. Febrile seizures that last less than 15 minutes do not cause any long-term health problems. However, if another one occurs, it is more likely to be prolonged, lasting longer than 15 minutes. A first febrile seizure that is prolonged does not increase the risk of having more. Even prolonged seizures are generally harmless on their own, but they do carry an increased risk of developing epilepsy.

WHO IS MORE LIKELY TO GET FEBRILE SEIZURES?

About 1 in every 25 children will have at least one febrile seizure. Young children between the ages of about six months and five years are the most likely to have febrile seizures. Children are at the greatest risk of having a febrile seizure at age two. The older a child is when the first febrile seizure occurs, the less likely that child is to have more, as there will be less time spent in the age group at risk. About 40 percent of children who have one febrile seizure will have another. Certain things increase the risk for more febrile seizures, including:

- **Young age**. Children who have their first febrile seizure when they are younger than 18 months are at an increased risk of having another one.
- **Family history**. Children whose family members had febrile seizures are more likely to have more than one seizure.
- **First sign of illness**. Children who have febrile seizures before exhibiting other symptoms of an illness are at greater risk of having multiple seizures.

- **Low temperature.** Children are more likely to have another febrile seizure if the first one is accompanied by a relatively low temperature.

HOW ARE FEBRILE SEIZURES DIAGNOSED AND TREATED?

Diagnosing Febrile Seizures

To diagnose febrile seizures in infants and children, health-care providers will review a child's medical history and perform a physical exam. They often test blood and urine to help pinpoint the cause of the fever. Keep in mind that dehydration from severe diarrhea or vomiting can cause seizures. Meningitis, an infection of the membranes surrounding the brain, can cause both fever and seizures that can look like febrile seizures but are much more serious. If meningitis is suspected, health-care providers may remove and test a small amount of the fluid that surrounds the brain and spinal cord. Most of the time, children who have febrile seizures will not need to be in the hospital. Health-care providers may recommend hospitalization if:

- the seizure is prolonged
- the child has a serious infection
- the child is younger than six months of age

Treating Febrile Seizures

Parents and caregivers should remain calm, take first aid measures, and carefully watch the child. During a febrile seizure, parents and caregivers should do the following:

- **Note the start time of the seizure.** If it lasts longer than five minutes, call an ambulance. The child should be taken right away to the nearest medical facility.
- **Call an ambulance if the seizure is less than five minutes, but the child does not seem to be recovering quickly.**
- **Gradually place the child on a protected surface, such as the floor, to prevent injury.** Do not restrain or hold a child during a convulsion.

- **Put the child on his or her side or stomach to prevent choking.** When possible, gently remove any objects from the child's mouth. Nothing should ever be placed in the child's mouth during a seizure. These objects can block the airway and make it hard to breathe.
- **Seek immediate medical attention if this is the child's first febrile seizure.** Once it is over, take the child to the doctor to check for the cause of the fever. This is especially urgent if the child shows these symptoms of meningitis, an infection over the brain surface, which can include a stiff neck, extreme lethargy, or a lot of vomiting.

Drugs that lower fevers, such as acetaminophen or ibuprofen, may provide comfort, but studies show that treating a fever does not lower the risk of febrile seizures. Health-care providers may recommend other medications to control seizures if needed.

HOW CAN YOU OR YOUR LOVED ONE HELP IMPROVE CARE FOR PEOPLE WITH FEBRILE SEIZURES?

Consider participating in a clinical trial so that clinicians and scientists can learn more about febrile seizures and related disorders. Clinical research uses human volunteers to help researchers learn more about a disorder and perhaps find better ways to safely detect, treat, or prevent disease. All types of volunteers are needed—those who are healthy or have an illness or disease—of all different ages, sexes, races, and ethnicities. This diversity ensures that study results apply to as many people as possible and that treatments will be safe and effective for everyone who will use them.[7]

---

[7] "Febrile Seizures," National Institute of Neurological Disorders and Stroke (NINDS), November 28, 2023. Available online. URL: www.ninds.nih.gov/health-information/disorders/febrile-seizures. Accessed March 14, 2024.

Section 25.4 | **Dizziness and Balance Problems**

Most people feel dizzy now and then. Kids, like adults, may occasionally feel lightheaded or unsteady. But if such feelings repeat or interfere with everyday life, it could be a sign of a balance disorder. Most balance problems are temporary and easy to treat, but these problems may also signal a more serious condition that could have a lasting effect. Learn to recognize the signs of dizziness or balance problems that may warrant a trip to a doctor. Experts have long suspected that dizziness and balance problems are often overlooked and untreated, but the scope of the problem was not fully understood. That is why the National Institutes of Health (NIH) supported the largest national survey to date to uncover information about these disorders in children. The study included data on nearly 11,000 kids aged 3–17.

The researchers found that more than one in 20 kids in the United States had a dizziness or balance problem, and only one-third of them received treatment in the previous year. "The findings suggest that dizziness and balance problems are fairly common among children," says Dr. James F. Battey Jr., a pediatrician and director of NIH's National Institute on Deafness and Other Communication Disorders (NIDCD). Our sense of balance is a complex process. It is managed by signals between the brain, ears, eyes, and sensors in the joints and other body parts. This intricate system helps your body monitor and maintain its position as you move throughout the day without you even having to think about it. But if any of these many sensory signals go wrong, it can weaken your sense of balance.

Balance disorders can make you stagger when walking. You might teeter or fall when trying to stand. Affected people might feel like they or the world around them is spinning or moving—a condition known as "vertigo." Other symptoms can include blurred vision, vomiting, diarrhea, confusion, and anxiety. Common causes of balance problems in children range from ear infections, severe headaches, and certain medications to more serious neurological disorders, head or neck injuries, and genetic conditions.

Balance disorders can be difficult to recognize and understand. They can be especially hard to diagnose in young children. Kids may not know the right words to describe their symptoms. Affected children may talk about a "spinning feeling." They may say their tummy or head feels bad or weird. They may walk unsteadily or seem clumsy. "Parents who notice dizziness and balance problems in their children should consult a health-care provider to rule out a serious underlying condition," Battey says.

Your child's pediatrician will likely ask questions about when the symptoms first appeared, how long they last, how often they occur, and what medications the child is taking. Your child's eyes and ears will be examined, and hearing and balance may be tested. You may be referred to a specialist, such as an otolaryngologist—a doctor with expertise in the ear, nose, and throat. Treatment will depend on the underlying cause. The good news is that most dizziness and balance problems in children are temporary and treatable. Still, it is important to check with a health professional if you notice any problems.

TELL YOUR DOCTOR

Dizziness and balance problems may be hard to spot in children. Younger kids may lack the vocabulary to describe their symptoms. Talk with a health-care provider if your child:

- falls frequently
- seems unsteady upon standing or walking
- feels as if the room is spinning around him/her
- feels as if moving when standing or sitting still
- feels as if he or she is falling
- feels lightheaded or as if he or she might faint
- says that vision becomes blurred[8]

[8] *NIH News in Health*, "Dizziness and Balance Problems in Kids," National Institutes of Health (NIH), March 4, 2016. Available online. URL: https://newsinhealth.nih.gov/2016/03/dizziness-balance-problems-kids. Accessed March 14, 2024.

Section 25.5 | **Constipation**

WHAT IS CONSTIPATION IN CHILDREN?

Constipation in children is a condition in which your child may have:

- fewer than two bowel movements a week
- stools that are hard, dry, or lumpy
- stools that are difficult or painful to pass

Your child may also tell you that they feel not all stool has passed. Some children have more bowel movements than others, so what is normal for one child may be different for another. Additionally, as children get older, their bowel movement patterns may change. Even an infant's bowel movements change a lot in the first few weeks and months of life. Constipation is not a disease but may be a symptom of another medical problem. In most cases, constipation in children lasts a short time and is not dangerous.

HOW COMMON IS CONSTIPATION IN CHILDREN?

Constipation is common in children of all ages. Almost one of every 20 visits children make to a doctor is because of constipation.

WHAT CAUSES CONSTIPATION IN CHILDREN?

Children most often get constipated from holding in their stool to avoid or delay having a bowel movement. When stool stays too long in the colon, the colon absorbs too much fluid from the stool. This causes the stool to become hard, dry, and difficult to pass.

Certain Medicines

Medicines and dietary supplements that can make constipation in children worse include the following:

- antacids that contain aluminum and calcium
- anticholinergics and antispasmodic
- anticonvulsants—used to prevent seizures
- iron supplements

- narcotic pain medicines
- some medicines used to treat depression

Certain Health and Nutrition Problems

Certain health and nutrition problems can cause constipation in children:

- not eating enough fiber
- not drinking enough liquids or dehydration
- Hirschsprung disease
- celiac disease
- disorders that affect your brain and spine, such as spina bifida
- spinal cord or brain injuries
- conditions that affect their metabolism, such as diabetes
- conditions that affect their hormones, such as hypothyroidism
- problems that can block or narrow the colon or rectum, including tumors

WHAT ARE THE SYMPTOMS OF CONSTIPATION IN CHILDREN?

Symptoms of constipation in children may include your child:

- having fewer than two bowel movements a week
- passing stools that are hard, dry, or lumpy
- having stools that are difficult or painful to pass
- telling you that he or she feels that not all stool has passed
- changing positions to avoid or delay having a bowel movement, including:
    - standing on tiptoes and then rocking back on his or her heels
    - clenching his or her buttocks
    - doing unusual, dance-like movements
- having a swollen abdomen, or bloating

- having daytime or nighttime wetting
- having a stool in his or her underwear that looks like diarrhea

If your child avoids or delays having a bowel movement, he or she may develop a fecal impaction.

WHAT ARE THE COMPLICATIONS OF CONSTIPATION IN CHILDREN?

Children with constipation that lasts for a short time usually do not have complications. However, avoiding or delaying a bowel movement may lead to:

- long-lasting constipation
- painful bowel movements
- bladder control problems
- fecal impaction

WHEN SHOULD YOUR CHILD SEE A DOCTOR?

Your child should see a doctor if his or her symptoms last for more than two weeks or do not go away with at-home treatment. Take your child to a doctor right away if he or she has constipation and any of the following symptoms:

- bleeding from his or her rectum
- blood in his or her stool
- bloating
- constant pain in his or her abdomen
- vomiting
- weight loss

WHAT MEDICAL TESTS DO DOCTORS USE TO FIND THE CAUSE OF CONSTIPATION IN CHILDREN?

Doctors do not normally need medical tests to diagnose constipation in children. However, in some cases, your child's doctor may use medical tests to help find the cause of constipation.

Lab Tests

Your child's doctor may look for signs of certain diseases and conditions that may be causing your child's constipation or are related to your child's constipation. The doctor may use one or more of the following lab tests:

- blood tests
- stool tests
- urine tests

Bowel Function Tests

If your child's constipation does not improve with changes in nutrition, the doctor may use bowel function tests, including colorectal transit studies. These tests help the doctor see how well stool moves through your child's colon.

Imaging Tests

In some cases, your child's doctor may use imaging tests of your child's abdomen to look for problems that may be causing his or her constipation. Imaging tests include the following:

- ultrasound
- x-rays
- computed tomography (CT) scan

HOW DO DOCTORS TREAT CONSTIPATION IN CHILDREN?

Your child's doctor may recommend giving your child an enema or laxative to help treat their constipation. Most laxatives are over-the-counter (OTC) medicines taken by mouth until your child's bowel movements are normal. The doctor may recommend stopping the laxative once your child has better eating and bowel habits. You should not give a child a laxative unless instructed to do so by a doctor. If your child is taking an OTC or prescription medicine or supplement that can cause constipation, the doctor may recommend stopping it, changing the dose, or switching to a different one. Talk with your child's doctor before stopping any medicines.

HOW CAN YOU PREVENT YOUR CHILD FROM BECOMING CONSTIPATED?

You can help prevent constipation in your child with the same things that treat constipation:

- Provide enough fiber in your child's diet.
- Have your child drink plenty of water and other liquids.
- Make having a bowel movement part of your child's routine.[9]

Section 25.6 | Vitamin K Deficiency Bleeding

Vitamin K is a substance that our body needs to form clots and stop bleeding. We get vitamin K from the food we eat, and some vitamin K is also made by the good bacteria that live in our intestines. Babies are born with very small amounts of vitamin K stored in their bodies, which can lead to serious bleeding problems if not supplemented.

WHAT IS VITAMIN K DEFICIENCY BLEEDING OR VITAMIN K DEFICIENCY BLEEDING?

Vitamin K deficiency bleeding (VKDB) occurs when babies cannot stop bleeding because their blood does not have enough vitamin K to form a clot. The bleeding can occur anywhere inside or outside the body. When it occurs inside the body, it can be difficult to notice. Commonly, a baby with VKDB will bleed into their intestines or brain, which can lead to brain damage and even death. Infants who do not receive the vitamin K shot at birth can develop VKDB at any time up to six months of age. There are three types of VKDB, based on the age of the baby when the bleeding problems start: early, classical, and late.

[9] "Definition and Facts for Constipation in Children," National Institute of Diabetes and Digestive and Kidney Diseases (NIDDK), May 15, 2018. Available online. URL: www.niddk.nih.gov/health-information/digestive-diseases/constipation-children/definition-facts. Accessed March 14, 2024.

WHY ARE BABIES MORE LIKELY TO HAVE VITAMIN K DEFICIENCY AND TO GET VITAMIN K DEFICIENCY BLEEDING?

All infants, regardless of sex, race, or ethnic background, are at higher risk for VKDB until they start eating regular foods, usually at age four to six months, and until the normal intestinal bacteria start making vitamin K. This is because:

- at birth, babies have very little vitamin K stored in their bodies because only small amounts pass to them through the placenta from their mothers
- the good bacteria that produce vitamin K are not yet present in the newborn's intestines
- breast milk contains low amounts of vitamin K, so exclusively breastfed babies do not get enough vitamin K from the breast milk, alone

WHAT CAN YOU DO TO PREVENT YOUR BABY FROM GETTING VITAMIN K DEFICIENCY AND VITAMIN K DEFICIENCY BLEEDING?

The good news is that VKDB is easily prevented by giving babies a vitamin K shot into a muscle in the thigh. One shot given just after birth will protect your baby from VKDB. To allow for immediate bonding and contact between the newborn and mother, the vitamin K shot can be delayed up to six hours after birth.

IS THE VITAMIN K SHOT SAFE?

Yes, many studies have shown that vitamin K is safe when given to newborns.

WHAT MIGHT CAUSE BABIES TO BE DEFICIENT IN VITAMIN K AND HAVE BLEEDING PROBLEMS?

Some things can put infants at a higher risk for developing VKDB. Babies at greater risk include the following:

- Babies who do not receive a vitamin K shot at birth. The risk is even higher if they are exclusively breastfed.
- Babies whose mothers used certain medications, such as isoniazid or medicines to treat seizures. These drugs interfere with how the body uses vitamin K.

- Babies who have liver disease often cannot use the vitamin K their body stores.
- Babies who have diarrhea, celiac disease, or cystic fibrosis (CF) often have trouble absorbing vitamins, including vitamin K, from the foods they eat.

HOW OFTEN ARE BABIES AFFECTED WITH VITAMIN K DEFICIENCY BLEEDING?

Since babies can be affected until they are six months old, healthcare providers divide VKDB into three types: early, classical, and late. Table 25.2 helps explain the following three different types.

- Early and classical VKDB are more common, occurring in 1 in 60 to 1 in 250 newborns, although the risk is much higher for early VKDB among those infants whose mothers used certain medications during the pregnancy.
- Late VKDB is rarer, occurring in 1 in 14,000 to 1 in 25,000 infants.
- Infants who do not receive a vitamin K shot at birth are 81 times more likely to develop late VKDB than infants who do receive a vitamin K shot at birth.

Table 25.2. Types of Vitamin K Deficiency Bleeding

Type of Vitamin K Deficiency Bleeding	When It Occurs	Characteristics
Early-onset	Within the first 24 hours after birth	• Severe • Mainly found in infants whose mothers used certain medications (such as medicines to treat seizures or isoniazid) that interfere with how the body uses vitamin K
Classical	Two days to 1 week after birth	• Bruising • Bleeding from the umbilical cord

Table 25.2. Continued

Type of Vitamin K Deficiency Bleeding	When It Occurs	Characteristics
Late-onset	One week to 6 months after birth, most commonly 2–8 weeks after birth	• 30–60 percent of infants have bleeding within the brain • Tends to occur in breastfed-only babies who have not received the vitamin K shot • Warning bleeds are rare

WHAT THINGS SHOULD YOU LOOK FOR IN YOUR BABY IF YOU THINK HE OR SHE MIGHT HAVE VITAMIN K DEFICIENCY BLEEDING?

Unfortunately, in the majority of cases of VKDB, there are no warning signs before a life-threatening event starts. Babies with VKDB might develop any of the following signs:

- bruises, especially around the baby's head and face
- bleeding from the nose or umbilical cord
- skin color that is paler than before (for darker-skinned babies, the gums may appear pale)
- after the first three weeks of life, the white parts of your baby's eyes may turn yellow
- a stool that has blood in it is black or dark and sticky (also called "tarry"), or vomiting blood
- irritability, seizures, excessive sleepiness, or a lot of vomiting may all be signs of bleeding in the brain

Remember, VKDB is easily preventable with just a single vitamin K shot at birth.[10]

[10] "What Is Vitamin K Deficiency Bleeding?" Centers for Disease Control and Prevention (CDC), July 24, 2023. Available online. URL: www.cdc.gov/ncbddd/vitamink/facts.html. Accessed March 14, 2024.

Chapter 26 | **Antibiotic Resistance**

WHAT ARE BACTERIA?

Bacteria are germs found inside and outside our bodies. Most germs are harmless, and some can even be helpful to humans, but some bacteria can cause infections, such as strep throat and urinary tract infections (UTIs).

WHAT IS AN ANTIBIOTIC?

Antibiotics are critical tools for preventing and treating infections caused by specific bacteria in people, animals, and crops. In health care, antibiotics are among our most powerful drugs for fighting life-threatening bacterial infections.

WHAT IS ANTIMICROBIAL RESISTANCE?

Antimicrobial resistance occurs when germs such as bacteria or fungi no longer respond to the drugs designed to kill them. This means these germs are not killed and continue to grow. It does not mean our body is resistant to antibiotics or antifungals. Antimicrobial resistance is a naturally occurring process. Bacteria and fungi are constantly finding new ways to avoid the effects of the antibiotic and antifungal drugs used to treat the infections they cause. Infections caused by antimicrobial-resistant germs are difficult, and sometimes impossible, to treat. In many cases, antimicrobial-resistant infections require extended hospital stays, additional follow-up doctor visits, and costly and toxic alternatives.

HOW CAN TAKING ANTIBIOTICS CONTRIBUTE TO ANTIMICROBIAL RESISTANCE?

Anytime antibiotics are used, they can contribute to antimicrobial resistance. Increases in antimicrobial resistance are driven by a combination of germs exposed to antibiotics, the spread of those germs, and their mechanisms of resistance. When antibiotics are needed, the benefits usually outweigh the risks of antimicrobial resistance. However, too many antibiotics are being used unnecessarily and misused, which threatens the usefulness of these important drugs.

For example, too many antibiotics are being prescribed unnecessarily to people in the United States. The Centers for Disease Control and Prevention (CDC) estimates that about 47 million antibiotic courses are prescribed for infections that do not need antibiotics, such as colds and the flu, in U.S. doctors' offices and emergency departments each year. This amounts to about 28 percent of all antibiotics prescribed in these settings.

Everyone has a role to play in improving antibiotic use. Appropriate antibiotic use helps fight antimicrobial resistance and ensures these lifesaving drugs will be available for future generations.

WHY SHOULD YOU CARE ABOUT ANTIMICROBIAL RESISTANCE?

Each year in the United States, at least 2.8 million people become infected with an antimicrobial-resistant infection, and more than 35,000 people die.

Antimicrobial resistance can affect any person at any stage of life. People receiving health care or those with weakened immune systems are often at higher risk for getting an infection.

Antimicrobial resistance jeopardizes advancements in modern health care that we have come to rely on, such as joint replacements, organ transplants, and cancer therapy. These procedures carry a significant risk of infection, and patients will not be able to receive them if effective antibiotics are not available. Beyond health care, antimicrobial resistance also affects the veterinary and agriculture industries.

HOW CAN YOU IMPROVE ANTIBIOTIC USE?

Taking antibiotics only when they are needed is an important way you can protect yourself and your family from antimicrobial resistance. Talk to your doctor about the best treatment if you are sick. Never pressure your doctor to prescribe an antibiotic. When antibiotics are not needed, they would not help you, and their side effects could still cause harm. Ask your doctor or pharmacist about steps you can take to feel better when an antibiotic is not needed.

If your doctor decides an antibiotic is the best treatment when you are sick, follow these instructions:

- Take the medication exactly as your doctor tells you.
- Do not share your medication with others.
- Do not save them for later. Talk to your pharmacist about safely discarding leftover medicines.
- Do not take antibiotics prescribed for someone else. This may delay the best treatment for you, make you even sicker, or cause side effects.
- Talk with your doctor and pharmacist if you have any questions about the antibiotics prescribed to you.

HOW CAN YOU PROTECT YOURSELF AND YOUR FAMILY FROM ANTIMICROBIAL RESISTANCE?

Other ways to protect yourself and your family from infections, including resistant infections:

- doing your best to stay healthy and keep others healthy
- cleaning hands
- covering coughs
- staying home when sick
- getting recommended vaccines, such as the flu vaccine[1]

If your child is sick, here are three important questions to ask your health-care professional.

[1] "Antimicrobial Resistance Questions and Answers," Centers for Disease Control and Prevention (CDC), November 15, 2022. Available online. URL: www.cdc.gov/antibiotic-use/antibiotic-resistance.html. Accessed March 28, 2024.

WHAT IS THE BEST TREATMENT FOR MY CHILD'S ILLNESS?

Your child can feel better without an antibiotic. Respiratory viruses usually go away in a week or two without treatment. Ask your health-care professional about the best way to feel better while your child's body fights off the virus (see Table 26.1).

Table 26.1. Questions to Ask Your Health-Care Professional

Common Condition	Common Cause			Are Antibiotics Needed?
	Bacteria	Bacteria or Virus	Virus	
Strep throat	✓			Yes
Whooping cough	✓			Yes
Urinary tract infection	✓			Yes
Sinus infection		✓		Maybe
Middle ear infection		✓		Maybe
Bronchitis/chest cold (in otherwise healthy children and adults)*		✓		No*
Common cold/runny nose			✓	
Sore throat (except strep)			✓	No
Flu			✓	No

**Studies show that in otherwise healthy children and adults, antibiotics for bronchitis would not help you feel better.*

WHAT CAN YOU DO TO HELP YOUR CHILD FEEL BETTER?

Pain relievers, fever reducers, saline nasal spray or drops, warm compresses, liquids, and rest may be the best ways to help your child feel better. Your health-care professional can tell you how to help relieve your child's symptoms.[2]

[2] "Questions to Ask Your Healthcare Professional," Centers for Disease Control and Prevention (CDC), August 31, 2018. Available online. URL: www.cdc.gov/antibiotic-use/community/pdfs/aaw/au_arent_always_the_answer_fs_508.pdf. Accessed March 28, 2024.

Chapter 27 | Pediatric Injury

Injuries are a leading cause of death and disability among U.S. children. Injuries in children can range from mild, which may not require a health-care provider visit or treatment, to severe, life-threatening, or fatal. Severe or life-threatening pediatric injury is sometimes called "pediatric trauma" and can result from a variety of unintentional and intentional causes, such as vehicle accidents, falls, poisoning, drowning, and suffocation.

WHAT IS PEDIATRIC INJURY?

Pediatric injury is a broad category that refers to physical harm to a child, typically defined as someone between one year and 18 years of age. Pediatric injuries have many different causes, severities, and effects.

- **Some injuries, such as insect bites, can be relatively mild and may not require medical attention**. Others, such as those from motor vehicle crashes, can be severe, life-threatening, or life-changing.
- **Injuries can be unintentional or accidental, such as those resulting from a fall off a bicycle**. They can also be intentional, such as homicides, suicides, maltreatment, and violence.
- **In some cases, injuries are so severe that they are fatal**. When they are not fatal, they may lead to lifelong physical or mental health problems and disabilities, requiring intense or specialized care.

WHAT IS PEDIATRIC EMERGENCY MEDICINE?

Pediatric emergency medicine focuses on the immediate care of infants, children, and adolescents with acute illnesses or injuries that require urgent medical attention. Treatment and care provided in hospital emergency departments are generally not long-term or continuing. Pediatric emergency medicine physicians consult with physicians from other specialties to resuscitate and stabilize children who are seriously ill or injured.

WHAT ARE EMERGENCY MEDICAL SERVICES FOR CHILDREN?

The Emergency Medical Services for Children (EMSC) program aims to reduce children's disability and death from severe illness or injury by increasing awareness and enhancing capabilities among prehospital, health systems, health-care providers, and the general public regarding the special physiological and psychological needs of children receiving emergency medical care.

WHAT IS PEDIATRIC CRITICAL CARE?

Children who have severe or life-threatening injuries need critical care, which includes constant monitoring and specialized treatments. Critical care occurs in hospital pediatric intensive care units (PICUs). PICUs are staffed by physicians with specialized training to care for children with traumatic injuries; these specialists are often called "pediatric intensivists."

Because injuries can affect many parts of the body at once, PICUs have access to various health-care providers who specialize in different types of medicine. These specialists may include emergency medicine physicians, surgeons, anesthesiologists, cardiologists, neurologists, and others. PICUs may also have access to pediatricians, nurses, social workers, psychologists, physical and occupational therapists, speech therapists, pharmacists, and others who help injured children and their families heal and recover.[1]

---

[1] "Pediatric Injury," *Eunice Kennedy Shriver* National Institute of Child Health and Human Development (NICHD), December 11, 2019. Available online. URL: www.nichd.nih.gov/health/topics/factsheets/pediatric. Accessed March 26, 2024.

INJURIES AMONG CHILDREN AND TEENS

Child unintentional injury death rates decreased by 11 percent from 2010 to 2019, but injury is still the leading cause of death for children and teens in the United States—and some are at higher risk. More than 7,000 children and teens aged 0–19 died because of unintentional injuries in 2019, which amounts to about 20 deaths each day. Leading causes of child unintentional injury include motor vehicle crashes, suffocation, drowning, poisoning, fires, and falls. Child injury is often preventable.

In 2018–2019, child unintentional injury death rates were highest among:

- male children
- babies under one year old and teens age 15–19 years
- American Indian and Alaska Native children and Black children

Despite overall decreases in child unintentional injury death rates from 2010 to 2019, rates increased among some groups:

- suffocation death rates increased by 20 percent among infants overall and 21 percent among Black children
- motor vehicle death rates among Black children increased by 9 percent, while rates among white children decreased by 24 percent
- poisoning death rates increased 50 percent among Hispanic children and 37 percent among Black children, while rates among white children decreased by 24 percent

Drowning was the leading cause of injury death for children aged one to four years. Drowning death rates were 2.6 times higher among Black children aged five to nine years and 3.6 times higher among Black children aged 10–14 years compared with white children of the same age.[2]

[2] "Injuries among Children and Teens," Centers for Disease Control and Prevention (CDC), September 22, 2021. Available online. URL: www.cdc.gov/injury/features/child-injury/index.html. Accessed March 26, 2024.

WHAT CAN BE DONE

States and communities can:

- align efforts with the National Action Plan (NAP) for Child Injury Prevention, released in 2012 by the Centers for Disease Control and Prevention (CDC) and more than 60 partner organizations
- strengthen data collection on child injury to identify problems and track progress
- use strategies shown to reduce injuries, such as graduated driver licenses, learn-to-swim programs, and prescription drug monitoring programs
- improve access to poison control centers, trauma center care, and preventive services such as cardiopulmonary resuscitation (CPR) and first aid training

Health-care systems can:

- use technology, such as electronic medical records, to improve the speed and quality of care for injured children, and to monitor the number and severity of injuries
- include child safety education for new parents and at all pediatric visits

Employers can:

- protect all employees, including youth, from workplace injuries by complying with existing safety standards and regulations
- provide proper safety training, education, and protective equipment for each job task

Everyone can:

- take steps to prevent child injury where you live, work, and play
- be a good role model—wear a seat belt, use a helmet, and follow other safety tips[3]

---

[3] "Child Injury," Centers for Disease Control and Prevention (CDC), January 29, 2020. Available online. URL: www.cdc.gov/vitalsigns/childinjury/index.html. Accessed March 26, 2024.

Chapter 28 | Childhood Mental Disorders

Chapter Contents

Section 28.1 | Understanding Mental Health in Children

WHAT IS CHILDREN'S MENTAL HEALTH?

Being mentally healthy during childhood means reaching developmental and emotional milestones and learning healthy social skills and how to cope when there are problems. Mentally healthy children have a positive quality of life (QOL) and can function well at home, in school, and in their communities. Mental disorders among children are described as serious changes in the way children typically learn, behave, or handle their emotions, causing distress and problems getting through the day.

Many children occasionally experience fears and worries or display disruptive behaviors. If symptoms are serious, persistent, and interfere with school, home, or play activities, the child may be diagnosed with a mental disorder. Mental health is not simply the absence of a mental disorder. Children who do not have a mental disorder might differ in how well they are doing, and children who have the same diagnosed mental disorder might differ in their strengths and weaknesses in how they are developing and coping, and in their quality of life. Understanding mental health as a continuum and identifying specific mental disorders are both ways to assess how well children are doing.

WHAT ARE COMMON CHILDHOOD MENTAL DISORDERS?

Among the more common mental disorders that can be diagnosed in childhood are attention deficit hyperactivity disorder (ADHD), anxiety (fears or worries), and behavior disorders. Other childhood disorders and concerns that affect how children learn, behave, or handle their emotions can include learning and developmental disabilities, autism, and risk factors such as substance use and self-harm.

WHAT ARE THE SYMPTOMS OF CHILDHOOD MENTAL DISORDERS?

Symptoms of mental disorders change over time as a child grows and may include difficulties with how a child plays, learns, speaks, and acts, or how the child handles their emotions. Symptoms often start in early childhood, although some disorders may develop during the teenage years. Diagnosis is often made during the school years and sometimes earlier; however, some children with a mental disorder may not be recognized or diagnosed as having one.

CAN CHILDHOOD MENTAL DISORDERS BE TREATED?

Childhood mental disorders can be treated and managed. There are many treatment options based on the best and most current medical evidence. Parents and doctors should work closely with everyone involved in the child's treatment—teachers, coaches, therapists, and other family members. Taking advantage of all available resources will help parents, health professionals, and educators guide the child toward success. Early diagnosis and appropriate services for children and their families can make a significant difference in the lives of children with mental disorders.

Get Help Finding Treatment

If you have concerns about a child, you can use the following resources to help you find a health-care provider familiar with treatment options:

- Psychologist Locator (http://locator.apa.org), a service of the American Psychological Association (APA) Practice Organization.
- Child and Adolescent Psychiatrist Finder (www.aacap.org/AACAP/Families_and_Youth/Resources/CAP_Finder.aspx), a research tool by the American Academy of Child and Adolescent Psychiatry (AACAP).
- Find a Cognitive Behavioral Therapist (www.findcbt.org/FAT), a search tool by the Association for Behavioral and Cognitive Therapies (ABCT).
- If you need help finding treatment facilities, visit FindTreatment.gov.

WHO IS AFFECTED?

Childhood mental disorders affect many children and families. Boys and girls of all ages and ethnic/racial backgrounds, living in all regions of the United States, experience mental disorders. Based on the National Research Council (NRC) and Institute of Medicine (IOM) report, it is estimated that in 2007, 13–20 percent of children living in the United States (up to one out of five children) experienced a mental disorder in a given year, costing individuals, families, and society an estimated $247 billion per year.

WHAT IS THE EFFECT OF MENTAL DISORDERS IN CHILDREN?

Mental health is important to overall health. Mental disorders are chronic health conditions—conditions that last a long time and often do not go away completely—that can continue through the lifespan. Without early diagnosis and treatment, children with mental disorders can have problems at home, in school, and in forming friendships. Mental disorders can also interfere with a child's healthy development, causing problems that can continue into adulthood.

PUBLIC HEALTH INCLUDES MENTAL HEALTH

Supporting children's mental health also includes making sure children meet developmental milestones, understanding what to do when there is a concern, supporting positive parenting strategies, and improving access to care. The Centers for Disease Control and Prevention (CDC) works with partner agencies to better understand mental health and mental disorders and their effect on children.

WHAT YOU CAN DO

- **Parents**. You know your child best. Talk to your child's health-care professional if you have concerns about the way your child behaves at home, in school, or with friends.
- **Youth**. It is just as important to take care of your mental health as it is to take care of your physical health. If you are angry, worried, or sad, do not be afraid to talk about your feelings and reach out to a trusted friend or adult.
- **Health-care professionals**. Early diagnosis and appropriate treatment based on updated guidelines are

very important. There are resources available to help diagnose and treat children's mental disorders.
- **Teachers/school administrators.** Early identification is important so that children can get the help they need. Work with families and health-care professionals if you have concerns about the mental health of a child in your school.[1]

Section 28.2 | Attention Deficit Hyperactivity Disorder

Attention deficit hyperactivity disorder (ADHD) is one of the most common neurobehavioral disorders of childhood. It is usually first diagnosed in childhood and often lasts into adulthood.

SIGNS AND SYMPTOMS OF ATTENTION DEFICIT HYPERACTIVITY DISORDER

It is normal for children to have trouble focusing and behaving at times. However, children with ADHD do not just grow out of these behaviors. The symptoms continue, can be severe, and can cause difficulty at school, at home, or with friends.

A child with ADHD might:
- have a hard time paying attention
- daydream a lot
- not seem to listen
- be easily distracted from schoolwork or play
- forget things
- be in constant motion or unable to stay seated
- squirm or fidget
- talk too much

[1] "What Is Children's Mental Health?" Centers for Disease Control and Prevention (CDC), July 26, 2023. Available online. URL: www.cdc.gov/childrensmentalhealth/basics.html. Accessed March 14, 2024.

- not be able to play quietly
- act and speak without thinking
- have trouble taking turns
- interrupt others

DIAGNOSIS OF ATTENTION DEFICIT HYPERACTIVITY DISORDER

Deciding if a child has ADHD is a process with several steps. There is no single test to diagnose ADHD, and many other problems, such as anxiety, depression, sleep problems, and certain types of learning disabilities, can have similar symptoms. One step in the process involves having a medical exam, including hearing and vision tests, to rule out other problems with symptoms similar to ADHD. Another part of the process may include a checklist for rating ADHD symptoms and taking a history of the child from parents, teachers, and sometimes the child.

TREATMENT FOR ATTENTION DEFICIT HYPERACTIVITY DISORDER

Attention deficit hyperactivity disorder can be successfully managed. Treatment options for ADHD include the following:

- behavior therapy, including training for parents
- medications
- school accommodations and interventions

In most cases, ADHD is best treated with a combination of behavior therapy and medication. For preschool-aged children (4–5 years old) with ADHD, behavior therapy, particularly training for parents, is recommended as the first line of treatment. What works best can depend on the child and family. Good treatment plans will include close monitoring, follow-ups, and making changes as needed along the way.

GET HELP

If you or your doctor has concerns about ADHD, you can take your child to a specialist such as a child psychologist or developmental pediatrician. You can also contact your local early intervention agency for children under age three or your public school for children aged three and older.[2]

Section 28.3 | Anxiety and Depression

Many children have fears and worries and may feel sad and hopeless from time to time. Strong fears may appear at different times during development. For example, toddlers are often very distressed about being away from their parents, even if they are safe and cared for. Although fears and worries are typical in children, persistent or extreme forms of fear and sadness could be due to anxiety or depression. Because the symptoms primarily involve thoughts and feelings, they are sometimes called "internalizing disorders."

ANXIETY

When a child does not outgrow the fears and worries typical in young children, or when there are so many fears and worries that they interfere with school, home, or play activities, the child may be diagnosed with an anxiety disorder. Examples of different types of anxiety disorders include the following:

- being very afraid when away from parents (separation anxiety)
- having extreme fear about a specific thing or situation, such as dogs, insects, or going to the doctor (phobias)
- being very afraid of school and other places where there are people (social anxiety)
- being very worried about the future and about bad things happening (general anxiety)

[2] National Center on Birth Defects and Developmental Disabilities (NCBDDD), "Is It ADHD?" Centers for Disease Control and Prevention (CDC), September 27, 2023. Available online. URL: www.cdc.gov/ncbddd/adhd/features/adhd.html. Accessed March 14, 2024.

- having repeated episodes of sudden, unexpected, intense fear that come with symptoms such as heart pounding, having trouble breathing, or feeling dizzy, shaky, or sweaty (panic disorder)

Anxiety may present as fear or worry but can also make children irritable and angry. Symptoms can include trouble sleeping, as well as physical symptoms such as fatigue, headaches, or stomachaches. Some anxious children keep their worries to themselves, so the symptoms can be missed.

DEPRESSION

Occasionally feeling sad or hopeless is a part of every child's life. However, some children experience sadness or loss of interest in activities they once enjoyed, or they may feel helpless or hopeless in situations they could typically change. When children persistently feel sadness and hopelessness, they may receive a diagnosis of depression. Examples of behaviors often seen in children with depression include the following:

- feeling sad, hopeless, or irritable a lot of the time
- not wanting to do or enjoy doing fun things
- showing changes in eating patterns—eating a lot more or a lot less than usual
- showing changes in sleep patterns—sleeping a lot more or a lot less than normal
- showing changes in energy—being tired and sluggish or tense and restless a lot of the time
- having a hard time paying attention
- feeling worthless, useless, or guilty
- showing self-injury and self-destructive behavior

Severe depression can lead a child to contemplate or plan for suicide. Among youth aged 10–24 years, suicide ranks among the leading causes of death. Some children may not openly discuss their feelings of helplessness and hopelessness and may not exhibit sadness. Depression can also manifest in behaviors such as causing trouble or appearing unmotivated, which may lead others to overlook or misinterpret the child's condition, labeling them as troublemakers or lazy.

TREATMENT FOR ANXIETY AND DEPRESSION

The first step in treatment is to consult a health-care provider, such as your child's primary care provider or a mental health specialist, to discuss undergoing an evaluation. The United States Preventive Services Task Force (USPSTF) recommends screening for anxiety in children aged 8–18 years and for depression in children affected by other conditions, like trauma. Specific symptoms, such as difficulty focusing, could indicate attention deficit hyperactivity disorder (ADHD). A thorough evaluation is crucial for accurate diagnosis and effective treatment planning. Collaboration with a health-care provider can help determine if medication should be included in the treatment regimen. A mental health professional can devise a therapy plan tailored to the child and family, which may involve child therapy, family therapy, or a combination of both. School involvement can also be integral to the treatment plan. For very young children, parental involvement in treatment is essential.

Cognitive-behavioral therapy (CBT) is a therapeutic approach used to address anxiety or depression, especially in older children. It focuses on transforming negative thoughts into more positive, effective ways of thinking, which can lead to improved behavior. Behavioral therapy for anxiety may involve teaching children strategies to cope with and manage anxiety symptoms while gradually exposing them to their fears to demonstrate that negative outcomes are unlikely. Treatment plans may also incorporate various methods to reduce stress and promote overall health, such as a balanced diet, physical activity, adequate sleep, consistent routines, and social support.

Get Help Finding Treatment

Here are tools to find a health-care provider familiar with treatment options:

- Psychologist Locator (http://locator.apa.org), a service of the American Psychological Association (APA) Practice Organization.

- Child and Adolescent Psychiatrist Finder (www.aacap.org/AACAP/Families_and_Youth/Resources/CAP_Finder.aspx), a research tool by the American Academy of Child and Adolescent Psychiatry (AACAP).
- Find a Cognitive Behavioral Therapist (www.findcbt.org/FAT), a search tool by the Association for Behavioral and Cognitive Therapies (ABCT).
- If you need help finding treatment facilities, visit FindTreatment.gov.
- Suicide and Crisis Lifeline: Call or text 988 or chat at 988lifeline.org

MANAGING SYMPTOMS: STAYING HEALTHY

Maintaining good health is crucial for all children and particularly beneficial for those dealing with depression or anxiety. Alongside receiving appropriate treatment, adopting a healthy lifestyle can contribute significantly to managing symptoms of depression or anxiety. Here are some healthy behaviors that may help:

- having a healthy eating plan centered on fruits, vegetables, whole grains, legumes (e.g., beans, peas, and lentils), lean protein sources, and nuts and seeds
- participating in physical activity for at least 60 minutes each day
- getting the recommended amount of sleep each night based on age
- practicing mindfulness or relaxation techniques

PREVENTION OF ANXIETY AND DEPRESSION

The exact reasons why some children develop anxiety or depression are not fully understood. Multiple factors may contribute, including biology and temperament. However, it is recognized that certain children are more susceptible to developing anxiety or depression when they encounter trauma, stress, maltreatment, bullying, or rejection by peers, or when their parents themselves experience anxiety or depression.[3]

---

[3] "Anxiety and Depression in Children," Centers for Disease Control and Prevention (CDC), July 25, 2023. Available online. URL: www.cdc.gov/childrensmentalhealth/depression.html. Accessed March 14, 2024.

Section 28.4 | Behavior or Conduct Problems

Children may occasionally argue, act aggressively, or display defiance toward adults. A behavior disorder may be diagnosed when these disruptive behaviors are unusual for the child's age, persist over time, or are particularly severe. These disorders, characterized by outwardly directed and disruptive behaviors, are often referred to as "externalizing disorders."

OPPOSITIONAL DEFIANT DISORDER

When children persistently act out in ways that seriously disrupt home, school, or peer interactions, they may receive a diagnosis of oppositional defiant disorder (ODD). Typically, ODD begins before the age of eight but generally no later than around 12 years old. Children with ODD are more likely to display oppositional or defiant behaviors towards familiar individuals, such as family members, regular caregivers, or teachers, and they exhibit these behaviors more frequently compared to their peers. Examples of ODD behaviors include the following:

- often being angry or losing one's temper
- often arguing with adults or refusing to comply with adults' rules or requests
- often resentful or spiteful
- deliberately annoying others or becoming annoyed with others
- often blaming other people for one's own mistakes or misbehavior

CONDUCT DISORDER

Conduct disorder (CD) is diagnosed when children exhibit an ongoing pattern of aggression toward others and serious violations of rules and social norms at home, school, and with peers. These rule violations may include breaking the law and can lead to arrest. Children with CD are at higher risk of injury and may experience difficulties in peer relationships. Examples of CD behaviors include the following:

- breaking serious rules, such as running away, staying out at night when told not to, or skipping school
- being aggressive in a way that causes harm, such as bullying, fighting, or being cruel to animals
- lying, stealing, or damaging other people's property on purpose

MANAGING SYMPTOMS: STAYING HEALTHY

Being healthy is crucial for all children and can be particularly significant for those with behavior or conduct problems. Alongside behavioral therapy and medication, adopting specific healthy lifestyle behaviors may mitigate challenging and disruptive behaviors your child might face. Here are some healthy behaviors that may help:

- engaging in regular physical activity, including aerobic and vigorous exercise
- eating a healthful diet centered on fruits, vegetables, whole grains, legumes (e.g., beans, peas, and lentils), lean protein sources, and nuts and seeds
- getting the recommended amount of sleep each night based on age
- strengthening relationships with family members

TREATMENT FOR DISRUPTIVE BEHAVIOR DISORDERS

Early initiation of treatment is crucial. Treatment effectiveness is maximized when it aligns with the specific needs of the child and their family. The initial step is to consult a health-care provider. A thorough assessment by a mental health professional may be necessary to establish an accurate diagnosis. Some behavioral signs, such as non-compliance with school rules, could indicate underlying learning issues requiring additional intervention. For younger children, the most well-supported treatment involves behavior therapy for parents, where a therapist teaches effective strategies to strengthen the parent-child relationship and manage the child's behavior. For school-age children and adolescents, a commonly utilized effective approach combines training and therapy involving the child, family, and school.

Get Help Finding Treatment

Here are tools to find a health-care provider familiar with treatment options:

- Psychologist Locator (http://locator.apa.org), a service of the American Psychological Association (APA) Practice Organization.
- Child and Adolescent Psychiatrist Finder (www.aacap.org/AACAP/Families_and_Youth/Resources/CAP_Finder.aspx), a research tool by the American Academy of Child and Adolescent Psychiatry (AACAP).
- Find a Cognitive Behavioral Therapist (www.findcbt.org/FAT), a search tool by the Association for Behavioral and Cognitive Therapies (ABCT).
- If you need help finding treatment facilities, visit FindTreatment.gov.

PREVENTION OF DISRUPTIVE BEHAVIOR DISORDERS

The reasons why some children develop disruptive behavior disorders remain uncertain. Numerous factors, including biological and social influences, likely contribute. Children face heightened risk when exposed to violence, criminal behavior, maltreatment, or inconsistent parenting. Parental mental health conditions such as substance use disorders (SUDs), depression, or attention deficit hyperactivity disorder (ADHD) also increase risk. Furthermore, the quality of early childhood care can influence the development of behavioral problems in children.[4]

[4] "Behavior or Conduct Problems in Children," Centers for Disease Control and Prevention (CDC), July 26, 2023. Available online. URL: www.cdc.gov/childrensmentalhealth/behavior.html. Accessed March 14, 2024.

Section 28.5 | Obsessive-Compulsive Disorder in Children

Many children occasionally experience troubling thoughts and feel compelled to act on them, even if their actions seem irrational. For instance, a child might fear bad luck unless they wear a specific piece of clothing. In some cases, these thoughts and urges persist despite efforts to ignore or dismiss them. When these unwanted thoughts occur frequently, accompanied by behaviors that consume significant time (more than an hour daily), disrupt activities, or cause distress, children may be diagnosed with obsessive-compulsive disorder (OCD). The distressing thoughts are termed "obsessions," and the repetitive behaviors are known as "compulsions."

SYMPTOMS OF OBSESSIVE-COMPULSIVE DISORDER

Having OCD means having obsessions, compulsions, or both. Examples of obsessive or compulsive behaviors include the following:

- Having unwanted thoughts, impulses, or images that occur over and over and which cause anxiety or distress.
- Having to think about or say something over and over (e.g., counting, or repeating words silently or out loud).
- Having to do something repeatedly (e.g., handwashing, placing things in a specific order, or checking the same things repeatedly, such as whether a door is locked).
- Having to do something over and over according to certain rules that must be followed exactly in order to make an obsession go away.

Children engage in these behaviors because they believe these actions will prevent harm or alleviate distress. However, these behaviors are often not logically connected to actual dangers, or they may be excessive, such as excessively frequent hand-washing.

A common misconception is that OCD solely manifests as extreme neatness and orderliness. While cleaning behaviors can be part of OCD, individuals with OCD often focus intensely on specific actions that must be repeated rather than on organization. Obsessions and compulsions can also evolve and vary over time.

TREATMENT FOR OBSESSIVE-COMPULSIVE DISORDER

The initial step in treatment is to consult with a health-care provider to schedule an evaluation. A thorough assessment by a mental health professional will determine whether the anxiety or distress stems from memories of a real traumatic event or other thoughts and beliefs. Additionally, the professional will assess for current or past tic disorders in individuals with OCD. Anxiety, depression, and disruptive behaviors may also co-occur with OCD.

Treatment options may include behavior therapy and medication. Cognitive behavioral therapy (CBT) is a type of behavior therapy that assists children in replacing negative thoughts with more constructive thinking patterns, leading to more effective behaviors. For OCD, behavior therapy often involves gradually exposing children to their fears in a controlled environment, helping them understand that negative outcomes do not typically occur when they resist their compulsions, thereby reducing their anxiety over time. While behavior therapy alone can be effective, some children benefit from a combination of behavior therapy and medication. Involvement of families and schools in the therapy process can help children manage stress, ensuring they receive supportive responses that do not inadvertently reinforce obsessions or compulsions.

Get Help Finding Treatment

Here are tools to find a health-care provider familiar with treatment options:

- Psychologist Locator (http://locator.apa.org), a service of the American Psychological Association (APA) Practice Organization.
- Child and Adolescent Psychiatrist Finder (www.aacap.org/AACAP/Families_and_Youth/Resources/CAP_Finder.aspx), a research tool by the American Academy of Child and Adolescent Psychiatry (AACAP).

- Find a Cognitive Behavioral Therapist (www.findcbt.org/FAT), a search tool by the Association for Behavioral and Cognitive Therapies.
- If you need help finding treatment facilities, visit FindTreatment.gov.

PREVENTION OF OBSESSIVE-COMPULSIVE DISORDER

The exact reasons why some children develop OCD are not fully understood, but biological and neurological factors likely play significant roles. Some children with OCD also have concurrent conditions like Tourette syndrome or other tic disorders. Research indicates that health issues during pregnancy and childbirth might increase the likelihood of OCD development, underscoring the importance of supporting women's health during pregnancy for various reasons, including reducing such risks.[5]

Section 28.6 | **Posttraumatic Stress Disorder**

All children may encounter highly stressful events that influence their thoughts and emotions. Typically, children recover promptly and effectively. However, severe stressors such as injury, the death or imminent death of a close family member or friend, or exposure to violence can have lasting effects on some children. These traumatic experiences may occur directly to the child or be witnessed happening to someone else. When children exhibit persistent symptoms lasting longer than one month following such stressors, causing distress or impairing their relationships and activities, they may receive a diagnosis of posttraumatic stress disorder (PTSD).

Examples of PTSD symptoms include the following:

- reliving the event over and over in thought or play
- nightmares and sleep problems

[5] "Obsessive-Compulsive Disorder in Children," Centers for Disease Control and Prevention (CDC), July 26, 2023. Available online. URL: www.cdc.gov/childrensmentalhealth/ocd.html. Accessed March 14, 2024.

- becoming very upset when something causes memories of the event
- lack of positive emotions
- intense ongoing fear or sadness
- irritability and angry outbursts
- constantly looking for possible threats, being easily startled
- acting helpless, hopeless, or withdrawn
- denying that the event happened or feeling numb
- avoiding places or people associated with the event

Children who have undergone traumatic stress may exhibit restlessness, fidgetiness, difficulty paying attention, and challenges in organization. These symptoms can sometimes be mistaken for those of attention deficit hyperactivity disorder (ADHD).

Examples of events that could cause PTSD include the following:

- physical, sexual, or emotional maltreatment
- being a victim or witness to violence or crime
- serious illness or death of a close family member or friend
- natural or man-made disasters
- severe car accidents

TREATMENT FOR POSTTRAUMATIC STRESS DISORDER

The initial step in treatment is to consult with a health-care provider to schedule an evaluation. For a PTSD diagnosis, symptoms must be linked to a specific triggering event. Because discussing the distressing event may be difficult for children, a health-care provider skilled in communicating with children and families is essential. Once diagnosed, the first priority is to create a sense of safety for the child through support from parents, friends, and school, and by minimizing exposure to potential traumatic events as much as possible.

Psychotherapy is a key treatment approach, involving methods such as talking, drawing, playing, or writing about the stressful event. This therapy can be conducted individually with the child, with the family, or in a group setting. Behavior therapy, particularly cognitive behavioral therapy (CBT), helps children modify their thoughts and emotions by initially changing their behaviors, thereby reducing fear and anxiety. In some cases, medication may also be prescribed to alleviate symptoms.

Get Help Finding Treatment

Here are tools to find a health-care provider familiar with treatment options:

- Psychologist Locator (http://locator.apa.org), a service of the American Psychological Association (APA) Practice Organization.
- Child and Adolescent Psychiatrist Finder (www.aacap.org/AACAP/Families_and_Youth/Resources/CAP_Finder.aspx), a research tool by the American Academy of Child and Adolescent Psychiatry (AACAP).
- Find a Cognitive Behavioral Therapist (www.findcbt.org/FAT), a search tool by the Association for Behavioral and Cognitive Therapies (ABCT).
- If you need help finding treatment facilities, visit FindTreatment.gov.

PREVENTION OF POSTTRAUMATIC STRESS DISORDER

The reasons why some children develop PTSD after experiencing stressful and traumatic events while others do not remain uncertain. Various factors, including biology and temperament, likely contribute. However, preventing risks such as maltreatment, violence, or injuries, and reducing the effect of unavoidable disasters on children, can help protect against PTSD.[6]

[6] "Posttraumatic Stress Disorder in Children," Centers for Disease Control and Prevention (CDC), July 26, 2023. Available online. URL: www.cdc.gov/childrensmentalhealth/ptsd.html. Accessed March 14, 2024.

Chapter 29 | Childhood Cancer

A cancer diagnosis is distressing at any age, particularly when the patient is a child. It is normal to have numerous questions, such as who will treat my child, will my child recover, and what does this mean for our family?

TYPES OF CANCER IN CHILDREN

In the United States in 2023, approximately 9,910 new cases of cancer are expected to be diagnosed among children from birth to 14 years, with about 1,040 children anticipated to succumb to the disease. Despite a 70 percent decline in cancer death rates for this age group from 1970 through 2020, cancer continues to be the primary cause of death from disease among children. The most frequently diagnosed types of cancer in children aged 0–14 years include leukemias, brain and other central nervous system (CNS) tumors, and lymphomas.

CAUSES OF CHILDHOOD CANCER

The causes of most childhood cancers remain unknown. Approximately 8–10 percent of childhood cancers are attributed to inherited mutations, genetic alterations that can be passed from parents to their children. Like cancers in adults, most childhood cancers are believed to arise from mutations in genes that disrupt normal cell growth regulation, leading to unchecked cell proliferation and cancer development. In adults, these mutations often result from aging and prolonged exposure to carcinogenic substances. However, pinpointing environmental factors contributing to childhood cancer has proven challenging due to its rarity and the difficulty in identifying early developmental exposures in children.

WHERE ARE CHILDREN WITH CANCER TREATED?

Children diagnosed with cancer are often treated at specialized children's cancer centers, which are hospitals or units within hospitals dedicated to providing comprehensive care for pediatric cancer patients. These centers feature a multidisciplinary team of healthcare professionals with specialized training in pediatric oncology/hematology, pediatric surgery, radiation oncology, rehabilitation, nursing, social work, and psychology. Clinical trials for various types of childhood cancers are frequently available at these centers, offering many patients the opportunity to participate in innovative research studies.

Most hospitals with expertise in pediatric oncology are affiliated with the Children's Oncology Group (COG), supported by the National Cancer Institute (NCI). COG is the world's largest organization conducting clinical research to enhance care and treatment for children with cancer. Families can locate COG-affiliated hospitals through the NCI's Cancer Information Service.

The National Institutes of Health (NIH) Clinical Center in Bethesda, Maryland, specifically houses the NCI's Pediatric Oncology Branch, where health professionals and scientists engage in translational research spanning basic science to clinical trials. Their efforts aim to improve outcomes for children, adolescents, and young adults with cancer and genetic tumor predisposition syndromes.

COPING WITH CANCER

Adjusting to a child's cancer diagnosis and maintaining resilience is a daunting challenge for every family member. The Support for Families When a Child Has Cancer resource (www.cancer.gov/

about-cancer/coping/caregiver-support/parents) provides guidance on discussing cancer with children, preparing them for potential changes, and supporting siblings. It also offers strategies for parents seeking support and tips for effective collaboration with the health-care team.

SURVIVORSHIP

It is crucial for childhood cancer survivors to receive follow-up care to monitor their health after completing treatment. All survivors should have a treatment summary and a survivorship care plan, as discussed in the Care for Childhood Cancer Survivors resource (www.cancer.gov/about-cancer/coping/survivorship/child-care). This resource also includes information on clinics specializing in follow-up care for individuals who have undergone childhood cancer treatment.

Survivors of any cancer may experience health issues months or years after treatment, known as "late effects." However, these effects are especially concerning for childhood cancer survivors due to potential long-term physical and emotional effects from treatment during childhood. The types of late effects vary depending on factors such as cancer type, age at treatment, specific treatments received, and other considerations. Information on managing these late effects can be found on the Care for Childhood Cancer Survivors page (www.cancer.gov/about-cancer/coping/survivorship/child-care).

Survivorship care and the adjustments that both parents and children may undergo are also addressed in the publication *Children with Cancer: A Guide for Parents* (www.cancer.gov/publications/patient-education/guide-for-parents).

RESEARCH

The NCI supports a wide array of research aimed at comprehending the causes, biology, and patterns of childhood cancers, as well as identifying optimal treatment strategies for children with cancer.

Within the realm of clinical trials, researchers are actively treating young cancer patients while learning from their experiences. Additionally, researchers are monitoring childhood cancer survivors to understand the health and other challenges they may encounter due to their cancer treatment.[1]

[1] "Childhood Cancers," National Cancer Institute (NCI), September 29, 2023. Available online. URL: www.cancer.gov/types/childhood-cancers. Accessed March 14, 2024.

Part 5 | **Healthy Infants and Toddlers (Ages 0–3)**

Chapter 30 | **Nutrition and Feeding**

Chapter Contents

PEOPLE AT RISK: CHILDREN UNDER FIVE

Children younger than five years are at an increased risk for foodborne illness and related health complications because their immune systems are still developing. Young children with developing immune systems cannot fight off infections as well as adults. In addition, young children produce less stomach acid that kills harmful bacteria, making it easier for them to get sick.

Foodborne illness (also called "food poisoning") can be particularly dangerous for young children because it often causes vomiting or diarrhea, or both. Since children's bodies are small, they can quickly lose a lot of body fluid and become dehydrated.

Food safety for young children depends on the food safety behaviors of their parents and caregivers. Handwashing is especially important. Children and those caring for them should wash hands often, especially before, during, and after preparing food and before eating.

In children under five years old, *Escherichia coli* (*E. coli*) infections are more likely to lead to hemolytic uremic syndrome (HUS), a severe complication that can cause chronic kidney disease (CKD), kidney failure, and death.

CHOOSE AND PREPARE SAFE FOOD

Learn about safer food choices for people with a higher risk for foodborne illness, including young children. If you prepare food for children under the age of five, you should always follow these four steps:

- **Clean**. Wash hands, utensils, and surfaces often. Germs can spread and survive in many places.
- **Separate**. Raw meat, poultry, seafood, and eggs can spread illness-causing bacteria to ready-to-eat foods, so keep them separate.
- **Cook**. Food is safely cooked only when the internal temperature is high enough to kill germs that can make you sick. See the safe minimum cooking temperatures

chart for how to safely prepare meat, seafood, chicken, and other foods.

- **Chill.** Refrigerate perishable food promptly. Bacteria that cause food poisoning multiply quickest between 40 °F (4 °C) and 140 °F (60 °C).

Follow these precautions when microwaving baby food:

- **Do not microwave baby foods in the jar.** Instead, transfer the food to a dish before microwaving it. This way, the food can be stirred and taste-tested for temperature.
- **Microwave four ounces of solid food in a dish for about 15 seconds on high power.** Always stir, let stand for 30 seconds, and taste-test before feeding. Food that is "baby-ready" should taste or feel lukewarm.
- **Do not heat baby-food meats, meat sticks, or eggs in the microwave.** Use the stovetop instead. These foods have a high-fat content, and since microwaves heat fats faster than other substances, these foods can cause splattering and overheating.

SAFE PREPARATION AND STORAGE OF INFANT FORMULA

How to Prepare Formula

- **Read instructions.** Carefully read and follow the instructions on the infant formula container.
- **Wash hands.** Wash your hands well before preparing bottles or feeding your baby.
- **Sanitize workspace.** Clean and sanitize the workspace where you will prepare the infant formula.
- **Clean bottles.** Use clean, sanitized bottles. Learn how to clean, sanitize, and store infant feeding items.
- **Use safe water.** If you use powdered infant formula, mix it with water from a safe source. If you are not sure if your tap water is safe for preparing infant formula, contact your local health department.

- **Measure water first**. Use the amount of water listed in the instructions for the infant formula container. Always measure the water first and then add the powder.
- **Extra precautions**. If your baby is younger than three months old, was born prematurely, or has a weakened immune system, you may want to take extra precautions in preparing your infant's formula to protect against *Cronobacter* infection, a rare but serious infection that can be caused by germs in powdered infant formula.
- **Timing**. Use prepared infant formula within two hours of preparation and within one hour from when feeding begins. If you do not start to use it within two hours, immediately store the bottle in the fridge and use it within 24 hours.
- **Discard leftovers**. Throw away the formula left in the bottle after feeding your baby.

Heating Breast Milk or Formula

Baby's milk or infant formula does not need to be warmed before feeding, but some people like to warm their baby's bottle. If you decide to warm the bottle, here is advice on how to warm it safely:

- **In hot tap water**. Place the bottle under hot, running tap water until the bottle reaches the desired temperature. This should take one to two minutes.
- **On the stove**. Heat water in a pan. Remove the pan from the heat and set the bottle in the hot water until the bottle is warm. When heating milk for the baby, always shake the liquid to even out the temperature and test it on the top of your hand—not the wrist (this is one of the areas least sensitive to heat)—before feeding. Milk that is baby-ready should feel lukewarm.

- **Avoid microwaves.** Never heat breast milk or infant formula in the microwave. Microwaves heat baby's milk and formula unevenly, which results in hot spots that can burn a baby's mouth and throat[1]

Section 30.2 | **Vitamins and Minerals**

Micronutrients are essential nutrients required in small amounts to maintain normal metabolism, growth, and physical health. For infants younger than six months of age, human milk or infant formula will supply the necessary micronutrients. After six months of age, complementary foods added to the diet will help supply the nutrient needs of growing infants. There are two types of micronutrients:

- vitamins
- minerals

VITAMINS

Vitamins are essential organic compounds. These noncaloric nutrients are needed in tiny amounts in the diet. They are vital to life and indispensable for bodily functions. Many vitamins act as facilitators, making it possible for the body to metabolize other nutrients.

Vitamin A

Vitamin A is essential for the following:

- formation and maintenance of healthy skin, hair, and mucous membranes
- proper vision
- bone growth
- healthy immune and reproductive systems

[1] Foodsafety.gov, "People at Risk: Children under Five," U.S. Department of Health and Human Services (HHS), September 21, 2023. Available online. URL: www.foodsafety.gov/people-at-risk/children-under-five. Accessed March 19, 2024.

Vitamin A deficiency can result from insufficient vitamin A intake, infection, or malnutrition. It can lead to varying severity of damage to the eyes, poor bone growth, loss of appetite, increased susceptibility to infections, and skin changes. Vitamin A deficiency is rare in the United States. Although there are no specific guidelines for infants, nursing mothers should increase their consumption of foods rich in vitamin A.

Vitamin D

Vitamin D is essential for the following:

- Skeletal health:
    - properly formed bones
    - utilization of calcium and phosphorus in the body
- Extraskeletal health:
    - enhancement of nearly all the cells in the immune system
    - improvement of muscle function and strength
    - promotion of heart health

An infant who does not receive sufficient vitamin D through diet, sun exposure, or supplementation can develop vitamin D deficiency. When this happens, the infant's intestines cannot absorb adequate amounts of calcium and phosphorus. As a result, mineralization of the infant's bones and teeth is impaired.

Rickets is an example of a vitamin D deficiency disease. Sometimes rickets has no symptoms, but often, it manifests as varying degrees of bone pain, swollen joints, poor growth, and bowing of the legs or knocked knees.

Vitamin E

Vitamin E, which is also identified as alpha-tocopherol, is an antioxidant and performs the following roles:

- It protects vitamin A and essential fatty acids from oxidation.
- It prevents the breakdown of tissues.

Vitamin E deficiency is rare because the vitamin is available in many foods. The transfer of vitamin E takes place from mother to infant in the last weeks of pregnancy. Premature babies who are born before that transfer takes place may be at risk for rupture of red blood cells (RBCs), leading to anemia.

Vitamin K

Vitamin K is vital for the following:

- proper blood clotting
- aiding in bone mineralization for bone formation

Babies are born with a very small amount of vitamin K stored in their bodies. Immediately, they must be given a vitamin K supplement to help their blood clot normally and avoid the risk of serious bleeding or hemorrhage. Infants who do not receive the vitamin K shot at birth can develop vitamin K deficiency bleeding (VKDB) at any time up to six months of age. An infant with VKDB may bleed into their intestines or brain, which can lead to brain damage and even death.

Vitamin B_1 (Thiamin)

Infants need vitamin B_1 for the following functions:

- to help the body release energy from carbohydrates during metabolism
- to support a healthy nervous system

Vitamin B_1 (thiamin) deficiency is rare but can occur in breastfed infants of thiamin-deficient mothers or when an infant's intestines do not absorb enough of the vitamin. This deficiency can cause a disease called "beriberi."

Vitamin B_2 (Riboflavin)

Vitamin B_2 (riboflavin) helps the body release energy from protein, fat, and carbohydrates during metabolism. Riboflavin deficiency has not been reported among infants in the United States, although breastfed infants whose mothers are on a vegan or macrobiotic diet that excludes dairy products, red meat, and poultry may be at risk. Riboflavin deficiency can inhibit growth. Symptoms of deficiency include skin changes and dermatitis, anemia, and lesions in the mouth.

Vitamin B_3 (Niacin)

Vitamin B_3 (niacin) helps the body release energy from protein, fat, and carbohydrates during metabolism. Niacin deficiency causes the disease pellagra. Symptoms include diarrhea, dermatitis, dementia, and ultimately death. The disease still occurs among poorly nourished people.

Vitamin B_6 (Pyridoxine)

Vitamin B_6 supports body systems in the following ways:

- It helps the body use protein to build tissues.
- It plays roles in immune function.
- It maintains normal nerve function.
- It synthesizes hemoglobin.
- It contributes to the regulation of blood glucose.

Vitamin B_6 deficiency can cause a form of anemia and weaken the immune response. Other symptoms include irritability, insomnia, depression, and greasy dermatitis.

Vitamin B_9 (Folate)

Vitamin B_9 is required for the following body functions:

- cell division
- growth and development of healthy blood cells
- formation of genetic material within every cell

Deficiencies of folate cause anemia, diminished immunity, and abnormal digestive function. Researchers have found that proper maternal folate intake protects infants from neural tube defects (NTDs), including spina bifida.

Vitamin B_{12} (Cobalamin)

Vitamin B_{12} is necessary to maintain:

- healthy blood cells
- proper functioning of the nervous system

The amount of vitamin B_{12} in an infant's body at birth is directly related to the mother's stores of vitamin B_{12} and to how many previous times she has been pregnant. After birth, the vitamin B_{12} intake of an infant who is exclusively breastfed depends on the mother's intake and stores of the vitamin. As long as the mother's diet has adequate amounts, the infant will receive adequate amounts through her milk. However, infants of breastfeeding mothers who follow strict vegetarian or vegan diets or eat very few dairy products, meat, or eggs are at risk for developing vitamin B_{12} deficiency by four to six months of age. Signs of deficiency include failure to thrive, movement disorders, delayed development, and megaloblastic anemia.

Vitamin C (Ascorbic Acid)

The major functions of vitamin C (ascorbic acid) include the following:

- forming collagen, a protein that gives structure to bones, cartilage, muscle, blood vessels, and other connective tissue
- maintaining capillaries, bones, and teeth
- healing wounds
- helping the body resist infections
- enhancing the absorption of iron

Vitamin C (ascorbic acid) deficiency can eventually lead to scurvy, a serious disease with the following symptoms in infants: poor bone growth, bleeding, and anemia.

MINERALS

Minerals come from inorganic, or nonliving, sources, such as soil and water. For an infant to grow and develop normally, an adequate supply of both major minerals and trace minerals is necessary.

Major minerals are not more important than trace minerals; both are essential. The distinction lies in their quantities in the body and dietary requirements. Major minerals are present in larger quantities in the body and, therefore, needed in greater amounts in the diet. Major minerals include calcium and phosphorus, while trace minerals include iron and zinc.

Calcium

Calcium plays an important role in the following body processes:

- bone and tooth development clotting
- intracellular signaling and hormonal secretion
- critical muscle and nerve function

Calcium deficiency is related to increased blood lead levels and perhaps increased vulnerability to the adverse effects of lead in the body. Infants at risk for lead poisoning should receive adequate calcium in their diet.

Iron

The following are the major functions of iron:

- proper formation and growth of healthy blood cells
- transportation of oxygen throughout the body
- prevention of iron deficiency anemia

To ensure that breastfeeding infants will not be affected by iron deficiency, the American Academy of Pediatrics (AAP) recommends the following:

- **For exclusively breastfed infants**. Iron in human milk is highly bioavailable, but it contains little iron. Therefore, infants who are exclusively breastfed may be at increased risk of iron deficiency after four months of age. Parents and caregivers should be encouraged to talk with their health-care providers about iron supplementation of 1 mg/kg per day of oral iron beginning at four months of age until appropriate iron-containing complementary foods are introduced into the diet.

- **For partially breastfed infants.** If more than half of the infant's daily feedings are from human milk and they are not receiving iron-containing complementary foods, the recommendation remains the same as for fully breastfed infants.
- **For infant formula-fed infants.** Iron-fortified formula should be used from birth through the entire first year of life.

The symptoms of iron deficiency anemia include irritability, pallor, lethargy, and poor food intake. Iron deficiency in infants and older children may be associated with irreversible behavioral abnormalities and abnormal functioning of the brain. Elevated blood lead levels may interfere with the utilization of iron, causing hypochromic normocytic anemia (lower than normal of paler RBCs).

Zinc

Zinc, an essential mineral, is needed in small quantities in the human body. It affects behavior and learning, assists in immune function, and is essential for wound healing, taste perception, and growth and development in infants. It works with proteins in every organ, helping more than 300 enzymes to perform the following functions:

- to make parts of the cell's genetic material
- to make heme in hemoglobin
- to help the pancreas with its digestive functions
- to help metabolize carbohydrates, protein, and fat
- to liberate vitamin A from storage in the liver
- to dispose of damaging free radicals

Daily adequate intake of this mineral is important because there is no storage system for zinc in the body.

Sodium

Sodium is a major part of the body's fluid and electrolyte balance system because it is the chief ion used to maintain the volume of fluid outside the cell. Sodium is also required for the following body functions:

- maintaining acid-base balance
- ensuring muscle contraction and nerve transmission

A deficiency of sodium would be harmful, but few diets lack sodium. Most foods include more salt than is needed. The kidneys filter the surplus sodium out of the blood and into the urine. The kidneys can also store sodium and release it into the bloodstream in the event of deficiency.

Fluoride

Fluoride is not considered an essential nutrient, but it is a beneficial mineral. If consumed at appropriate levels, fluoride decreases the susceptibility of the teeth to dental caries (tooth decay). When allowed to come in contact with teeth and to some extent when consumed before teeth erupt, this mineral is incorporated into the mineral portion of the teeth. Once fluoride is an integral part of the tooth structure, teeth are stronger and more resistant to decay.[2]

Section 30.3 | **Mealtime**

Mealtime can be a fun, rewarding, and sometimes messy time for you and your child. The healthy mealtime patterns you establish now will help promote healthy habits in the future.

SIGNS YOUR CHILD IS HUNGRY OR FULL

Even before your child can talk, they will show signs of hunger or fullness using sounds and movements. Crying is often a late sign of hunger. Look for other signs of hunger listed below, so you can put

[2] Food and Nutrition Service (FNS), "Infant Nutrition and Feeding," U.S. Department of Agriculture (USDA), April 15, 2019. Available online. URL: https://wicworks.fns.usda.gov/sites/default/files/media/document/infant-feeding-guide.pdf. Accessed March 19, 2024.

your child to the breast or bottle while they are still calm. As your child gets older, they will develop more specific signs for hunger and fullness. Understanding these signs is important to help you know when and how often to feed your child.

Following are some examples of signs your child may show for hunger and fullness when he or she is a newborn to 5 months old and signs your child may start to show between 6 and 23 months old.

Birth to Five Months Old

- Your child may be hungry if he or she:
  - puts hands to mouth
  - turns head toward breast or bottle
  - puckers, smacks, or licks lips
  - has clenched hands
- Your child may be full if he or she:
  - closes his or her mouth
  - turns his or her head away from the breast or bottle
  - relaxes hands

6–23 Months Old

- Your child may be hungry if he or she:
  - reaches for or points to food
  - opens his or her mouth when offered a spoon or food
  - gets excited when he or she sees food
  - uses hand motions or makes sounds to let you know he or she is still hungry
- Your child may be full if he or she:
  - pushes food away
  - closes his or her mouth when food is offered
  - turns his or her head away from the food
  - uses hand motions or makes sounds to let you know he or she is full

Let your child decide how much they want to eat. They do not need to finish a bottle or all the food in the jar or on the plate. Food is not a good reward or punishment. Talk to your child's doctor or nurse if you are concerned about how much or how little they are eating.

MEALTIME ROUTINES AND TIPS

Mealtime can be a messy and fun learning experience when feeding your 6- to 24-month-old child. Your child may have about three meals and two to three snacks every day. Having a routine can help children know what to expect when it is time for meals or snacks.

Here are some routines and tips for mealtimes:

- Clean:
    - Wash your child's hands before mealtime.

Tip: To help with cleanup, put newspaper or a plastic mat on the floor under your child's high chair or booster seat.

- Be safe:
    - Sit your child in a safe place. A high chair or booster seat are good options.
    - Strap your child into the high chair or booster seat.
    - Watch children at all times to make sure they are safe.

Tip: Learn important food safety steps to keep your child safe from foodborne illness.

- Focus:
    - Face your child toward you or other family members at the table.
    - Limit distractions. Avoid letting television (TV), videos, cell phones, or pets distract your child from eating. These can also distract you too. Focus on your child during mealtimes.
    - Talk with your child during mealtimes, and it is important for your child to have your attention.

Tip: Mealtimes do not have to be long. Mealtimes can last 10 or 15 minutes or for as long as your child can pay attention.

- Family meals:
  - Sitting down as a family for mealtime can teach your child how to eat and help your child develop social skills.
  - Give your child healthy food options at each meal.

Tip: If you want your child to try new foods, model healthy eating. It can help your child learn what to do.

- Amount:
  - Let your child decide how much to eat. Your child does not have to finish all the food on the plate or drink all the liquid in the cup or bottle.

Tip: Watch your children for signs that they are hungry or full.

FINGERS, SPOONS, FORKS, AND CUPS

Your child is learning a lot about food and how to eat and drink. At first, you may need to help your child eat. After children are about 12 months old, they will quickly get better at using spoons, forks, and cups.

Fingers

Your child will start to use fingers to pick up food. This helps your baby develop fine motor skills. Offer your baby finger foods that are small enough to pick up and soft enough to chew. Here are some examples:

- small cooked noodles
- small pieces of bread
- small pieces of soft, ripe peeled fruit or soft cooked vegetables
- small slices of mild cheese or crackers

By the time children are 12 months old, they should be able to easily feed themselves with their fingers.

Spoons and Forks

At first, babies learn how to swallow solid foods such as pureed or mashed foods you feed them from a spoon.

- Most babies can swallow a spoonful of pureed foods without choking when they are around six months old.
- Babies can start to use a spoon by themselves at around 10–12 months old.
- Your child will continue to get better at using tools such as spoons and forks. Give your child a chance to use spoons and forks even if it is messy.

Cups

Children can start learning how to use a cup without a lid when they are nine months old.

- When children are about 12 months old, they can hold a cup with two hands.
- Give your child a chance to use a cup—be ready for some spills.
- Talk with your child's doctor or nurse if you have any questions about things your baby can do at this age.[3]

Section 30.4 | **Breastfeeding Guidelines and Recommendations**

WHAT ARE THE BENEFITS OF BREASTFEEDING?

Breastfeeding is beneficial for both infants and mothers. Breast milk is the best source of nutrition for most infants. As an infant grows, breast milk changes to meet their nutritional needs. Breastfeeding can also help protect both the infant and mother against certain illnesses and diseases.

---

[3] "Mealtime," Centers for Disease Control and Prevention (CDC), April 11, 2022. Available online. URL: www.cdc.gov/nutrition/infantandtoddlernutrition/mealtime/index.html. Accessed March 19, 2024.

Benefits to Infants

Infants who are breastfed have a lower risk of:

- asthma
- obesity
- type 1 diabetes
- severe lower respiratory disease
- acute otitis media (AOM; ear infections)
- sudden infant death syndrome (SIDS)
- gastrointestinal infections (diarrhea/vomiting)
- necrotizing enterocolitis (NEC) for preterm infants

Benefit to Mothers

Mothers who breastfeed their infants have a lower risk of:

- breast cancer
- ovarian cancer
- type 2 diabetes
- high blood pressure (HBP)[4]

WHAT ARE THE RECOMMENDATIONS FOR BREASTFEEDING?

In the United States, the American Academy of Pediatrics (AAP) recommends the following:

- **First six months after birth**. Infants should be fed breast milk exclusively for the first six months after birth. Exclusive breastfeeding means the infant does not receive any additional foods (except vitamin D) or fluids unless medically recommended.
- **After the first six months and until the infant is one year old**. The mother continues breastfeeding while gradually introducing solid foods into the infant's diet.
- **After one year**. Breastfeeding can be continued if mutually desired by the mother and her infant.

[4] "Frequently Asked Questions (FAQs)," Centers for Disease Control and Prevention (CDC), August 4, 2022. Available online. URL: www.cdc.gov/breastfeeding/faq/index.htm#benefits. Accessed March 19, 2024.

The World Health Organization (WHO) promotes, as a global public health recommendation, the following:

- **First six months after birth.** Infants should be exclusively breastfed for the first six months after birth to achieve optimal growth, development, and health.
- **After the first six months.** To meet their evolving nutritional requirements, infants should receive nutritionally adequate and safe complementary foods while breastfeeding continues for up to two years of age or beyond.

Recommendations to Support Breastfeeding

According to the Centers for Disease Control and Prevention (CDC), the majority of new mothers start out breastfeeding, but only a minority still exclusively breastfeed by the time their infants are six months old. Many factors influence successful breastfeeding, including support from health-care providers, family and community, and the workplace. The *2011 Surgeon General's Call to Action to Support Breastfeeding* (www.hhs.gov/surgeongeneral/reports-and-publications/breastfeeding/index.html) makes 20 recommendations to support new mothers in their decision to breastfeed.[5]

WHAT ARE HUMAN MILK BANKS?

Human milk banks are a service established to collect milk from donors and process, screen, store, and distribute donated milk to meet the specific needs of individuals for whom human milk is prescribed by licensed health-care providers. When possible, human milk banks also serve healthy infants who have been adopted or are not able to receive their mother's milk. Milk banks accept donations directly at their deposit sites or arrange for safe, overnight transportation of human milk at no cost to the donor.

---

[5] "What Are the Recommendations for Breastfeeding?" *Eunice Kennedy Shriver* National Institute of Child Health and Human Development (NICHD), January 31, 2017. Available online. URL: www.nichd.nih.gov/health/topics/breastfeeding/conditioninfo/recommendations. Accessed March 19, 2024.

IS IT SAFE FOR FAMILIES TO BUY BREAST MILK ON THE INTERNET?

The AAP and the U.S. Food and Drug Administration (FDA) recommend avoiding internet-based milk-sharing sites and instead suggest contacting milk banks. Research has shown that some milk samples sold online have been contaminated with a range of bacteria. Nonprofit donor human milk banks, where processed human milk comes from screened donors, have a long safety record in North America. All member banks of the Human Milk Banking Association of North America (HMBANA) must operate under specific evidence-based guidelines that require extensive testing and processing procedures, as well as self-reported health information and a health statement from both the donor's health-care provider and the infant's health-care provider. Because most of the milk from milk banks is given to hospitalized and fragile infants, milk banks may not have enough to serve healthy infants at all times.

HOW CAN A MOTHER CONTINUE TO PROVIDE BREAST MILK TO HER INFANT AFTER RETURNING TO WORK OR SCHOOL?

Being prepared to return to work or school can help a mother ease the transition and continue to breastfeed after her maternity leave is over. The Office on Women's Health (OWH) provides information for making this transition easier (www.womenshealth.gov/breastfeeding/breastfeeding-home-work-and-public/breastfeeding-and-going-back-work). When a mother is away from her infant, she can pump or hand express her breast milk so that her infant can drink breast milk from a bottle. The PUMP Act, an extension of the FLSA, requires employers to support breastfeeding mothers by providing reasonable break time and a clean, private space that is not a bathroom to express their breast milk for one year after each child's birth.

ARE THERE RISKS TO BREASTFEEDING IN POOLS OR SPLASH PADS?

No scientific study has examined the health and safety of breastfeeding babies while in the water. It is unlikely that breastfeeding in the water presents any more risks for babies and young children (zero to four years old) than the risks associated with regular pool or splash pad use for this age group. These risks include swallowing water, exposure to swimming-related illnesses, issues regulating body temperature, and drowning. The CDC is not aware of any risks to other swimmers related to breastfeeding in pool or splash pad water.[6]

Section 30.5 | Weaning or Complementary Feeding

At some point, either you or your child will be ready to stop breastfeeding. Weaning from breastfeeding is the process of transitioning a baby's diet from breast milk to other foods and drinks.

WHEN TO WEAN

When to wean is a personal decision and will be different for everyone. Each child may be ready to wean, or stop breastfeeding, at different ages. Some children will gradually show more interest in eating solid foods and less interest in breastfeeding, while others may want to stop breastfeeding more suddenly. Mothers may also be ready to wean at different times. This is a personal decision. If you and your child have decided it is time to wean and your child is younger than 12 months old:

- give your child infant formula in place of breast milk

If you and your child have decided it is time to wean and your child is 12 months or older:

- give your child fortified cow's milk in place of breast milk (He or she does not need infant or toddler formula.)

[6] See footnote [4].

HOW TO WEAN

To make the process easier for you and your child, wean over several weeks or more. As you gradually stop breastfeeding, your body will start producing less breast milk, and eventually, your body will no longer make breast milk. Weaning gradually can help your child:

- get used to the taste of infant formula (for your child younger than 12 months old) or fortified cow's milk (for your child 12 months or older)
- adjust to drinking from a bottle or cup

Start weaning by replacing one breast milk feeding a day with a bottle of infant formula (for your child younger than 12 months) or with a cup of fortified cow's milk (for your child 12 months or older). Continue to replace more breast milk feedings with infant formula or fortified cow's milk over time.[7]

WHEN, WHAT, AND HOW TO INTRODUCE SOLID FOODS

The *U.S. Dietary Guidelines for Americans* and the American Academy of Pediatrics (AAP) recommend introducing foods other than breast milk or infant formula when children are about six months old. Introducing foods before four months old is not recommended. Every child is different, so how do you know if your child is ready for foods other than breast milk or infant formula? Look for the following signs that your child is developmentally ready. Your child:

- sits up alone or with support
- is able to control the head and neck
- opens the mouth when food is offered
- swallows food rather than pushes it back out onto the chin
- brings objects to the mouth
- tries to grasp small objects, such as toys or food
- transfers food from the front to the back of the tongue to swallow

[7] "Weaning," Centers for Disease Control and Prevention (CDC), July 9, 2021. Available online. URL: www.cdc.gov/nutrition/InfantandToddlerNutrition/breastfeeding/weaning.html. Accessed March 19, 2024.

What Foods Should be Introduced to the Child First?

The AAP states that for most children, you do not need to give foods in a specific order. Your child can begin eating solid foods at about six months old. By the time they are seven or eight months old, your child can eat a variety of foods from different food groups. These foods include infant cereals, meat or other proteins, fruits, vegetables, grains, yogurts and cheeses, and more.

If your child is eating infant cereals, it is important to offer a variety of fortified infant cereals such as oats, barley, and multigrain instead of only rice cereal. Providing only infant rice cereal can increase the risk of exposure to arsenic.

How Should a Parent Introduce Their Child to Foods?

Let your child try one single-ingredient food at a time initially. This helps you see if your child has any problems with that food, such as allergies. Wait three to five days between each new food. Before you know it, your child will be on their way to eating and enjoying many new foods. Introduce potentially allergenic foods when other foods are introduced.

Potentially allergenic foods include cow's milk products, eggs, fish, shellfish, tree nuts, peanuts, wheat, soy, and sesame. Drinking cow's milk or fortified soy beverages is not recommended until your child is older than 12 months, but other cow's milk products, such as yogurt, can be introduced before 12 months. If your child has severe eczema or an egg allergy, talk with your child's doctor or nurse about when and how to safely introduce foods with peanuts.

HOW MUCH AND HOW OFTEN TO FEED

From 6 to 12 months old, breast milk and/or infant formula remains the main source of nutrition for your child, but solid foods will gradually begin to make up a bigger part of their diet. As you start to introduce food, it can be hard to know how much to give your child to eat. Children's bellies are small and cannot hold a lot of food. Here are things to keep in mind:

- **Start small.** Give one or two tablespoons of food and watch for signs that he or she is still hungry or full.

- **Balance**. Solid foods are introduced over time and will gradually become a bigger part of his or her diet.
- **Feeding**. Give your child something to eat or drink about every two to three hours or about five or six times a day. This will give your child about three meals and two to three snacks every day.

As your child gets older, they may eat different amounts of food each day. This is normal. Beginning around 12 months old, your child grows more slowly than when they were younger. Your child may even go a couple of days without eating much at all. Over the course of a week, your child should get all the foods and nutrients they need.

FOODS AND DRINKS TO ENCOURAGE

Healthy eating patterns your child starts now will help promote healthy habits in the future. It is important to provide foods that match your child's eating skills. Initially, foods may need to be soft, mashed, or bite-sized.

Encourage Your Child to Eat

Offer your child a variety of fruits, vegetables, whole grains, meats, and yogurt or cheeses. Create a rainbow of different-colored foods on your child's plate. Here are a few examples:

- **Fruits**. Bananas, strawberries, pears, oranges, melons, or avocados.
- **Vegetables**. Cooked spinach, carrots, beans, peas, lentils, yams, or beets.
- **Whole grains**. Whole grain breads, crackers, or pastas.
- **Proteins**. Soft, small pieces of beef, lamb, chicken, fish, turkey, eggs, or tofu.
- **Dairy**. Pasteurized cheeses or yogurts, including soy-based yogurt.

Once your child is 12 months old, they may be eating more of the foods that you eat. Eating a healthy diet sets a good example for your toddler. Continue to offer a variety of healthy options and allow your child to choose what to eat.

Encourage Your Child to Drink

When your child is between 6 and 12 months old, you can offer your child:

- water (4–8 ounces per day)
- breast milk (if you are still breast-feeding) or infant formula

Once your child is 12 months old, you can begin offering plain whole cow's milk or fortified unsweetened soy beverages.

COW'S MILK AND MILK ALTERNATIVES

Your growing child needs vitamins and minerals such as vitamin D and calcium to build strong bones. Pasteurized whole cow's milk and soy beverages fortified with vitamin D are good sources of vitamin D and calcium. Most cow's milk sold in the United States is fortified with vitamin D.

Choose milk or milk alternatives that are unflavored and unsweetened. Flavored cow's milk and fortified soy beverages can have added sugars, which your child does not need.

When Should a Parent Introduce Their Child to Cow's Milk?

At 12 months old (but not before), your child can be introduced to cow's milk. Before your child is 12 months old, cow's milk may put them at risk for intestinal bleeding. It also contains too many proteins and minerals for your baby's kidneys to handle and does not have the right amount of nutrients your baby needs.

How Much and How Often?

Cow's milk or fortified soy beverages can be part of a child's balanced and diverse diet but not the only component. The *U.S. Dietary Guidelines for Americans* recommend that children aged 12–23 months get 1⅔ to 2 cup equivalents of dairy a day, including cow's milk, yogurt, cheese, fortified soy beverages, and soy-based yogurt. If your child drinks too much cow's milk, they may not be hungry for other foods with important nutrients. Some experts say that consuming too much cow's milk can make it harder for your child's body to absorb the iron they need from foods.

Continue to follow your child's cues to determine when they are hungry or full. Talk with your child's doctor or nurse if you have questions about adding cow's milk or fortified soy beverages to their diet.

Whole Cow's Milk or Lower Fat Cow's Milk

Children can drink unflavored, unsweetened whole cow's milk. Whole cow's milk is the same as lower-fat cow's milk except that it is higher in fat. It is important for young children to get fat in their diet for healthy growth and development. If your child has excessive weight gain or a family history of obesity, high cholesterol or triglycerides, or cardiovascular disease, talk to your child's doctor or nurse about the type of cow's milk to give.

Raw Milk

Raw milk and raw milk products from cows, goats, and sheep can carry harmful bacteria and other germs that can make your child very sick and can be life-threatening. Raw milk can also be called "unpasteurized milk." Do not give your child raw or unpasteurized milk.

Milk Alternatives

Milk alternatives can include beverages made from plants, such as soy, oat, rice, coconut, cashew, and almond.[8]

[8] "Foods and Drinks for 6–24 Month Olds," Centers for Disease Control and Prevention (CDC), December 1, 2021. Available online. URL: www.cdc.gov/nutrition/infantandtoddlernutrition/foods-and-drinks/index.html. Accessed March 19, 2024.

Chapter 31 | Vaccination and Immunization for Infants and Toddlers

Chapter Contents

Different vaccines work in various ways, but each helps the body's immune system learn how to fight germs. It typically takes a few weeks for protection to develop after vaccination, but that protection can last a lifetime. Some vaccines, such as those for tetanus or seasonal flu, require occasional booster doses to maintain the body's defenses.

STRENGTHENING YOUR BABY'S IMMUNE SYSTEM

Immunity is the body's way of preventing disease. Because a baby's immune system is not fully developed at birth, babies face a greater risk of becoming infected and getting seriously ill. Vaccines help teach the immune system how to defend against germs. Vaccination protects your baby by helping build up their natural defenses.

Children are exposed to thousands of germs every day through the food they eat, the air they breathe, and the things they put in their mouths. Babies are born with immune systems that can fight most germs, but some germs cause serious or even deadly diseases that a baby cannot handle. For those, babies need the help of vaccines. Vaccines use very small amounts of antigens to help your child's immune system recognize and learn to fight serious diseases. Antigens are the parts of a germ that cause the body's immune system to go to work.

VACCINE INGREDIENTS

Nowadays, vaccines use only the ingredients they need to be as safe and effective as possible. A vaccine could include any of these kinds of ingredients:

- **Adjuvants**. Adjuvants, such as aluminum salts, help boost the body's response to a vaccination (they are also found in antacids, antiperspirants, etc.).
- **Stabilizers**. Stabilizers, such as sugars or gelatin, help keep a vaccine effective after it is manufactured (they are naturally present in the body and found in foods such as Jell-O®).

- **Formaldehyde.** It helps prevent bacterial contamination during manufacturing. Formaldehyde is naturally present in the body at levels higher than vaccines (it is also found in the environment, preservatives, and household products).
- **Thimerosal.** It is a preservative used in the vaccine manufacturing process. It is no longer used to make any vaccine except multidose vials of the flu vaccine. Single-dose vials of the flu vaccine are available as an alternative.

VACCINES ARE SAFE

Before a new vaccine is ever given to people, extensive lab testing is done. Once testing in people begins, it can still take years before clinical studies are complete and the vaccine is licensed. After a vaccine is licensed, the U.S. Food and Drug Administration (FDA), the Centers for Disease Control and Prevention (CDC), the National Institutes of Health (NIH), and other federal agencies continue routine monitoring and investigate any potential safety concerns.

MILD SIDE EFFECTS ARE EXPECTED

Vaccines, such as medicine, can have some side effects. However, most people who get vaccinated experience only mild side effects or none at all. The most common side effects include fever, tiredness, body aches, and redness, swelling, and tenderness at the injection site. Mild reactions usually resolve on their own within a few days. Serious, long-lasting side effects are extremely rare. The CDC tracks and investigates reports of serious side effects to ensure they are monitored and understood.

WHY YOUR CHILD SHOULD GET VACCINATED

Vaccines can prevent common diseases that used to seriously harm or even kill infants, children, and adults. Without vaccines, your child is at risk of becoming seriously ill or even dying from childhood diseases such as measles and whooping cough. It is always better to prevent a disease than to treat one after it occurs.

- Vaccination is a safe, highly effective, and easy way to help keep your family healthy.
- The recommended vaccination schedule balances when a child will likely be exposed to a disease and when a vaccine will be most effective.
- Vaccines are tested to ensure they can be given safely and effectively at the recommended ages.[1]

Section 31.2 | **Common Questions about Vaccines**

DO INFANTS HAVE NATURAL IMMUNITY?

Babies may get some temporary protection from the mother during the last few weeks of pregnancy, but only for diseases to which the mother is immune. Breastfeeding may also protect your baby temporarily from minor infections, such as colds. These antibodies do not last long, leaving your baby vulnerable to disease.

WHAT ARE THE RISKS AND BENEFITS OF VACCINES?

Vaccines can prevent infectious diseases that once killed or harmed many infants, children, and adults. Without vaccines, your child is at risk of getting seriously ill and suffering pain, disability, and even death from diseases such as measles and whooping cough. The main risks associated with getting vaccines are side effects, which are almost always mild (redness and swelling at the injection site) and go away within a few days. Serious side effects after vaccination, such as a severe allergic reaction, are very rare, and doctors and clinic staff are trained to deal with them. The disease prevention

[1] "Making the Vaccine Decision: Addressing Common Concerns," Centers for Disease Control and Prevention (CDC), July 19, 2023. Available online. URL: www.cdc.gov/vaccines/parents/why-vaccinate/vaccine-decision.html. Accessed March 11, 2024.

benefits of getting vaccines are much greater than the possible side effects for almost all children. The only exceptions are cases in which a child has a serious chronic medical condition, such as cancer or a disease that weakens the immune system, or has had a severe allergic reaction to a previous vaccine dose.

WHAT ARE THE COMMON SIDE EFFECTS OF VACCINES?

Vaccines, like any medication, may cause some side effects. Most of these side effects are very minor, such as soreness where the shot was given, fussiness, or a low-grade fever. These side effects typically last only a couple of days and are treatable. For example, you can apply a cool, wet washcloth to the sore area to ease discomfort.

CAN VACCINES OVERLOAD YOUR BABY'S IMMUNE SYSTEM?

Vaccines do not overload the immune system. Every day, a healthy baby's immune system successfully fights off thousands of germs. Antigens are parts of germs that cause the body's immune system to go to work to build antibodies, which fight off diseases.

The antigens in vaccines come from the germs themselves, but the germs are weakened or killed, so they cannot cause serious illness. Even if babies receive several vaccinations in one day, vaccines contain only a tiny fraction of the antigens they encounter every day in their environment. Vaccines give your child the antibodies they need to fight off serious vaccine-preventable diseases.

WHY DO VACCINES START SO EARLY?

The recommended schedule protects infants and children by providing protection early in life before they come into contact with life-threatening diseases. Children receive vaccinations early because they are susceptible to diseases at a young age.

SHOULD YOUR CHILD GET SHOTS IF THEY ARE SICK?

Talk with your child's doctor, but children can usually get vaccinated even if they have a mild illness such as a cold, earache, mild fever, or diarrhea. If the doctor says it is okay, your child can still get vaccinated.

IF YOU ARE BREASTFEEDING, DO YOU VACCINATE YOUR BABY ON SCHEDULE?

Yes, even breastfed babies need to be protected with vaccines at the recommended ages. The immune system is not fully developed at birth, which puts newborns at greater risk for infections. Breast milk provides important protection from some infections as your baby's immune system develops. For example, babies who are breastfed have a lower risk of ear infections, respiratory tract infections, and diarrhea. However, breast milk does not protect children against all diseases. Even in breastfed infants, vaccines are the most effective way to prevent many diseases.

CAN YOU WAIT TO VACCINATE YOUR BABY SINCE THEY ARE NOT IN CHILDCARE?

No, even young children who are cared for at home can be exposed to vaccine-preventable diseases, so it is important for them to get all their vaccines at the recommended ages. Children can catch these illnesses from any number of people or places, including parents, siblings, visitors to their home, playgrounds, or even grocery stores. Regardless of whether your baby is cared for outside the home, your baby comes into contact with people throughout the day, some of whom may have a vaccine-preventable disease. Many of these diseases can be especially dangerous to young children, so it is safest to vaccinate your child at the recommended ages.

CAN YOU WAIT UNTIL YOUR CHILD GOES TO SCHOOL TO CATCH UP ON IMMUNIZATIONS?

No. Before entering school, young children can be exposed to vaccine-preventable diseases. Children under the age of five are especially susceptible to diseases because their immune systems have not built up the necessary defenses to fight infection.

WHY DO ADOLESCENTS NEED VACCINES?

Vaccines are recommended throughout our lives to protect against serious diseases. As protection from childhood vaccines wears off, adolescents need vaccines that will extend protection. Adolescents need protection from additional infections as well, before the risk of exposure increases.

WHY ARE MULTIPLE DOSES NEEDED FOR EACH VACCINE?

Getting every recommended dose of each vaccine provides your child with the best protection possible. Depending on the vaccine, your child will need more than one dose to build high enough immunity to help prevent disease or to boost immunity that fades over time. Your child may also receive more than one dose to make sure they are protected if they did not get immunity from a first dose or to protect them against germs that change over time, such as the flu. Every dose is important because each protects against an infectious disease that can be especially serious for infants and very young children.[2]

Section 31.3 | **Before, during, and after the Shots**

Prepare for your child's doctor vaccine visit and know what to do to support your child during and after your child is vaccinated.

BEFORE THE VISIT

- Read about the vaccines your child is getting.
    - Read vaccine materials you received from your child's health-care professional and write down any questions you may have.

[2] "Common Questions about Vaccines," Centers for Disease Control and Prevention (CDC), August 7, 2023. Available online. URL: www.cdc.gov/vaccines/parents/FAQs.html. Accessed March 12, 2024.

- Get a list of vaccines your child may need; use the quick vaccine assessment tool (www2a.cdc.gov/vaccines/childquiz).
- Learn more about the benefits and risks of the vaccines that your child will receive by reviewing the Vaccine Information Statements (www.cdc.gov/vaccines/hcp/vis/index.html). You can also request Vaccine Information Statements at the doctor's office.
- Find your child's personal immunization record (www.cdc.gov/vaccines/parents/records/keeping-track.html) and bring it to your appointment. An up-to-date record tells your doctor exactly what shots your child has already received.

- Be ready to support your child during the vaccine visit. Pack your child's favorite toy, book, or blanket to comfort them during vaccinations. If your child is older and you can have a chat, do the following:
  - Be honest with your child. Explain that shots can pinch or sting, but that it will not hurt for long.
  - Engage other family members, especially older siblings, to support your child.
  - Avoid telling scary stories or making threats about shots.
  - Remind your child that vaccines can keep him or her healthy.

AT THE DOCTOR'S OFFICE

If you have questions about vaccination, ask your child's doctor or health-care professional. Your child's doctor will give you Vaccine Information Statements (www.cdc.gov/vaccines/hcp/vis/current-vis.html) for the vaccines that your child will be getting that day. Vaccine Information Statements include information about the risks and benefits of each vaccine. If your doctor does not give you one, you can request one.

MAKE SHOTS EASIER ON YOUR CHILD

For babies and younger children, do the following:

- Distract and comfort your child by cuddling, singing, or talking softly.
- Smile and make eye contact with your child. Let your child know that everything is ok.
- Comfort your child with a favorite toy or book. A blanket that smells familiar will also help.
- Hold your child firmly on your lap, whenever possible.

Once your child has received all the shots, be especially supportive. Hold and cuddle your child. A soothing voice, praise, and hugs will help reassure the child that everything is okay. Additionally, babies can be soothed through swaddling, skin-to-skin contact, and breastfeeding. If older than six months, babies can also be given a sweet beverage.

For older children and adolescents, do the following:

- Point out interesting things in the room to help create distractions.
- Tell or read stories.
- Support your child if he or she cries.
- Never scold a child for not "being brave."
- Take deep breaths with your child to help "blow out" the pain.

Fainting (syncope) can be common among adolescents immediately after getting shots. To help prevent injuries from a fall while fainting, your preteen or teen should stay seated for 15 minutes after the shot. Before you leave the appointment, ask your child's doctor for advice on using a non-aspirin pain reliever and other steps you can take at home to comfort your child.

AFTER THE SHOTS

Sometimes children experience mild reactions from shots, such as pain at the injection site, a rash, or a fever. These reactions are normal and will soon go away. These tips will help you identify and minimize mild side effects:

- Read the Vaccine Information Sheet(s) your child's doctor gave you to learn about side effects your child may experience.
- Use a cool, damp cloth to help reduce redness, soreness, and/or swelling in the place where the shot was given.
- Reduce fever with a lukewarm water sponge bath.
- Offer liquids more often. It is normal for some children to eat less during the 24 hours after getting vaccines.
- Ask your child's doctor if you can give your child a nonaspirin pain reliever.
- Pay extra attention to your child for a few days. If you see something that concerns you, call your child's doctor.[3]

Section 31.4 | **Immunization Schedule: Birth to Two Years**

VACCINES SHORTLY AFTER BIRTH

Whether you are becoming a parent for the first time or you have been here before, your baby's birth is an exciting time. This is also the first time your infant will be vaccinated—your first opportunity to protect your child from serious diseases.

Hepatitis B

FIRST DOSE OF THREE

Hepatitis B (HepB) is an infectious and potentially serious disease that can cause liver damage and liver cancer. There is no cure for HepB. Mothers can unknowingly pass the hepatitis B virus (HBV) to their babies at birth, which is why babies should get their first dose within 24 hours of birth.

[3] "Before, During, and After Shots," Centers for Disease Control and Prevention (CDC), August 5, 2019. Available online. URL: www.cdc.gov/vaccines/parents/visit/index.html. Accessed March 12, 2024.

If you have HepB, your baby should get the first shot of the HepB vaccine within 12 hours of birth. An additional medicine called "hepatitis B immune globin" (HBIG) can help protect your newborn against HepB. HBIG provides your baby's body with extra help to fight the virus immediately after birth.

VACCINES AT ONE TO TWO MONTHS

During the first months of your baby's life, routine vaccines can help protect your child from a variety of serious or potentially fatal diseases. At one to two months, your baby should receive vaccines to protect them from the following diseases:

Diphtheria, Tetanus, and Whooping Cough (Pertussis)

FIRST DOSE OF FIVE

The diphtheria, tetanus, and pertussis (DTaP) vaccine provides the best protection from three serious diseases: diphtheria, tetanus, and whooping cough (pertussis). All three of these diseases can be deadly for people of any age, and whooping cough is especially dangerous for babies.

Haemophilus influenzae Type B Disease

FIRST DOSE OF THREE OR FOUR

Haemophilus influenzae (flu) type B (Hib) disease is a serious illness caused by the bacteria Hib. Babies and children younger than five years old are most at risk for Hib disease. It can cause lifelong disability and be deadly. Doctors recommend that your child get three or four doses of the Hib vaccine, depending on the brand.

Hepatitis B

SECOND DOSE OF THREE

Hepatitis B is an infectious and potentially serious disease that can cause liver damage and liver cancer. If babies are infected at birth, HepB can be a lifelong, chronic infection. There is no cure for HepB, but the HepB vaccine is the best way to prevent it.

Pneumococcal Disease

FIRST DOSE OF FOUR

Pneumococcal disease can cause potentially serious and even deadly infections. The pneumococcal conjugate vaccine protects against the bacteria that cause pneumococcal disease.

Polio (Inactivated Polio Vaccine)

FIRST DOSE OF FOUR

Polio is a disabling and life-threatening disease caused by poliovirus, which can infect the spinal cord and cause paralysis. It most often affects children younger than five years old. Polio was eliminated in the United States through vaccination, and continued use of the polio vaccine has kept this country polio-free.

Rotavirus

FIRST DOSE OF TWO OR THREE

Rotavirus can be very dangerous, even deadly, for babies and young children. Doctors recommend that your child get two or three doses of the rotavirus vaccine (depending on the brand).

VACCINES AT FOUR MONTHS

Now that your baby is four months old, they have likely started getting their childhood vaccines, and they are ready for another checkup. Routine doctor visits help ensure that your baby receives their second doses of important vaccines at the right time. At four months, your baby should receive vaccines to help protect against the following diseases:

Diphtheria, Tetanus, and Whooping Cough (Pertussis)

SECOND DOSE OF FIVE

Diphtheria, tetanus, and pertussis (DTaP) vaccine is the best protection from three serious diseases: diphtheria, tetanus, and whooping cough (pertussis). All three of these diseases can be deadly for people of any age, and whooping cough is especially dangerous for babies.

Haemophilus influenzae Type B Disease

SECOND DOSE OF THREE OR FOUR

The Hib disease is a serious illness caused by the bacteria Hib. Babies and children younger than five years old are most at risk for Hib disease. It can cause lifelong disability and be deadly. Doctors recommend that your child get three or four doses of the Hib vaccine, depending on the brand.

Pneumococcal Disease

SECOND DOSE OF FOUR

Pneumococcal disease can cause potentially serious and even deadly infections. The pneumococcal conjugate vaccine protects against the bacteria that cause pneumococcal disease.

Polio (Inactivated Polio Vaccine)

SECOND DOSE OF FOUR

Polio is a disabling and life-threatening disease caused by poliovirus, which can infect the spinal cord and cause paralysis. It most often affects children younger than five years old. Polio was eliminated in the United States through vaccination, and continued use of the polio vaccine has kept this country polio-free.

Rotavirus

SECOND DOSE OF TWO OR THREE

Rotavirus can be very dangerous, even deadly for babies and young children. Doctors recommend that your child get two or three doses of the rotavirus vaccine (depending on the brand).

VACCINES AT SIX MONTHS

At six months old, your baby is ready for another round of vaccines, including their first flu shot. As your little one continues to grow and develop, help protect them from these potentially serious diseases.

Diphtheria, Tetanus, and Whooping Cough (Pertussis)

THIRD DOSE OF FIVE

A DTaP vaccine is the best protection from three serious diseases: diphtheria, tetanus, and whooping cough (pertussis). All three of these diseases can be deadly for people of any age, and whooping cough is especially dangerous for babies.

Haemophilus influenzae Type B Disease

THIRD DOSE OF FOUR

The Hib disease is a serious illness caused by the bacteria Hib. Babies and children younger than five years old are most at risk for Hib disease. It can cause lifelong disability and be deadly. Doctors recommend that your child get three or four doses of the Hib vaccine, depending on the brand.

Influenza (Flu)

YEARLY

Flu is a respiratory illness caused by influenza viruses. It spreads easily and can cause serious illness, especially in children younger than five years and children of any age with certain chronic conditions, including asthma. Everyone six months of age and older should get a flu vaccine every year, ideally by the end of October.

Pneumococcal Disease

THIRD DOSE OF FOUR

Pneumococcal disease can cause potentially serious and even deadly infections. The pneumococcal conjugate vaccine protects against the bacteria that cause pneumococcal disease.

Polio (Inactivated Polio Vaccine)

THIRD DOSE OF FOUR

Polio is a disabling and life-threatening disease caused by poliovirus, which can infect the spinal cord and cause paralysis. It most often affects children younger than five years old. Polio was eliminated in the United States through vaccination, and continued use of the polio vaccine has kept this country polio-free.

Rotavirus

THIRD DOSE OF THREE

Rotavirus can be very dangerous, even deadly for babies and young children. Doctors recommend that your child gets two or three doses of the rotavirus vaccine (depending on the brand).

VACCINES AT 7–11 MONTHS

There are no specific age-based vaccinations during this age range, but talk to your child's doctor about annual flu vaccination and any vaccines that needed third doses due at this time.

Influenza (Flu)

YEARLY

Influenza is a respiratory illness caused by influenza viruses. Flu spreads easily and can cause serious illness, especially in children younger than five years and children of any age with certain chronic conditions, including asthma. Everyone six months of age and older should get a flu vaccine every year by the end of October.

VACCINES AT 12–23 MONTHS

As your child enters their toddler stage, they will start becoming aware of themselves and their surroundings. As a parent, make sure you are aware of their next vaccines. Between 12 and 23 months of age, your baby should receive vaccines to protect them from the following diseases.

Chickenpox

FIRST DOSE OF TWO

Chickenpox (varicella) is a very contagious disease known for its itchy, blister-like rash and fever. While chickenpox is a mild disease for many, it can be serious and even life-threatening, especially in babies, teenagers, pregnant women, and people with weakened immune systems.

Diphtheria, Tetanus, and Whooping Cough (Pertussis)

FOURTH DOSE OF FIVE

A vaccine is the best protection from three serious diseases: diphtheria, tetanus, and whooping cough (pertussis). All three of these diseases can be deadly for people of any age, and whooping cough is especially dangerous for babies.

Haemophilus influenzae Type B Disease

THIRD DOSE OF THREE OR FOURTH DOSE OF FOUR

The Hib disease is a serious illness caused by the bacteria Hib. Babies and children younger than five years old are most at risk for Hib disease. It can cause lifelong disability and be deadly. Doctors recommend that your child get three or four doses of the Hib vaccine, depending on the brand.

Hepatitis A

FIRST DOSE OF TWO

Hepatitis A (HepA) can be a serious, even fatal, liver disease caused by the hepatitis A virus (HAV). Children with the virus often do not have symptoms, but they often pass the disease to others, including their unvaccinated parents or caregivers.

Hepatitis B

THE THIRD DOSE OF THREE BETWEEN 6 AND 18 MONTHS

Hepatitis B is an infectious and potentially serious disease that can cause liver damage and liver cancer. If babies are infected at birth, HepB can be a lifelong, chronic infection. There is no cure for HepB, but the HepB vaccine is the best way to prevent it.

Influenza (Flu)

YEARLY

Flu is a respiratory illness caused by influenza viruses. It spreads easily and can cause serious illness, especially in children younger than five years and children of any age with certain chronic conditions, including asthma. Everyone six months of age and older should get a flu vaccine every year, ideally by the end of October.

Measles, Mumps, and Rubella

FIRST DOSE OF TWO

The measles, mumps, and rubella (MMR) vaccine helps prevent three diseases: measles, mumps, and rubella (German measles). These diseases are contagious and can be serious.

Pneumococcal Disease

FOURTH DOSE OF FOUR

Pneumococcal disease can cause potentially serious and even deadly infections. The pneumococcal conjugate vaccine protects against the bacteria that cause pneumococcal disease.

Polio (Inactivated Polio Vaccine)

THIRD DOSE OF FOUR BETWEEN 6 AND 18 MONTHS

Polio is a disabling and life-threatening disease caused by poliovirus, which can infect the spinal cord and cause paralysis. It most often sickens children younger than five years old. Polio was eliminated in the United States with vaccination, and continued use of polio vaccine has kept this country polio-free.

VACCINES AT TWO TO THREE YEARS

Your toddler has spent the last two to three years exploring and discovering their world. It is important for your child to get the flu vaccine so they can keep exploring and be better protected from the flu.

Influenza (Flu)

YEARLY

Flu is a respiratory illness caused by influenza viruses. It spreads easily and can cause serious illness, especially in children younger than five years and children of any age with certain chronic conditions, including asthma. Everyone six months of age and older should get a flu vaccine every year, ideally by the end of October.

CARE FOR YOUR CHILD AFTER VACCINATIONS

Give Your Child Extra Care and Attention

- Pay extra attention to your child for a few days. If you see something that concerns you, call your child's doctor.
- Read the Vaccine Information Sheet(s) (www.cdc.gov/vaccines/hcp/vis/index.html) your child's doctor gave you to learn about side effects your child may experience.

Treat Mild Reactions

Sometimes children have mild reactions from vaccines, such as pain at the injection site or a rash. These reactions, also called "side effects," are normal and will soon go away.

- Use a cool, damp cloth to help reduce redness, soreness, and/or swelling at the injection site.
- Reduce fever with a cool sponge bath.
- Ask your child's doctor if you can give your child a nonaspirin pain reliever.[4]

[4] "Vaccines Shortly after Birth," Centers for Disease Control and Prevention (CDC), July 10, 2023. Available online. URL: www.cdc.gov/vaccines/parents/by-age/newborn-birth.html. Accessed March 12, 2024.

Chapter 32 | Safe Sleep Practices

There are about 3,400 sleep-related deaths among U.S. babies each year. The Centers for Disease Control and Prevention (CDC) supports the recommendations issued by the American Academy of Pediatrics (AAP) to reduce the risk of all sleep-related infant deaths, including sudden infant death syndrome (SIDS). Parents and caregivers can help create a safe sleep area for babies by taking the following steps:

- **Place your baby on his or her back for all sleep times—naps and at night**. Even if a baby spits up during sleep, their anatomy and gag reflex help prevent them from choking while sleeping on their back. Babies who sleep on their backs are much less likely to die of SIDS than babies who sleep on their sides or stomachs.
- **Use a firm, flat (not at an angle or inclined) sleep surface, such as a mattress in a safety-approved crib covered only by a fitted sheet**. Some parents and caretakers might feel they should place their baby on a soft surface to help them be more comfortable while sleeping. However, soft surfaces can increase the risk of sleep-related death. A firm sleep surface helps reduce the risk of SIDS and suffocation.
- **Keep your baby's sleep area (e.g., a crib or bassinet) in the same room where you sleep, ideally until your baby is at least six months old**. Accidental suffocation or strangulation can happen when a baby is sleeping in an adult bed or other unsafe sleep surfaces. Sharing a room with your baby is much safer than bed-sharing

and may decrease the risk of SIDS by as much as 50 percent. Placing the crib close to your bed so the baby is within view and reach can also help make it easier to feed, comfort, and monitor your baby.
- **Keep soft bedding such as blankets, pillows, bumper pads, and soft toys out of your baby's sleep area.** Additionally, do not cover your baby's head or allow your baby to get too hot. Some parents may feel they should add sheets or blankets to the crib to keep their baby warm and comfortable while sleeping. However, sheets, comforters, and blankets can increase the risk of suffocation or overheating. If you are worried about your baby getting cold during sleep, you can dress them in sleep clothing, such as a wearable blanket, also known as a "sleep sack." Weighted products, such as weighted sleepers, weighted swaddles, weighted sleep sacks, and weighted blankets, are not safe for infants.[1]

There have been dramatic improvements in reducing baby deaths during sleep since the 1990s, when recommendations were introduced to place babies on their backs for sleep. However, since the late 1990s, the decline has slowed. Other recommended safe sleep practices today include eliminating hazards such as keeping blankets, pillows, bumper pads, and soft toys out of the sleep area.

Recommendations also include room sharing but not bed sharing. These practices can help lower the risk of sleep-related infant deaths, including SIDS, accidental suffocation, and deaths from unknown causes. Not all caregivers follow these recommendations. Health-care providers can counsel caregivers on safe sleep practices during pregnancy and baby care visits.[2]

[1] "Helping Babies Sleep Safely," Centers for Disease Control and Prevention (CDC), September 29, 2023. Available online. URL: www.cdc.gov/reproductivehealth/features/baby-safe-sleep/index.html. Accessed March 12, 2024.

[2] "Safe Sleep for Babies—Eliminating Hazard," Centers for Disease Control and Prevention (CDC), January 9, 2018. Available online. URL: www.cdc.gov/vitalsigns/pdf/2018-01-vitalsigns.pdf. Accessed March 12, 2024.

Chapter 33 | **Infant and Toddler Hygiene**

Chapter Contents

Section 33.1 | How to Clean, Sanitize, and Store Infant Feeding Items

WHAT ARE INFANT FEEDING ITEMS?

Infant feeding items include bottles and the nipples, rings, and caps that go with them. Certain bottles may also include valves or membranes. Some infants may be fed with a syringe, medicine cup, spoon, or supplemental nursing system.

CAN YOU USE A BLENDER, WHISK, OR SPOON TO MIX FORMULA?

The safest method of mixing formula is by shaking or swirling the formula and water inside the feeding bottle. Blenders can be difficult to clean, and blenders used to prepare infant formula have been linked to illnesses among babies. Whisks and spoons are easier to clean, but they may still increase the risk of introducing germs into your baby's milk.

CLEANING

How Often Should Baby Bottles Be Cleaned?

Bottles should be cleaned after every feeding. If your baby does not finish drinking a bottle within two hours, throw away the unfinished formula. Germs can grow quickly if breast milk or formula is added to a partially used bottle or if a used bottle is only rinsed rather than cleaned.

How Do You Clean Infant Feeding Items in the Dishwasher?

- **Take apart**. Separate all bottle parts (e.g., bottles, nipples, caps, rings, valves).
- **Rinse**. Rinse bottle parts and any other feeding items by holding them under running water. The water can be warm or cold.
- **Wash**. Place bottle parts and other feeding items in the dishwasher. (Be sure to place small items inside a closed-top basket or mesh laundry bag, so they do not end up

in the dishwasher filter.) If possible, run the dishwasher using hot water and a heated drying cycle (or sanitizing setting); this can help kill more germs.
- **Remove from dishwasher**. Wash your hands with soap and water before removing and storing cleaned items.

How Do You Clean Infant Feeding Items by Hand?

- **Wash hands**. Wash your hands well with soap and water for 20 seconds.
- **Take apart**. Separate all bottle parts (e.g., bottles, nipples, caps, rings, valves).
- **Rinse**. Rinse bottle parts and any other feeding items by holding them under running water. Do not set them in the sink. The water can be warm or cold.
- **Wash feeding items.**
- **Rinse again**. Rinse by holding items under running water or by holding completely under fresh water in a separate basin that is used only for cleaning infant feeding items.
- **Allow to air-dry**. Place bottle parts, wash basin, and bottle brush on a clean, unused dish towel or paper towel in an area protected from dirt and dust. Allow to air dry thoroughly.
- **Clean wash basin and bottle brush**. Rinse the wash basin and brush well and allow them to air-dry after each use. Wash them every few days, either in a dishwasher with hot water and a heated drying cycle (if they are dishwasher-safe) or by hand with soap and warm water.

How Do You Clean Brushes and Basins Used to Wash Bottles?

You can clean brushes and basins in a dishwasher if they are dishwasher-safe or wash them by hand with soap and hot water. They can be sanitized with one of the following methods: boil, steam, or soak in a bleach solution if recommended by the item's manufacturer. If you steam an item, be sure the entire item fits in the steamer.

Do You Need to Clean Infant Formula Containers?

No studies have shown that babies have become sick from contamination on the outside of an infant formula container. Also, powdered infant formula is less likely to become contaminated if it stays dry. Avoid using liquid cleaners on infant formula containers to help prevent contaminating the powdered formula inside the container.

If you want to clean the formula container, use a disinfectant wipe or paper towel sprayed with disinfectant to clean the outside of the container and lid before it is opened for the first time. Do not submerge the container or place it under running water. Wait until the surfaces are completely dry before opening the container. Do not clean the inside of the infant formula container.

Do You Need to Clean Infant Formula Scoops?

When powdered formula stays dry, it is less likely to get contaminated. To keep liquids away from the powdered formula, do not clean the formula scoop unless it gets dirty. If the scoop is dropped on the floor or otherwise soiled, clean it as carefully as you would your baby's bottles and allow it to air-dry completely before placing it back in the formula container.

SANITIZING

How Do You Sanitize Infant Feeding Items for Extra Protection?

It is important to note that if you use a dishwasher with hot water and a heated drying cycle (or sanitizing setting) to clean infant feeding items, a separate sanitizing step is not necessary.

- **For extra germ removal, sanitize feeding items at least once daily**. Sanitizing is particularly important when your baby is younger than two months, was born prematurely, or has a weakened immune system. Daily sanitizing of feeding items may not be necessary for older, healthy babies if those items are cleaned carefully after each use.

- **Before sanitizing, make sure you have cleaned feeding items, bottle brushes, and wash basins using one of the methods above.** Sanitize all items (even the bottle brush and wash basin) by boiling, steaming, or bleaching.

How Often Should Baby Bottles Be Sanitized?

If your baby is less than two months old, was born prematurely, or has a weakened immune system due to illness (such as HIV) or medical treatment (such as chemotherapy for cancer), sanitizing feeding items daily (or more often) is particularly important. For older, healthy babies, daily sanitizing may not be necessary if feeding items are cleaned carefully after each use.

STORAGE

How Should You Store Infant Feeding Items Safely?

Allow the clean feeding items, bottle brushes, and wash basins to air-dry thoroughly before storing to help prevent germs and mold from growing. Once the items are completely dry, put them back together and store them in a clean, protected area to prevent contamination.

- **Wash hands.** Wash hands well with soap and water.
- **Put back together.** Put together the clean, dry bottle parts.
- **Store safely.** Place reassembled bottles and other feeding items, wash basin, and dry bottle brush in a clean, protected area, such as inside a closed kitchen cabinet that is used only to store clean dishes.

Why Should You Air-Dry Infant Feeding Items on a Clean Towel Instead of Using a Drying Rack?

Air-drying infant feeding items on a clean dish towel or paper towel is probably more hygienic than using a drying rack. Drying racks may trap moisture, allow mold and germs to grow, and be difficult to clean. If you prefer to use a drying rack, use it to dry only your infant's feeding items. Every few days (or at least daily if your baby is less than two months old, was born prematurely, or has a weakened immune system), be sure to wash, sanitize, and allow the drying rack to dry thoroughly to reduce contamination.[1]

Section 33.2 | **Diaper Hygiene**

DIAPER-CHANGING STEPS FOR CHILDCARE SETTINGS

The following are the diaper-changing steps for childcare settings:

- Prepare:
  - Cover the diaper changing surface with a disposable liner.
  - If you use diaper cream, dispense it onto a tissue now.
  - Bring your supplies (e.g., clean diaper, wipes, diaper cream, gloves, plastic or waterproof bag for soiled clothing, extra clothes) to the diapering area.
- Clean the child:
  - Place the child on a diapering surface and unfasten the diaper.
  - Clean the child's diaper area with disposable wipes. Always wipe front to back!
  - Keep soiled diaper/clothing away from any surfaces that cannot be easily cleaned. Securely bag soiled clothing.
- Remove trash:
  - Place used wipes in the soiled diaper.
  - Discard the soiled diaper and wipes in the trash can.
  - Remove and discard gloves, if used.

[1] "How to Clean, Sanitize, and Store Infant Feeding Items," Centers for Disease Control and Prevention (CDC), February 21, 2023. Available online. URL: www.cdc.gov/hygiene/childcare/clean-sanitize.html. Accessed March 12, 2024.

- Replace the diaper:
  - Slide a fresh diaper under the child.
  - Apply diaper cream, if needed, with a tissue or a freshly gloved finger.
  - Fasten the diaper and dress the child.
- Wash the child's hands:
  - Wash the child's hands with soap and water and place him or her in a safe, supervised area.
- Clean up:
  - Remove the liner from the changing surface and discard in the trash can.
  - Wipe up any visible soil with damp paper towels or a baby wipe.
  - Wet the entire surface with disinfectant; make sure you read and follow the directions on the disinfecting spray, fluid, or wipe. Choose a disinfectant appropriate for the surface material.
- Wash your hands:
  - Wash your hands thoroughly with soap and water.

DIAPER-CHANGING STEPS AT HOME

Protect yourself and your children from germs by following these diapering steps:

- Clean the child:
  - Keep a hand on the child for safety at all times.
  - Place the child on a diapering surface and unfasten the diaper.
  - Clean the child's diaper area with fresh baby wipes. Remember to always wipe from front to back!
  - Keep dirty diaper/clothing away from any surfaces that cannot be easily cleaned.
- Remove the dirty disposable diaper:
  - Set the used baby wipes in the dirty diaper.
  - Place the dirty diaper and used baby wipes in a plastic-lined, lidded trash can.
- Replace the diaper:
  - Slide a fresh diaper under the child.

    - Apply diaper cream, if needed.
    - Fasten the diaper and dress the child.
- Wash the child's hands:
    - Wash the child's hands with soap and water and place him or her in a safe, supervised area.
- Clean the diapering surface, especially if there were any spills or leaks of diaper contents:
    - If the diapering surface is waterproof, wipe up any visible soil with damp paper towels or a baby wipe. Then scrub with a disinfectant spray or wipe and allow the surface to air-dry.
    - If the diapering surface has a fabric cover, remove the soiled cover and replace it with a fresh one.
- Wash your hands:
    - Wash your hands thoroughly with soap and water.[2]

[2] "Diaper Changing Steps for Childcare Settings," Centers for Disease Control and Prevention (CDC), July 5, 2022. Available online. URL: www.cdc.gov/hygiene/childcare/childcare.html. Accessed March 12, 2024.

Chapter 34 | Oral Health

Chapter Contents

Section 34.1 | Safely Soothing Teething Pains

Teething is a normal but potentially painful experience for infants and toddlers. Well-meaning parents and caregivers may turn to medications and products that could be harmful. Soothing children's gums with prescription or over-the-counter (OTC) drugs, homeopathic drugs, or teething jewelry marketed for relieving teething pain may seem like good options. However, these products can be dangerous and can lead to serious injury or even death. This also applies to older children with special needs who may use teething jewelry for sensory stimulation.

The American Academy of Pediatrics (AAP) recommends alternative ways to treat teething pain, including rubbing infants' gums with a clean finger or providing a teething ring made of firm rubber to chew on. For children with sensory stimulation needs, parents and caregivers should talk to their child's health-care provider about safer options. On average, children begin teething around four to seven months and have a total of 20 baby teeth by age three. According to the AAP, occasional symptoms of teething include mild irritability, a low-level fever, drooling, and an urge to chew something hard.

THE RISKS OF TEETHING BRACELETS, NECKLACES, AND OTHER JEWELRY

Teething jewelry includes necklaces, bracelets, and other items worn by either an adult or a child. It is used by parents and caregivers and marketed to relieve an infant's teething pain. It may also be marketed for use by people with special needs, such as autism or attention deficit hyperactivity disorder (ADHD), to provide sensory stimulation or redirect chewing on clothes or body parts.

The beads of the jewelry may be made from materials such as amber, wood, marble, or silicone. Jewelry marketed for teething is not the same as teething rings or teethers, which are made of hard plastic or rubber and are not wearable by an adult or a child. There are serious risks associated with using jewelry marketed for relieving teething pain, such as choking, strangulation, injury to the mouth, and infection. Other concerns include potential injury to the mouth or infection if a piece of the jewelry irritates or pierces the child's gums.

TEETHING CREAMS AND GELS ALSO HAVE RISKS

Parents and caregivers might try to relieve a teething baby by rubbing numbing medications on the child's gums. However, the U.S. Food and Drug Administration (FDA) warns against using any sort of topical medication to treat teething pain in children, including prescription or OTC creams and gels, or homeopathic teething tablets. They offer little to no benefit and are associated with serious risk.

The use of benzocaine gels, sprays, ointments, solutions, and lozenges for mouth and gum pain can lead to a serious—and sometimes fatal—condition called "methemoglobinemia," in which the oxygen-carrying capacity of red blood cells is greatly reduced. Prescription and OTC benzocaine oral health-care drug products are also widely used in adults. Doctors and dentists often use sprays containing benzocaine to numb the mucous membranes of the mouth and throat or to suppress the gag reflex during medical and surgical procedures, such as transesophageal echocardiograms, endoscopy, intubation, and feeding tube replacements. However, benzocaine sprays are not FDA-approved for these uses.

WHAT YOU CAN DO TO EASE TEETHING PAIN

If your child's gums are swollen and tender, gently rub or massage the gums with your finger or give your child a teething ring made of firm rubber to chew. Ensure the teething ring is not frozen; if the object is too hard, it can hurt your child's gums. Parents should supervise their children so they do not accidentally choke on the teething ring.

Parents and caregivers of children with special needs who may require sensory stimulation should talk to their child's health-care provider about safer options and treatment. Jewelry marketed for relieving teething pain and providing sensory stimulation can lead to serious injuries, including strangulation and choking.

The FDA continues to closely monitor the use of teething jewelry and other teething pain relief products and is evaluating whether other actions are necessary to address the risks associated with these products as part of its commitment to protecting public health, especially when it comes to the health and safety of children.[1]

Section 34.2 | Dental Care for Baby Teeth and Gums

Healthy teeth are important—even baby teeth. Children need healthy teeth to help them chew and to speak clearly. And, baby teeth hold space for adult teeth.

PROTECT YOUR BABY'S TEETH WITH FLUORIDE

Fluoride protects teeth from tooth decay and can even heal early decay. Fluoride is in the drinking water of many towns and cities. Ask a dentist or doctor if your water has fluoride in it. If it does not, ask about other kinds of fluoride, such as fluoride varnish or drops, that can help keep your baby's teeth healthy.

CHECK AND CLEAN YOUR BABY'S TEETH

- **Check your baby's teeth**. Healthy teeth should be all one color. If you see spots or stains on the teeth, take your baby to a dentist.
- **Clean your baby's teeth**. Clean them as soon as they come in with a clean, soft cloth or a baby's toothbrush. Clean the teeth at least once a day. It is best to clean them right before bedtime.

At about the age of two (or sooner if a dentist or doctor suggests it), you should start putting fluoride toothpaste on your child's

[1] "Safely Soothing Teething Pain and Sensory Needs in Babies and Older Children," U.S. Food and Drug Administration (FDA), May 23, 2018. Available online. URL: www.fda.gov/consumers/consumer-updates/safely-soothing-teething-pain-and-sensory-needs-babies-and-older-children. Accessed March 13, 2024.

toothbrush. Use only a tiny bit of toothpaste, no bigger than a grain of rice.

FEED YOUR BABY HEALTHY FOOD

- Choose foods without a lot of sugar in them.
- Give your child fruits and vegetables for snacks.
- Save cookies and other treats for special occasions.

DO NOT PUT YOUR BABY TO BED WITH A BOTTLE

Milk, formula, juice, and other drinks such as soda all contain sugar. If sugary liquids stay on your baby's teeth too long, it can lead to tooth decay, which can cause pain for your baby. Avoid putting your baby to bed with a bottle at night or at nap time. If you do put your baby to bed with a bottle, fill it only with water.

Here are some other things you can do:

- Between feedings, do not give your baby a bottle or sippy cup filled with sweet drinks to carry around.
- Near his or her first birthday, teach your child to drink from an open cup.
- If your baby uses a pacifier, do not dip it in anything sweet such as sugar or honey.

TAKE YOUR CHILD TO THE DENTIST

Your child should have a dental visit by his or her first birthday. At this visit, the dentist will do the following:

- Check your child's teeth.
- Show you the best way to clean your child's teeth.
- Talk to you about other things such as a healthy diet and fluoride that can keep your child's mouth healthy.[2]

[2] "A Healthy Mouth for Your Baby," National Institute of Dental and Craniofacial Research (NIDCR), July 1, 2019. Available online. URL: www.nidcr.nih.gov/sites/default/files/2019-10/a-healthy-mouth-for-your-baby.pdf. Accessed March 13, 2024.

Chapter 35 | Safe and Healthy Childcare Services

When it comes to finding childcare, you want a program that is convenient, open when you need it, and within your budget. Most importantly, you need a childcare program that ensures children are safe, healthy, and learning. To make sure the program can support your child, family, and your ability to work, it is important to choose a quality childcare program.

Quality childcare offers children supportive, nurturing relationships with trusted teachers and positive, diverse learning experiences. For children from birth to the age of five years, quality childcare settings can prepare your child for school. In these early years, children's brains develop quickly. The experiences they have during this time will influence how they learn and develop in the years to come. These experiences will also encourage the skills and attitudes children need to succeed in school and throughout life.

GETTING STARTED: SIMPLE STEPS FOR FINDING AND CHOOSING CHILDCARE

Finding the right childcare can sometimes be a stressful experience. There is a lot of information to consider, and it may feel overwhelming at times. Here are some simple steps that can guide your childcare search and ensure you have all the information needed to make the best choice for your child.

Learn the Basics

- Understand your childcare options.
- Learn how childcare programs are licensed and regulated to ensure children's health and safety.
- Learn about additional quality standards that help programs go beyond licensing requirements to provide high-quality care to help children learn, grow, and get ready for school.

Search for Childcare Programs in Your Area

Use your state or territory's online childcare search tool. States and territories are required to have an online childcare list or search to help you find childcare. To find your state or territory's online childcare search, visit the "Find childcare" (https://childcare.gov) now page.

INVESTIGATE

Review the information your state or territory provides about childcare providers on their online childcare search or childcare consumer education website. This information can help you make informed childcare choices.

LICENSING STATUS

Check to see if the program is licensed, registered, certified, or legally license-exempt. Also, verify if the program's license has been suspended or revoked.

QUALITY RATINGS

Childcare quality ratings are how states measure and improve childcare program quality. States use these ratings to share information about the quality of programs in a way that is helpful and understandable.

Contact Each Program

Ask these questions to help determine if the program meets your child and family's needs:

- Are they licensed? If not, are they legally licensed-exempt?
- Do they have space for your children?
- What are their hours of operation?
- What is the cost of care?
- If you receive childcare financial assistance from your state or territory, ask if they accept childcare assistance payments.
- When can you schedule a time to visit (in-person or virtually)?

Consider All the Information You Found

- How did you feel when you called and visited the program? Did you feel welcome?
- Were the children happy and engaged in age-appropriate activities? Are you confident your child will be happy and safe there?
- Which provider made you feel most comfortable?

LOOK, LISTEN, AND ASK: CHOOSING QUALITY CHILDCARE TIP SHEETS

Choosing a childcare program for your child is an important decision. You need to feel comfortable with your choice and be confident that your child is in a safe and caring environment. When looking for childcare, visit each setting in person to ensure the program is the right fit for your child. Visiting allows you to see firsthand how the program operates, what your child will experience during a typical day, and how the teachers interact and work with children. It also allows you to see what the classrooms and play spaces look like and gives you a chance to ask questions. The Look, Listen, and Ask tip sheets are short tools to help guide your childcare program visits. They are designed to help you learn more about the program. There is a tip sheet for each kind of childcare setting:

- Look, Listen, and Ask: Tips for Choosing a Quality Childcare Center (https://childcare.gov/sites/default/files/2022-04/Choosing-a-Child-Care-Center.pdf)
- Look, Listen, and Ask: Tips for Choosing a Family Childcare Home (https://childcare.gov/sites/default/files/2022-04/Choosing-a-Family-Child-Care-Home.pdf)
- Look, Listen, and Ask: Tips for Choosing Quality Before-School and Afterschool Care (https://childcare.gov/sites/default/files/2022-04/Choosing-Before-and-After-School-Care.pdf)
- Look, Listen, and Ask: Tips for Choosing a Quality School Vacation or Summer Program (https://childcare.gov/sites/default/files/2022-04/Choosing-Vacation-and-Summer-Programs.pdf)

YOUR RESPONSIBILITIES ONCE YOU FIND CARE

You and your childcare provider should work as partners to support your child's well-being. Building a strong relationship with your childcare provider is one of the best ways to help ensure your child is happy, safe, and learning while in care. Talking with your child's caregivers and visiting and participating in activities at your child's program send a strong message. It tells both your child and your child's caregiver that you are interested in what your child is doing and that learning is important. Here are some ways to stay involved and ensure care meets your child's needs.

STAY CONNECTED WITH YOUR CHILD

It is important to stay connected with your child so that you can understand what they do at childcare and how they feel about it.

- **Ask your child how they feel about their day**. For example, "Did you have a happy or sad day? Why?"

- **Ask your child what they do during the day**. For example, "I had to read many things today at work and had fun talking to my coworkers. What did you do today? What was the best part? What was not your favorite? Who did you play with?"
- **Ask your child how they interacted with the caregiver**. Listen carefully to what they say. For example, "What did you do today with Ms. Anne? Did you have fun? Do you like seeing Ms.Anne?"
- **Observe your child's behavior during drop-off and pick-up times**. Talk with your caregiver about any changes or concerning behavior.
- **If your child says they do not want to return, ask them why they feel that way**. For example, "Do you have fun playing with the other kids? Do you like your teachers? What part of the day is not your favorite?" Be sure to follow up with the caregiver to discuss.[1]

[1] ChildCare.gov, "How Do I Find and Choose Quality Childcare?" Administration for Children and Families (ACF), March 24, 2022. Available online. URL: https://childcare.gov/consumer-education/choosing-quality-childcare. Accessed March 14, 2024.

Chapter 36 | **Physical Activity for Preschoolers**

WHAT CAN YOU DO TO GET—AND KEEP—YOUR CHILD ACTIVE?

As a parent, you can help shape your child's attitudes and behaviors regarding physical activity. Knowing the recommendations is a great place to start. Encourage your child to be physically active for 60 minutes or more each day, with activities ranging from informal, active play to organized sports. Here are some ways you can do this:

- Encouraging lots of safe and unstructured movement and play can help build a strong foundation for an active lifestyle.
- Set a positive example by leading an active lifestyle yourself.
- Include physical activity in your family's daily routine by taking family walks or playing active games together.
- Give your children equipment that encourages physical activity.
- Take young people to places where they can be active, such as public parks, community baseball fields, or basketball courts.
- Be positive about the physical activities in which your child participates and encourage them to be interested in new activities.
- Make physical activity fun. Fun activities can be anything your child enjoys, either structured or nonstructured. Activities can range from team or individual sports to recreational activities such as

walking, running, skating, bicycling, swimming, playground activities, or free-time play.
- Instead of watching television (TV) after dinner, encourage your child to find fun activities to do on their own or with friends and family, such as walking, playing chase, or riding bikes.
- Always provide protective equipment such as helmets, wrist pads, or knee pads for activities such as riding bicycles or scooters, skateboarding, roller skating, rock-wall climbing, and other activities where there may be a high risk of injuries. Ensure that activities are appropriate for your child's age.

WHAT IF YOUR CHILD HAS A DISABILITY?

Physical activity is important for all children. It is best to talk with a doctor before your child begins a physical activity routine. Try to get advice from a professional with experience in physical activity and disability. They can provide guidance on the amounts and types of physical activity that are appropriate for your child's abilities.[1]

PLAY TIME CAN BE ACTIVE TIME!

Good activity habits begin early in your child's life. As early as infancy, you can help your child grow lifelong healthy play habits. Your child learns from you, so while you help your child be active, try to do the same activities!

For Your Infant

- **Keep your baby active with tummy time and time spent out of the swing or bouncy chair**. This will give your child plenty of chances to stretch, reach, and kick, so your child can reach important milestones such as crawling and sitting up.

[1] "Making Physical Activity a Part of a Child's Life," Centers for Disease Control and Prevention (CDC), June 28, 2023. Available online. URL: www.cdc.gov/physicalactivity/basics/adding-pa/activities-children.html. Accessed March 13, 2024.

- **Avoid putting a TV in your baby's room**. The more you talk to and play with your baby, the more likely he will be healthy as he grows.

For Your Toddler

- **Even very active toddlers need physical activity**. Keep moving by dancing, jumping, and walking together.
- **Try to limit screen time to two hours or less a day**. Children with lots of active playtime outside and indoors are likelier to stay healthy and active as they grow up.

For Your Preschooler

- **Help your child stay active and learn by spending time outdoors**. This encourages physical activity and promotes learning.
- **Try to limit TV, video games, and computer time to two hours or less a day**. Children who watch more than two hours of TV daily are more likely to be overweight as they age.

For Yourself and Your Family

- **When you spend time being active, your child learns healthy habits from you**. Your actions serve as a positive example for your child's behavior.
- **Set playtime, mealtime, and bedtime routines to make daily life easier to handle**. Consistent routines help create a structured and manageable environment.
- **Talk with your child's pediatrician, early care and education staff, and other parents**. This can provide you with ideas for making playtime active time.[2]

[2] "Healthy Habits Start Early," Early Childhood Learning and Knowledge Center (ECLKC), September 25, 2023. Available online. URL: https://eclkc.ohs.acf.hhs.gov/sites/default/files/pdf/active-play-family-tips.pdf. Accessed April 22, 2024.

Part 6 | **Healthy Children (Ages 4–11)**

Chapter 37 | **Diet and Nutrition for Children**

Healthy eating in childhood and adolescence is important for proper growth and development and to prevent various health conditions. The *Dietary Guidelines for Americans*, 2020–2025 (www.dietaryguidelines.gov) recommend that people aged two years or older follow a healthy eating pattern that includes the following:

- a variety of fruits and vegetables
- whole grains
- fat-free and low-fat dairy products
- a variety of protein foods
- oils

These guidelines also recommend that individuals limit calories from solid fats (major sources of saturated and trans-fatty acids) and added sugars and reduce sodium intake. Unfortunately, most children and adolescents do not follow the recommendations set forth in the *Dietary Guidelines for Americans*.[1]

HEALTHY EATING

What Should Your Child Eat and Drink?

Just like adults, children need to consume foods and beverages packed with nutrients. Also, like adults, children should consume just enough calories to fuel their daily living and activities. The *Dietary Guidelines for Americans*, 2020–2025, suggest balancing

[1] "Childhood Nutrition Facts," Centers for Disease Control and Prevention (CDC), August 5, 2022. Available online. URL: www.cdc.gov/healthyschools/nutrition/facts.htm. Accessed March 13, 2024.

calories consumed with physical activity. The guidelines also recommend improving eating habits to promote health, reduce disease risk, and reduce overweight and obesity. Americans aged two years and older are encouraged to consume various healthy foods and beverages. The suggested items include the following:

- fruits, vegetables, unsalted nuts and seeds, and whole grains
- fat-free or low-fat dairy products, including milk, yogurt, cheese, and/or fortified nondairy beverages
- a variety of protein foods, including seafood, lean meats and poultry, eggs, beans, peas, nuts, seeds, and soy products

What Foods and Beverages Should Be Limited?

Youth and adults are also encouraged to get less:

- refined grains
- added sugars
- saturated fats such as lard, butter, and margarine, which are often solid at room temperature
- salt

Added sugars, solid fats, and salt often occur in pizzas, chips, crackers, sodas, sugar-sweetened drinks, desserts such as cookies or cake, and fast foods. If children and teens consume these foods and beverages, these items should be limited in a healthy eating plan. Another step is to ensure your children have breakfast to spark the energy they need to focus in school. Some studies suggest that eating breakfast regularly may decrease children's chances of developing obesity.

How Can You Help Your Child Eat Better?

USE LESS FAT, SALT, AND SUGAR

Here are some ideas to help you and your child follow a healthy eating plan:

- **Cook with fewer solid fats.** Use olive or canola oil instead of butter or margarine. Bake or roast foods instead of frying. "Oven-frying" recipes that involve little or no oil can give foods a crunchy texture.

- **Choose and prepare foods with less salt**. Keep the saltshaker off the table. Have cut-up fruits and vegetables on hand for snacks instead of salty snacks such as chips or crackers.
- **Limit your child's intake of sugar**. Choose hot or cold cereals with no added sugar or low sugar.
- **Fill half of your child's plate with fruits and vegetables.**

SERVE NUTRIENT-RICH FOODS AND BEVERAGES

Many foods and beverages are particularly rich in key nutrients and vitamins—such as potassium, calcium, vitamin D, and dietary fiber—that are important to your children's health and development. Here are some ideas for boosting your children's intake of these nutrients:

- **Offer more fruit for breakfast, snacks, and desserts**. Add dark green, red, and orange vegetables to stews and soups. Add beans (black, kidney, pinto), peas, and lentils to casseroles and salads.
- **Serve more low-fat milk and milk products**. If your child cannot digest much lactose, called "lactose intolerance," serve lactose-free milk, cheese, or yogurt. Your child can also try nondairy drinks, such as soy, almond, or rice drinks enriched with calcium or vitamin D.
- **Serve fresh, frozen, or canned salmon, shrimp, and light tuna**. For young children, you may serve safe types of seafood one to two times a week in child-sized portions, starting with one-ounce portions at the age of two.
- **Replace the refined grains (bread, pasta, rice) your child eats with whole grains**. Eat more bran. Check Nutrition Facts labels to find products high in dietary fiber. Look at the ingredients list to be sure that whole grains are one of the first items.

THINK ABOUT THE DRINK

- Serve more water.
- Offer low-fat or fat-free milk instead of whole milk.
- Avoid serving sugar-sweetened beverages and fruit-flavored drinks.
- Offer fresh fruit, which has more fiber than juice; if serving juice, offer small portions of 100 percent fruit juice.

OFFER HEALTHY SNACKS

Snacks, along with meals, can help children get enough nutrients to stay healthy. Buy or prepare single-serving snacks for younger children to help them get just enough to satisfy their hunger.

Try to keep healthy food in the house for snacks and meals for the whole family. Offer such snacks as the following:

- sliced apples, oranges, pears, and carrots
- whole-grain bread served with low-fat cheese, favorite spread, or roasted veggies
- fresh, frozen, or canned vegetables[2]

BENEFITS OF HEALTHY EATING

Healthy eating can help individuals achieve and maintain a healthy body weight, consume important nutrients, and reduce the risk of developing health conditions such as the following:

- high blood pressure (HBP)
- heart disease
- type 2 diabetes
- cancer
- osteoporosis
- iron deficiency
- dental caries (cavities)[3]

---

[2] "Helping Your Child: Tips for Parents and Other Caregivers," National Institute of Diabetes and Digestive and Kidney Diseases (NIDDK), October 1, 2019. Available online. URL: www.niddk.nih.gov/health-information/weight-management/healthy-eating-physical-activity-for-life/helping-your-child-tips-for-parents. Accessed March 13, 2024.

[3] See footnote [1].

SMART SNACKS IN SCHOOL

Smart Snacks in School refers to the national nutrition standards for foods and beverages sold outside the federal reimbursable school meal programs during the school day. These items are called "competitive foods" because they can compete with participation in school meal programs. As of the 2014–2015 school year, all competitive foods and beverages sold during the school day must meet or exceed Smart Snacks in School nutrition standards, which include limits on fat, sugar, sodium, and calorie content. These standards are the minimum requirement for schools, but states and local education agencies can continue to implement stronger nutrition standards for all competitive foods in schools.[4]

[4] "Smart Snacks and School Vending Machines," Centers for Disease Control and Prevention (CDC), May 1, 2023. Available online. URL: www.cdc.gov/healthyschools/nutrition/smartsnacks.htm. Accessed March 13, 2024.

Chapter 38 | Vaccination and Immunization for Children

Chapter Contents

Section 38.1 | Vaccines for Children Program

Your children may be able to get no-cost vaccines through the Vaccines for Children (VFC) program of the Centers for Disease Control and Prevention (CDC) at health-care providers' offices, pharmacies, and health clinics enrolled in the VFC program. The VFC program helps ensure all children have a better chance of getting their recommended vaccinations on schedule. Vaccinating on time means healthier children, families, and communities. Vaccines provided by the VFC program protect babies, young children, and adolescents from preventable diseases.

CHILDREN WHO ARE ELIGIBLE FOR THE VACCINES FOR CHILDREN PROGRAM

Children aged 18 years or younger who meet at least one of the following requirements are eligible for the VFC program:

- American Indian or Alaska Native
- Medicaid-eligible
- uninsured
- underinsured

Additional Information on Children Who Are Underinsured

Underinsured means that your child has health insurance, but the insurance policy:

- does not cover any vaccines
- does not cover certain recommended vaccines, or
- does cover recommended vaccines but has a fixed dollar limit or cap for payment

Underinsured children are only eligible to receive vaccines at Federally Qualified Health Centers (FQHCs) or Rural Health Clinics (RHCs). FQHCs and RHCs provide health care to medically underserved areas and meet certain criteria under Medicare and Medicaid programs. However, through a deputization agreement, FQHCs/RHCs can choose to delegate their VFC program authority for vaccinating underinsured children to other VFC program–enrolled provider locations (usually public health department clinics) as agents of the FQHC/RHC.

DO YOU NEED PROOF OF A CHILD'S ELIGIBILITY?

You do not have to show any proof that your child is eligible for free vaccines using the VFC program. However, your doctor is required to ask and document the following:

- Is your child on Medicaid?
- Does your child have any health insurance coverage? Does the insurance cover vaccines?
- Is your child of American-Indian or Alaskan-Native heritage?

Many doctors will already have this information in your child's medical record or as part of normal business records, but if your child's insurance or Medicaid status changes, you need to inform the doctor's office of those changes.

WHAT IS THE COST OF VACCINES PROVIDED BY THE VACCINES FOR CHILDREN PROGRAM?

There is no cost for the vaccines given by VFC program providers to eligible children. This means that no one can charge a fee for the vaccine itself.

VACCINES COVERED THROUGH THE VACCINES FOR CHILDREN PROGRAM

The VFC program covers all vaccines included in the pediatric immunization schedules that are determined by the Advisory Committee on Immunization Practices (ACIP):

- recommended immunizations for children from birth through six years old (www.cdc.gov/vaccines/parents/downloads/parent-ver-sch-0-6yrs.pdf)
- recommended immunizations for children from 7 through 18 years old (www.cdc.gov/vaccines/schedules/downloads/teen/parent-version-schedule-7-18yrs.pdf)

The vaccines offered through the VFC program protect children from these preventable diseases:

- coronavirus disease 2019 (COVID-19)
- dengue
- diphtheria
- *Haemophilus influenzae* type b (Hib)
- hepatitis A (HepA)
- hepatitis B (HePB)
- human papillomavirus (HPV)
- influenza (flu)
- measles
- meningococcal
- mumps
- pertussis (whooping cough)
- pneumococcal
- polio
- rotavirus
- respiratory syncytial virus (RSV)
- rubella (German measles)
- tetanus (lockjaw)
- varicella (chickenpox)

If your child is behind on their vaccine schedule, they can catch up on their routine vaccines through the VFC program. Call or visit your provider to discuss how your child can get back on schedule.

LOCATIONS OF VACCINES FOR CHILDREN PROGRAM PROVIDERS

You can get vaccines for your child at any private doctor, private clinic, hospital, public health clinic, community health clinic, school, or pharmacy that is an enrolled VFC program provider. Over 37,000 providers are enrolled in the VFC program nationwide.

- **Health-care providers**. Most pediatricians in the United States and its territories are VFC program–enrolled providers. Birthing hospitals can also be VFC program providers to administer RSV and HepB vaccines to infants. Talk to your child's doctor to see if they are a provider.

- **Schools**. In some states, schools are enrolled. Talk to your child's school to see if they are a VFC program provider.
- **Departments of health**. Your state or territory health department is responsible for managing the VFC program where you reside. Each state or territory has a VFC program coordinator who is responsible for enrolling providers and monitoring their participation in the program.
- **FQHCs and RHCs**. FQHCs and RHCs may be enrolled in the VFC program.

To find a VFC program provider near you, contact your state or local health department (www.cdc.gov/publichealthgateway/healthdirectories) to see if your state has a searchable website for VFC program providers.[1]

Section 38.2 | **Immunization Schedule: 4–11 Years**

VACCINES AT 4–6 YEARS

Growing up means more school days and playdates, which also means more opportunities for spreading germs and getting sick. As your child enters school age and interacts with more kids, help protect them from diseases by keeping their vaccinations up to date. At four to six years of age, your child should receive vaccines to protect them from the following diseases.

Chickenpox (Varicella)

SECOND DOSE OF TWO

Chickenpox is a very contagious disease known for its itchy, blister-like rash and fever. While chickenpox is mild for many, it can be

[1] "Vaccines for Children Program (VFC) Information for Parents," Centers for Disease Control and Prevention (CDC), December 19, 2023. Available online. URL: www.cdc.gov/vaccines/programs/vfc/parents/index.html. Accessed March 14, 2024.

serious and even life-threatening, especially in babies, teenagers, pregnant women, and people with weakened immune systems.

Diphtheria, Tetanus, and Whooping Cough (Pertussis)

FIFTH DOSE OF FIVE

The diphtheria, tetanus, and pertussis (DTaP) vaccine is the best protection from three serious diseases: diphtheria, tetanus, and whooping cough (pertussis). All three of these diseases can be deadly for people of any age, and whooping cough is especially dangerous for babies.

Influenza (Flu)

YEARLY

Flu is a respiratory illness caused by influenza viruses. Flu spreads easily and can cause serious illness, especially in children younger than five years and children of any age with certain chronic conditions, including asthma. Everyone six months of age and older should get a flu vaccine every year, ideally by the end of October.

Measles, Mumps, and Rubella

SECOND DOSE OF TWO

The measles, mumps, and rubella (MMR) vaccine helps prevent three diseases: measles, mumps, and rubella (German measles). These diseases are contagious and can be serious.

Polio (IPV)

FOURTH DOSE OF FOUR

Polio is a disabling and life-threatening disease caused by the poliovirus, which can infect the spinal cord and cause paralysis. It most often sickens children younger than five years old. Polio was eliminated in the United States with vaccination, and continued use of the polio vaccine has kept the country polio-free.

Care for Your Child after Vaccinations

GIVE YOUR CHILD EXTRA CARE AND ATTENTION

- Pay extra attention to your child for a few days. If you see something that concerns you, call your child's doctor.
- Read the Vaccine Information Sheet(s) your child's doctor gave you to learn about side effects your child may experience.

TREAT MILD REACTIONS

Sometimes children have mild reactions from vaccines, such as pain at the injection site or a rash. These reactions, also called "side effects," are normal and will soon go away.

- Use a cool, damp cloth to help reduce redness, soreness, and/or swelling at the injection site.
- Reduce fever with a cool sponge bath.
- Ask your child's doctor if you can give your child a nonaspirin pain reliever.

Vaccines before School

Your child will typically need a certificate of immunization to enroll in school. Your state may also require children entering school to be vaccinated against certain diseases, such as whooping cough (pertussis). If you are unsure of your state's school immunization requirements, check with your child's doctor, your child's school, or your state's health department. Your doctor's office or health-care clinic should be able to provide a record of your child's immunizations. You can also ask if your doctor has recorded the vaccines your child has received in your state's immunization registry.

VACCINES AT 7–10 YEARS

Your child may be learning to become more independent at this stage. As they develop friendships and become more social, the flu vaccine can help keep your child from getting sick with the flu and missing school days with their friends.

Human Papillomavirus

TWO DOSES

Human papillomavirus (HPV) is a common virus that can cause several cancers in men and women. Although typically given to children aged 11–12 years, the HPV vaccine can be given as early as nine years to help protect them against cancers caused by HPV infection. For best protection, most children in this age group will need two shots of the HPV vaccine, 6–12 months apart.

Influenza (Flu)

YEARLY

Flu is a respiratory illness caused by influenza viruses. Flu spreads easily and can cause serious illness, especially in children younger than five years and in children of any age with certain chronic conditions, including asthma. Everyone six months of age and older should get a flu vaccine every year, ideally by the end of October.

Vaccines Your Child May Have Missed

Now is a good time for your child to catch up on any missed vaccines. Make an appointment for your child to get caught up if they have not received vaccines to protect against any of the following diseases:

- chickenpox (varicella)
- hepatitis A (HepA)
- hepatitis B (HepB)
- measles, mumps, and rubella (MMR)
- polio (IPV)
- tetanus, diphtheria, and pertussis (whooping cough) (Tdap)

Care for Your Child after Vaccinations

GIVE YOUR CHILD EXTRA CARE AND ATTENTION

- Pay extra attention to your child for a few days. If you see something that concerns you, call your child's doctor.

- Read the Vaccine Information Sheet(s) your child's doctor gave you to learn about side effects your child may experience.

TREAT MILD REACTIONS

Sometimes children have mild reactions from vaccines, such as pain at the injection site or a rash. These reactions, also called "side effects," are normal and will soon go away.

- Use a cool, damp cloth to help reduce redness, soreness, and/or swelling at the injection site.
- Reduce fever with a cool sponge bath.
- Ask your child's doctor if you can give your child a nonaspirin pain reliever.

VACCINES AT 11–12 YEARS

Although your 11- or 12-year-old is getting closer to their teen years, they are still dependent on you. Help them stay healthy by keeping them up to date with the recommended vaccines. Your preteen should receive routinely recommended vaccines to protect them from the following diseases:

Human Papillomavirus

TWO DOSES

HPV is a common virus that can cause several cancers in men and women. HPV vaccination is recommended at ages 11–12 years to help protect against cancers caused by HPV infection. For best protection, most children in this age group will need two shots of the HPV vaccine, 6–12 months apart.

Influenza (Flu)

YEARLY

Flu is a respiratory illness caused by influenza viruses. Flu spreads easily and can cause serious illness, especially in children younger than five years and in children of any age with certain chronic conditions, including asthma. Everyone six months of age and older should get a flu vaccine every year, ideally by the end of October.

Meningococcal Disease

FIRST DOSE OF TWO

Meningococcal disease refers to any illness caused by a type of bacteria called "*Neisseria meningitidis*." These bacteria can cause meningococcal meningitis or bloodstream infections, which can be serious, even deadly. The meningococcal vaccine called "MenACWY" helps protect against four types of bacteria that cause meningococcal disease (serogroups A, C, W, and Y).

Tetanus, Diphtheria, and Whooping Cough (Pertussis)

FIRST DOSE

A tetanus, diphtheria, and pertussis (whooping cough) (Tdap) booster shot protects older children from three serious diseases—diphtheria, tetanus, and whooping cough (pertussis). While people of any age in the United States can get all three of these potentially deadly diseases, whooping cough is most common. Preteens and teens who get whooping cough may cough for 10 weeks or more, possibly leading to rib fractures from severe coughing.

Benefits of Vaccinating Your Child Now

- Protects against dangerous diseases, including infections, where the risk of exposure increases as adolescents get older.
- Boosts protection from several diseases as protection from early childhood vaccines wears off.

When to Vaccinate Your Child

You can take advantage of any visit to your child's doctor to get recommended vaccines, including during sports physicals or annual checkups before the school year. Ask the doctor or nurse every year if there are any vaccines that your child may need. If your child has serious allergies, including allergies to yeast, latex, or chicken eggs, inform the doctor or nurse before your child gets any shots.

After Vaccination

Sometimes children have mild reactions from vaccines, called "side effects." After vaccination, your preteen might experience the following:

- **Redness and soreness**. Use a cool, damp cloth to help reduce redness, soreness, and/or swelling at the injection site.
- **Fainting after getting a shot**. Although rare, fainting after any vaccine is more common among adolescents. Sitting or lying down when getting a shot and then for about 15 minutes after the shot can help prevent fainting.

Serious side effects are rare.[2]

[2] "Vaccines by Age," Centers for Disease Control and Prevention (CDC), May 10, 2019. Available online. URL: www.cdc.gov/vaccines/parents/by-age/index.html. Accessed March 14, 2024.

Chapter 39 | Oral Hygiene

Chapter Contents

Section 39.1 | **Brushing Your Child's Teeth**

TIPS FOR BRUSHING YOUR CHILD'S TEETH

Brushing is one of the main ways you can keep your child's teeth healthy. You should brush your child's teeth with fluoride toothpaste twice each day to help prevent tooth decay (cavities). Begin brushing as soon as your child's first tooth appears. Tips for brushing your child's teeth include the following:

- **Brush your child's teeth after breakfast and before bed.**
- **Use a child-sized toothbrush with soft bristles and fluoride toothpaste.**
    - For children under the age of three, use a small smear of fluoride toothpaste.
    - For children aged three to six, use fluoride toothpaste the size of a pea.
- **Young children like to do things by themselves.** It is good to let children brush their teeth while an adult watches. However, children under the age of seven or eight cannot brush their teeth well yet. An adult needs to brush the child's teeth too.
- **Find a position where your child is comfortable, and you can see your child's teeth while you brush.** For example, sit on the floor with your baby's or young child's head in your lap. Alternatively, stand behind your child in front of a mirror.
- **Gently brush your child's teeth using small circles.** Brush all surfaces of the teeth, including the insides and outsides.
- **After brushing, have your child spit out the remaining toothpaste but not rinse.** The small amount of toothpaste that stays in your child's mouth is good for the teeth.
- **If you are having trouble brushing your child's teeth, use a timer, a counting game, or a song while**

brushing. You can also ask the staff at your child's dental clinic for help.[1]

BRUSHING AT THE CLASSROOM TABLE

A quick and structured approach to daily brushing in the classroom is to have children brush at the table as a group. There are many benefits of brushing at the table as a group:

- It provides a calm, orderly way to teach children how to brush.
- It takes less time when all children brush together and is less messy than brushing at the sink.
- It allows teachers to serve as role models by brushing their own teeth with children.
- It allows teachers sitting at the table with children to observe and encourage each child or make changes to their brushing method.
- It is less likely that children will pass bacteria (germs) from one toothbrush to another. Bacteria can easily spread when children rinse their toothbrushes under the same stream of water or if they play with their toothbrushes and the bristles touch each other.
- It provides an opportunity to include math and science concepts.[2]

[1] "Brushing Your Child's Teeth," Early Childhood Learning and Knowledge Center (ECLKC), April 26, 2023. Available online. URL: https://eclkc.ohs.acf.hhs.gov/sites/default/files/pdf/brushing-teeth.pdf. Accessed March 14, 2024.
[2] "Brushing at the Classroom Table," Early Childhood Learning and Knowledge Center (ECLKC), November 9, 2022. Available online. URL: https://eclkc.ohs.acf.hhs.gov/oral-health/brush-oral-health/brushing-teeth-classroom-table. Accessed March 14, 2024.

Section 39.2 | Managing Tooth Decay: Reversal and Cavity Prevention

You probably know that a dental cavity is a hole in a tooth. But did you know that a cavity is the result of a tooth decay process that happens over time? Did you know that you can interrupt and even reverse this process to avoid a cavity?

WHAT ARE INSIDE OUR MOUTHS?

Our mouths are full of bacteria. Hundreds of different types live on our teeth, gums, tongue, and other places in our mouths. Some bacteria are helpful, but others can be harmful, such as those that play a role in the tooth decay process. Tooth decay is the result of an infection with certain types of bacteria that use sugars in food to make acids. Over time, these acids can create a cavity in the tooth.

WHAT GOES ON INSIDE OUR MOUTHS ALL DAY?

Throughout the day, a tug of war takes place inside our mouths. On one team are dental plaque—a sticky, colorless film of bacteria—plus foods and drinks that contain sugar or starch (such as milk, bread, cookies, candy, soda, juice, and many others). Whenever we eat or drink something that contains sugar or starch, the bacteria use them to produce acids. These acids begin to eat away at the tooth's hard outer surface, or enamel. On the other team are the minerals in our saliva (such as calcium and phosphate) plus fluoride from toothpaste, water, and other sources. This team helps enamel repair itself by replacing minerals lost during an "acid attack." Our teeth go through this natural process of losing minerals and regaining minerals all day long.

HOW DOES A CAVITY DEVELOP?

When a tooth is exposed to acid frequently—for example, if you eat or drink often, especially foods or drinks containing sugar and starches—the repeated cycles of acid attacks cause the enamel to continue to lose minerals. A white spot may appear where minerals have been lost. This is a sign of early decay. Tooth decay can be stopped or reversed at this point. Enamel can repair itself by using minerals from saliva and fluoride from toothpaste or other sources. But if the tooth decay process continues, more minerals are lost. Over time, the enamel is weakened and destroyed, forming a cavity. A cavity is permanent damage that a dentist has to repair with a filling.

HOW CAN WE AVOID A CAVITY?

Fluoride is a mineral that can prevent tooth decay from progressing. It can even reverse or stop early tooth decay. Fluoride works to protect teeth by:

- preventing mineral loss in tooth enamel and replacing lost minerals
- reducing the ability of bacteria to make acid

You can get fluoride by:

- drinking fluoridated water from a community water supply
- brushing with a fluoride toothpaste

If the dentist thinks your child needs more fluoride, he or she may:

- apply a fluoride gel or varnish to tooth surfaces
- prescribe fluoride tablets
- recommend using a fluoride mouth rinse

KEEP AN EYE ON HOW OFTEN YOUR CHILD EATS, AS WELL AS WHAT THEY EAT

Your child's diet is important in preventing cavities. Remember, every time we eat or drink something that contains sugar or starches, bacteria in our mouth use the sugar and starch to produce acids. These acids begin to eat away at the tooth's enamel. Our saliva can help fight off this acid attack. But if we eat frequently throughout the day—especially foods and drinks containing sugar and starches—the repeated acid attacks will win the tug of war, causing the tooth to lose minerals and eventually develop a cavity. That is why it is important to keep an eye on how often your children eat as well as what they eat.

- **Limit between-meal snacks**. This reduces the number of acid attacks on teeth and gives teeth a chance to repair themselves.
- **Save candy, cookies, soda, and other sugary drinks for special occasions**.
- **Limit fruit juice**. Follow the Daily Juice Recommendations (www.healthychildren.org/English/healthy-living/nutrition/Pages/Fruit-Juice-and-Your-Childs-Diet.aspx) from the American Academy of Pediatrics (AAP).
- **Make sure your child does not eat or drink anything with sugar in it after bedtime tooth brushing**. Saliva flow decreases during sleep. Without enough saliva, teeth are less able to repair themselves after an acid attack.

MAKE SURE YOUR CHILD BRUSHES

Be sure to supervise young children when they brush. Here is what you should know:

- **For children aged three to six, you put the toothpaste on the brush**. Use only a pea-sized amount of fluoride toothpaste. (In children under the age of two, dental experts recommend that you do not use fluoride toothpaste unless a doctor or dentist tells you to.)
- **Encourage your child to spit out the toothpaste rather than swallow it**.
- **Children under the age of six tend to swallow much of the toothpaste on their brush**. If children regularly consume higher-than-recommended amounts of fluoride during the teeth-forming years, their permanent teeth may develop white lines or flecks called "dental fluorosis." Fluorosis is usually mild; in many cases, only a dental professional would notice it.

- **If your child is younger than six, you will need to help your child brush.** Young children cannot get their teeth cleaned by themselves. Try brushing your child's teeth first and then let them finish.

TAKE YOUR CHILD TO THE DENTIST FOR REGULAR CHECKUPS

Visit a dentist regularly for cleanings and an examination. During the visit, the dentist or hygienist will:

- remove dental plaque
- check for any areas of early tooth decay
- show you and your child how to thoroughly clean the teeth
- apply a fluoride gel or varnish, if necessary
- schedule your next regular checkup[3]

SCHOOL DENTAL SEALANT PROGRAMS

Dental sealants are a quick, easy, and painless way to prevent most cavities that children get in the permanent back teeth, where 9 in 10 cavities occur. Children aged 6–11 years without sealants have almost three times more first-molar cavities than children with sealants. School dental sealant programs are an effective way to deliver this highly effective preventive intervention to millions of children who might not receive regular dental care. Increasing sealant use among low-income children can greatly reduce tooth decay. As a parent, ask your child's dentist to apply sealants when appropriate. If your child's school has a sealant program, sign your child up to participate. If they do not, ask your child's school to start one.[4]

[3] "The Tooth Decay Process: How to Reverse It and Avoid a Cavity," National Institute of Dental and Craniofacial Research (NIDCR), August 1, 2022. Available online. URL: www.nidcr.nih.gov/health-info/tooth-decay/more-info/tooth-decay-process. Accessed March 14, 2024.

[4] "Children's Dental Health," Centers for Disease Control and Prevention (CDC), January 30, 2023. Available online. URL: www.cdc.gov/oralhealth/publications/features/childrens-dental-health.html. Accessed March 14, 2024.

Chapter 40 | Managing Food Allergy and Intolerance

A food allergy is a reaction to food or drink, where the body mistakenly interprets some part of it as a danger and activates the immune system. Between 4 and 8 percent of children in the United States have at least one food allergy, and although the exact reason is unknown, they are on the rise in the United States and other parts of the world. Some children are more prone to food allergies than others, such as those who have eczema or asthma. The tendency to be allergic also seems to run in families. Children who are severely allergic do not have to eat a certain food to have a reaction. They can have reactions to food particles in the air or on surfaces that they touch. This is why some situations require a complete ban on a specific type of food.

Not all food allergies are the same. Some are more common than others, and some lead to severe reactions such as anaphylaxis, while others usually do not. It is important to learn more about specific kinds of food allergies and how to care for children who have them.

IMMUNOGLOBULIN E-MEDIATED FOOD ALLERGIES

Immunoglobulin E (IgE) is an antibody that, when working properly, helps the body respond to parasites or other harmful organisms. IgE tells the body to release histamine, which causes sneezing or hives. When the body releases too much histamine, a child may experience:

- itching
- swelling of the mouth and throat
- trouble breathing
- anaphylaxis, a medical emergency, which includes the abovementioned symptoms, low blood pressure, and faintness/unconsciousness

Children can react differently to the same foods on different days. The response depends on how the food was prepared, how much the child eats, or whether the child is ill. For example, a child who is allergic to eggs may have a runny nose one day and experience swelling of the throat and difficulty breathing on another. About 90 percent of all allergies are responses to eight foods:

- peanuts
- eggs
- milk
- wheat
- soy
- tree nuts (e.g., almonds, Brazil nuts, cashews, hazelnuts, pecans, pistachios, and walnuts)
- fish
- shellfish (e.g., shrimp, crab, crayfish, lobster, oysters, clams)

Many children who are allergic to milk, eggs, soy, and wheat lose their food allergy later—some by the age of three and 85 percent by the age of 10. A smaller number of children with food allergies never lose their allergy. Most often, these are children with allergies to tree nuts, fish, shellfish, and peanuts.

OTHER TYPES OF FOOD ALLERGIES

The allergies listed below are not common compared to IgE-mediated allergies and usually do not lead to respiratory symptoms.

These are more likely to cause gastrointestinal symptoms such as nausea, vomiting, diarrhea, or gassiness.

Food Protein-Induced Enterocolitis Syndrome

This allergy may show up in infants when they begin to eat solid food or formula. The infants seem to have a severe "stomach bug" with projectile vomiting and, later, diarrhea. The symptoms start within a few hours of eating the solid food to which they are allergic. Food protein-induced enterocolitis syndrome does not usually occur when an infant is exclusively breastfed.

Oral Allergy Syndrome

Some children who have pollen allergies may also have a reaction to certain foods. Trace amounts of pollen can exist on the skin of certain fruits and vegetables. For example, a child allergic to ragweed can have allergic symptoms around the mouth and in the throat when they eat certain melons. Symptoms can include itching or tingling of the lips, tongue, and roof of the mouth or throat. There may also be hives around the mouth where the food comes into contact with the skin, swelling of the lips or tongue, and throat tightness. Very rarely, symptoms may go beyond the mouth and throat or result in anaphylaxis.

Eosinophilic Esophagitis

This is a swallowing disorder caused by allergies to food or pollen. A child with this type of allergy may have problems with swallowing, vomiting, reflux, and poor weight gain. Children with this allergy may also have asthma or eczema.

Allergic Proctocolitis

Allergic proctocolitis is an allergy to formula or breast milk that affects infants in their first year of life. The symptoms include blood-streaked, watery, green, and mucus-filled stools, diarrhea, vomiting, anemia, and fussiness.

FOOD ALLERGY DIAGNOSES, FOOD INTOLERANCES, AND OTHER CONSIDERATIONS

- **Food allergies are diagnosed by a physician or other health-care worker**. Consider asking for medical documentation of food allergies, including:
  - symptoms to look for
  - actions to take when symptoms appear
  - recommended medications (e.g., antihistamines or epinephrine autoinjector)
  - instructions on giving the medication
- **Symptoms of food allergies and intolerances often overlap**. Sometimes families believe their child has a food allergy when it is actually an intolerance. An intolerance means that a child has trouble digesting a particular food. Foods that commonly cause intolerances are milk, gluten, and certain dyes. Intolerances may cause vomiting, diarrhea, and stomach pain, but they do not cause allergic reactions or anaphylaxis. Caregivers should understand whether a child has an intolerance or an allergy so that staff alertness and emergency procedures can focus on children who are most at risk. Asking families to provide a list of food intolerances and preferences separately from food allergies shows that staff take their needs seriously. Openness to accommodating intolerances as well as food preferences creates trust with families and focuses emergency procedures on the children who need them.
- **Celiac disease is an autoimmune disease, not an allergy or an intolerance**. It requires total avoidance of gluten, which is different from a food allergy or intolerance. A child with celiac disease can become seriously ill if not diagnosed and treated effectively, so specific information and training of staff is critical.[1]

---

[1] "Caring for Children with Food Allergies," Early Childhood Learning and Knowledge Center (ECLKC), December 1, 2023. Available online. URL: https://eclkc.ohs.acf.hhs.gov/publication/caring-children-food-allergies. Accessed March 14, 2024.

IDEAS FOR PARENTS

As a parent, you can be involved in your child's school by:

- attending meetings, workshops, or training events offered by the school
- communicating with school staff and other parents
- volunteering for school events or in your child's classroom
- reinforcing healthy messages and practices your child learns at school
- helping make decisions about health in the school
- being part of community activities supported by the school

Here are some specific ideas for how you can support your child's school in addressing food allergies:

- Have an ongoing conversation with your child to discuss their food allergies, their feelings about having food allergies, and if they feel safe and supported at school.
- Work with your child's health-care provider to establish a current emergency care plan and for timely completion of required school forms.
- Provide emergency medication to the school nurse or other school health official.
- Ensure that there is a current individualized health-care plan and assist with setting goals.
- Communicate with your child's teachers, counselors, and school health services staff about your child's food allergies and how they are coping while at school.
- Work with teachers and other staff to identify nonfood rewards for your child, thereby reducing exposure to allergens.
- Talk with school nutrition services about your child's allergies and advanced menu viewing.
- Volunteer with your child, or get involved at school health events to educate staff and other families about food allergies.

- Join a group, such as the PTA, school wellness committee, or school health advisory council, that addresses the needs of a supportive and healthy school environment.
- Share research-based websites or written materials about food allergies with teachers, nurses, and administrators, when possible (e.g., www.cdc.gov/healthyschools/foodallergies/index.htm).[2]

[2] "Children and Adolescents with Food Allergies—How Can You Help," Centers for Disease Control and Prevention (CDC), November 5, 2015. Available online. URL: www.cdc.gov/healthyschools/parentsforhealthyschools/pdf/P4HS_Allergies.pdf. Accessed March 14, 2024.

Chapter 41 | **Positive Parenting Tips**

Chapter Contents

Section 41.1 | Building Healthy Relationships with Children

Parents have an important job. Raising kids is both rewarding and challenging. You are likely to get a lot of advice along the way, from doctors, family, friends, and even strangers. But every parent and child is unique. Being sensitive and responsive to your kids can help you build positive, healthy relationships together.

"Being a sensitive parent and responding to your kids cuts across all areas of parenting," says Arizona State University's Dr. Keith Crnic, a parent-child relationship expert. "What it means is recognizing what your child needs in the moment and providing that in an effective way."

"This can be especially critical for infants and toddlers," he adds. Strong emotional bonds often develop through sensitive, responsive, and consistent parenting in the first years of life. For instance, holding your baby lovingly and responding to their cries helps build strong bonds.

BUILDING BONDS

Strong emotional bonds help children learn how to manage their own feelings and behaviors and develop self-confidence. They create a safe base from which children can explore, learn, and relate to others.

Experts call this type of strong connection between children and their caregivers "secure attachment." Securely attached children are more likely to be able to cope with challenges such as poverty, family instability, parental stress, and depression.

An analysis shows that about 6 out of 10 children in the United States develop secure attachments to their parents. The 4 out of 10 kids who lack such bonds may avoid their parents when they are upset or resist their parents if they cause them more distress. Studies suggest that this can make kids more prone to serious behavior problems. Researchers have been testing programs to help parents develop behaviors that encourage secure attachment.

BEING AVAILABLE

Modern life is full of things that can influence your ability to be sensitive and responsive to your child. These include competing priorities, extra work, lack of sleep, and distractions such as mobile devices. Some experts are concerned about the effects that distracted parenting may have on emotional bonding and children's language development, social interaction, and safety.

If parents are inconsistently available, kids can become distressed and feel hurt, rejected, or ignored. They may have more emotional outbursts and feel alone. They may even stop trying to compete for their parents' attention and start to lose emotional connections to their parents.

"There are times when kids really do need your attention and want your recognition," Crnic explains. Parents need to communicate that their kids are valuable and important, and children need to know that parents care about what they are doing, he says.

It can be tough to respond with sensitivity during tantrums, arguments, or other challenging times with your kids. "If parents respond by being irritable or aggressive themselves, children can mimic that behavior, and a negative cycle then continues to escalate," explains Dr. Carol Metzler, who studies parenting at the Oregon Research Institute.

According to Crnic, kids start to regulate their own emotions and behavior around the age of three. Up until then, they depend more on you to help them regulate their emotions, whether to calm them or help get them excited.

"They are watching you to see how you do it and listening to how you talk to them about it," he explains. "Parents need to be good self-regulators. You are not only trying to regulate your own emotions at the moment, but helping your child learn to manage their emotions and behavior."

As kids become better at managing their feelings and behavior, it is important to help them develop coping skills, such as active problem-solving. These skills can help them feel confident in handling what comes their way.

"When parents engage positively with their children, teaching them the behaviors and skills they need to cope with the world, children learn to follow rules and regulate their own feelings," Metzler says.

"As parents, we try really hard to protect our kids from the experience of bad things," Crnic explains. "But if you protect them all the time and they are not in situations where they deal with difficult or adverse circumstances, they are not able to develop healthy coping skills."

He encourages you to allow your kids to have more of those experiences and then help them learn how to solve the problems that emerge. Talk through the situation and their feelings. Then work with them to find solutions to put into practice.

MEETING NEEDS

As children grow up, it is important to remember that giving them what they need does not mean giving them everything they want. "These two things are very different," Crnic explains. "Really hone in on exactly what is going on with your kid at the moment. This is an incredibly important parenting skill, and it is linked to so many great outcomes for kids."

Think about where a child is in life and what skills they need to learn at that time. Perhaps they need help managing emotions, learning how to behave in a certain situation, thinking through a new task, or relating to friends.

"You want to help kids become confident," Crnic says. "You do not want to aim too high where they cannot get there or too low where they have already mastered the skill." Another way to boost confidence while strengthening your relationship is to let your kid take the lead.

"Make some time to spend with your child that is not highly directive, where your child leads the play," advises Dr. John Bates, who studies children's behavior problems at Indiana University Bloomington. "Kids come to expect it, and they love it, and it really improves the relationship."

Bates also encourages parents to focus on their child's actual needs instead of sticking to any specific parenting principles. It is never too late to start building a healthier, more positive relationship with your child, even if things have gotten strained and stressful.

"Most importantly, make sure that your child knows that you love them and are on their side," Metzler says. "For older children, let them know that you are genuinely committed to building a stronger relationship with them and helping them be successful."

By being a sensitive and responsive parent, you can help set your kids on a positive path, teach them self-control, reduce the likelihood of troublesome behaviors, and build a warm, caring parent-child relationship.

TIPS FOR CONNECTING WITH YOUR KIDS

- Catch kids showing good behavior and offer specific praise.
- Give children meaningful jobs at home and positive recognition afterward.
- Do not be overly critical; help them improve their skills one step at a time.
- Use kind words, tones, and gestures when giving instructions or making requests.
- Spend some time daily in warm, positive, loving interactions with your kids.
- Brainstorm solutions to problems at home or school together.
- Set rules for yourself for mobile device use and other distractions; for example, check your phone after your child goes to bed.
- Ask about your child's concerns, worries, goals, and ideas.
- Participate in activities that your child enjoys.[1]

[1] *NIH News in Health*, "Positive Parenting—Building Healthy Relationships with Your Kids," National Institutes of Health (NIH), September 7, 2017. Available online. URL: https://newsinhealth.nih.gov/special-issues/parenting/positive-parenting. Accessed March 14, 2024.

Section 41.2 | Positive Parenting Tips for Preschoolers

DEVELOPMENTAL MILESTONES

Skills such as naming colors, showing affection, and hopping on one foot are called "developmental milestones." Developmental milestones are things most children can do by a certain age. Children reach milestones in how they play, learn, speak, behave, and move (such as crawling, walking, or jumping). As children grow into early childhood, their world will begin to open up. They will become more independent and begin to focus more on adults and children outside the family. They will want to explore and ask more about the surrounding things. Their interactions with family and those around them will help shape their personality and their own ways of thinking and moving.

During this stage, children should be able to ride a tricycle, use safety scissors, notice a difference between girls and boys, help dress and undress themselves, play with other children, recall part of a story, and sing a song.

POSITIVE PARENTING TIPS

The following are some things you, as a parent, can do to help your preschooler during this time:

- **Continue to read to your child.** Nurture their love for books by taking them to the library or bookstore.
- **Let your child help with simple chores.**
- **Encourage your child to play with other children.** This helps the child to learn the value of sharing and friendship.
- **Be clear and consistent when disciplining your child.** Explain and show the behavior that you expect from her. Whenever you tell your child no, follow up with what they should be doing instead.
- **Help your child develop good language skills by speaking to him or her in complete sentences and using "grown-up" words.** Help the child use the correct words and phrases.

- **Help your child through the steps to solve problems when he or she is upset.**
- **Give your child a limited number of simple choices, such as what to wear, when to play, and what to eat for a snack.**

CHILD SAFETY FIRST

As your child becomes more independent and spends more time in the outside world, it is important that you and your child are aware of ways to stay safe. Here are a few tips to protect your child:

- **Tell your child why it is important to stay out of traffic.** Tell them not to play in the street or run after stray balls.
- **Be cautious when letting your child ride his or her tricycle.** Keep your child on the sidewalk and away from the street, and always have your child wear a helmet.
- **Check outdoor playground equipment.** Make sure there are no loose parts or sharp edges.
- **Watch your child at all times, especially when they are playing outside.**
- **Be safe in the water.** Teach your child to swim, but watch out at all times when they are in or around any body of water (this includes kiddie pools).
- **Teach your child how to be safe around strangers.**
- **Keep your child in a forward-facing car seat with a harness until they reach the top height or weight limit allowed by the car seat's manufacturer.** Once your child outgrows the forward-facing car seat with a harness, it will be time for them to travel in a booster seat but still in the back seat of the vehicle.

HEALTHY BODIES

- **Eat meals with your child whenever possible.** Let your child see you enjoying fruits, vegetables, and whole grains at meals and snacks. Your child should eat and drink only a limited amount of food and beverages that contain added sugars, solid fats, or salt.

- **Keep television sets out of your child's bedroom**. Set screen time limits for your child to no more than one hour per day of quality programming at home, school, or after-school care, and develop a media use plan for your family.
- **Provide your child with age-appropriate play equipment, such as balls and plastic bats, but let your preschooler choose what to play with**. This will make moving and being active fun for your preschooler.
- **Make sure your child gets the recommended amount of sleep each night: for preschoolers aged three to five years, 10–13 hours per 24 hours (including naps).**[2]

Section 41.3 | **Positive Parenting Tips for Middle Childhood**

DEVELOPMENTAL MILESTONES

Middle childhood brings many changes in a child's life. By this time, children can dress themselves, catch a ball more easily using only their hands, and tie their shoes. Having independence from family becomes more important now. Events such as starting school bring children this age into regular contact with the larger world. Friendships become increasingly important. Physical, social, and mental skills develop quickly at this time. This is a critical period for children to develop confidence in all areas of life, such as through friends, schoolwork, and sports.

Here is some information on how children develop during middle childhood.

[2] National Center on Birth Defects and Developmental Disabilities (NCBDDD), "Preschoolers (3–5 Years of Age)," Centers for Disease Control and Prevention (CDC), February 22, 2021. Available online. URL: www.cdc.gov/ncbddd/childdevelopment/positiveparenting/preschoolers.html. Accessed March 15, 2024.

Emotional/Social Changes

Children in this age group might:

- show more independence from parents and family
- start to think about the future
- understand more about their place in the world
- pay more attention to friendships and teamwork
- want to be liked and accepted by friends

Thinking and Learning

Children in this age group might:

- show rapid development of mental skills
- learn better ways to describe experiences and talk about thoughts and feelings
- have less focus on one's self and more concern for others

POSITIVE PARENTING TIPS

The following are some things you, as a parent, can do to help your child during this time:

- **Show affection for your child.** Recognize their accomplishments.
- **Help your child develop a sense of responsibility by asking them to help with household tasks, such as setting the table.**
- **Talk with your child about school, friends, and things they look forward to in the future.**
- **Talk with your child about respecting others.** Encourage them to help people in need.
- **Help your child set their own achievable goals, so they will learn to take pride in themselves and rely less on approval or rewards from others.**
- **Help your child learn patience by letting others go first or finishing a task before going out to play.** Encourage them to think about possible consequences before acting.

- **Make clear rules and stick to them, such as how long your child can watch television or when they have to go to bed. Be clear about what behavior is acceptable and what is not.**
- **Do fun things together as a family, such as playing games, reading, and going to events in your community.**
- **Get involved with your child's school.** Meet the teachers and staff and understand their learning goals and how you and the school can work together to help your child do well.
- **Continue reading to your child.** As your child learns to read, take turns reading to each other.
- **Use discipline to guide and protect your child, rather than punishment to make them feel bad about themselves.** Follow up any discussion about what not to do with a discussion of what to do instead.
- **Praise your child for good behavior.** It is best to focus praise more on what your child does ("you worked hard to figure this out") than on traits they cannot change ("you are smart").
- **Support your child in taking on new challenges.** Encourage them to solve problems, such as a disagreement with another child, independently.
- **Encourage your child to join school and community groups, such as team sports, or to take advantage of volunteer opportunities.**

CHILD SAFETY FIRST

More physical ability and more independence can put children at risk for injuries from falls and other accidents. Motor vehicle crashes are the most common cause of death from unintentional injury among children this age. Here are some tips to keep your child safe:

- Protect your child properly in the car.
- Teach your child to watch out for traffic and how to be safe when walking to school, riding a bike, and playing outside.

- Make sure your child understands water safety and always supervise them when swimming or playing near water.
- Supervise your child when they are engaged in risky activities, such as climbing.
- Talk with your child about how to ask for help when they need it.
- Keep potentially harmful household products, tools, equipment, and firearms out of your child's reach.

HEALTHY BODIES

As parents, you can help make schools healthier by:

- working with your child's school to limit access to foods and drinks with added sugar, solid fat, and salt that can be purchased outside the school lunch program
- ensuring your child has one hour or more of physical activity each day
- keeping TV sets out of your child's bedroom. Set limits for screen time at home, school, or after-school care, and develop a media use plan for your family
- practicing healthy eating habits and physical activity early. Encourage active play and be a role model by eating healthy at family mealtimes and having an active lifestyle
- making sure your child gets the recommended amount of sleep each night: for school-age children 6–12 years, 9–12 hours per 24 hours (including naps)[3]

---

[3] National Center on Birth Defects and Developmental Disabilities (NCBDDD), "Middle Childhood (6–8 Years of Age)," Centers for Disease Control and Prevention (CDC), February 22, 2021. Available online. URL: www.cdc.gov/ncbddd/childdevelopment/positiveparenting/middle.html. Accessed March 15, 2024.

Chapter 42 | **Role of Family Structure in Child Development**

It is normal for young children to test the limits. That is how they learn what is right and wrong. However, it can be frustrating and really test our patience as parents! One way to keep control and help children learn is to create structure. The structure is created by consistent routines and rules. Rules teach children what behaviors are okay and not okay, and routines teach children what to expect throughout the day.

WHEN CAN YOU START CREATING A STRUCTURE WITH ROUTINES AND RULES?

Creating structure at any age can help your child and you. Children can begin learning routines and rules at a very young age. You can start with routines for important activities of the day, such as meals, bedtime, or in the morning.

EXAMPLES OF FAMILY ROUTINES

The following are examples of routines and daily schedules of parents with toddlers and preschoolers. Some parents find it helpful to have extremely detailed schedules, while others find it helpful to have a general idea of the day's activities. You can decide what will work best for you and your family.

Family with a Three-and-a-Half-Year-Old

DAILY SCHEDULE

- Wake up around 6:20 a.m.
- Get out of bed by 6:30 a.m.
- Go potty, get dressed, brush teeth, and leave by 6:50 a.m.
- Eat breakfast or a snack in the car.
- Pick up from daycare around 4:00 p.m.
- Have playtime from 4:00 p.m. to 5:00 p.m.
- Prepare dinner around 5:00 p.m. and eat around 5:45 p.m.
- Bath around 6:30 p.m.
- Read or do something together, such as a game or art project, around 7:00 p.m. Go potty, brush your teeth, and go to bed by 8:00 p.m.
- Read a story and be quiet/asleep by 8:30 p.m.

Family with Three Kids, Twins Aged Four- and a Two-Year-Old

DAILY SCHEDULE

- Wake up at 7:00 a.m. and have milk.
- Watch cartoons until breakfast at 8:00 a.m.
- Get dressed for the day.
- Have a snack at 10:00 a.m.
- Have lunch at noon, followed by a nap at 12:30 p.m.
- Have dinner at 5:30 p.m.
- Bath at 6:00 p.m., followed by a story and a few songs in the bedroom.
- Off the lights by 6:45 or 7:00 p.m.
- Prepare dinner around 5:00 p.m. and eat around 5:45 p.m.
- Bath around 6:30 p.m.
- Read or do something together, such as a game or art project, around 7:00 p.m.
- Go potty, brush teeth, and go to bed by 8:00 p.m.
- Read a story and be quiet/asleep by 8:30 p.m.

Family with Two Kids, a 17-Month-Old and a 3-Year-Old

PRESCHOOL DAYS

- **7:30 to 8:00 a.m**. Get kids out of bed.
- **8:00 a.m**. Eat breakfast, no screen time.
- **8:15 a.m**. Get kids dressed for preschool, brush teeth and hair, and play until 8:35 a.m.
- **8:40 a.m**. Leave the house for preschool.
- **12:00 noon**. Pick up kids from preschool.
- **12:20 p.m**. Have lunch and read a book before nap.
- **1:00 p.m**. Nap time (plan the afternoon during this time, including starting dinner).
- **3:30 to 4:00 p.m**. Get up from a nap and have a snack.
- **4:00 to 5:15 p.m**. Play.
- **5:30 p.m**. Watch a television show while parents cook/finish dinner.
- **6:00 to 6:15 p.m**. Dinner.
- **6:30 p.m**. Bath time, brush teeth, and get pajamas on.
- **7:00 p.m**. Do something fun together, letting children lead.
- **7:15 p.m**. Book and cuddle time.
- **7:30 to 7:45 p.m**. Lights-out.

NONPRESCHOOL DAYS

- **8:00 a.m**. Get kids out of bed.
- **8:30 a.m**. Eat breakfast.
- **9:00 to 10:00 a.m**. Kids play inside or watch television while parents get ready for the day.
- **10:15 a.m**. Get kids dressed and ready for any activities for the day.
- **10:30 a.m**. Have snacks on the way to activity.
- **10:30 a.m. to 12:15 p.m**. Activity.
- **12:30 p.m**. Lunch.
- **1:00 p.m**. Nap time.
- **3:30 to 4:00 p.m**. Get up from a nap and have a snack.
- **4:00 to 5:15 p.m**. Play.

- **5:30 p.m**. Watch a television show while parents cook/finish dinner.
- **6:00 to 6:15 p.m**. Dinner.
- **6:30 p.m**. Bath time, brush teeth, and get pajamas on.
- **7:00 p.m**. Do something fun together, letting children lead.
- **7:15 p.m**. Book and cuddle time.
- **7:30 to 7:45 p.m**. Lights-out.[1]

CREATING RULES

Family rules help create structure. A family rule is a specific, clear statement about behaviors you expect from your child. Rules work best when there is consistency, predictability, and follow-through.

WHY ARE FAMILY RULES IMPORTANT?

Family rules help children understand what behaviors are okay and not okay. As children grow, they will be in places where they must follow rules. Following rules at home can help children learn to follow the rules in other places. It is normal for children to break the rules and test limits. Consistent follow-through with consequences when rules are broken helps your child have a clear understanding of the importance of rules. Remember, young kids sometimes break the rules because they simply forget. Not all broken rules occur because kids are testing the limits. However, our responses should be the same no matter the reason for breaking the rule.

WHY SHOULD ALL FAMILY MEMBERS KNOW AND FOLLOW THE RULES?

For family rules to work well, everyone must know, understand, and follow the rules. By doing this, children do not get mixed messages about what is okay or not. For example, you know screen time should be limited for young children, and you want dinner

---

[1] "Building Structure," Centers for Disease Control and Prevention (CDC), November 5, 2019. Available online. URL: www.cdc.gov/parents/essentials/toddlersandpreschoolers/structure/building.html. Accessed March 15, 2024.

time to be family time, so you set a family rule that no screens are allowed during dinner. If another caregiver checks their phone during dinner, your child may be confused. Your child's behavior will be better if all caregivers support the rules in the same way. This is true for parents, grandparents, or any other caregivers in your child's life.

WHAT IS A GOOD NUMBER OF FAMILY RULES FOR TODDLERS AND PRESCHOOLERS?

The number of rules you set depends on your child's ability to understand and remember. It is also hard for parents to consistently enforce lots of new rules. For young children, focus on only two or three of the most important rules at any one time. As your child learns a rule and follows it consistently, you can add new rules.[2]

[2] "Creating Rules," Centers for Disease Control and Prevention (CDC), November 5, 2019. Available online. URL: www.cdc.gov/parents/essentials/toddlersandpreschoolers/structure/rules.html. Accessed March 15, 2024.

Chapter 43 | **Physical Education and Physical Activity for Children**

Physical education is the foundation of a Comprehensive School Physical Activity Program. It is an academic subject characterized by a planned, sequential K–12 curriculum (course of study) based on the national standards for physical education. Physical education provides cognitive content and instruction designed to develop motor skills, knowledge, and behaviors for physical activity and physical fitness. Supporting schools in establishing daily physical education can provide students with the ability and confidence to be physically active for a lifetime.

There are many benefits of physical education in schools. When students get physical education, they can:

- increase their level of physical activity
- improve their grades and standardized test scores
- stay on task in the classroom

Increased time spent in physical education does not negatively affect students' academic achievement.[1]

The Physical Activity Guidelines for Americans, 2nd edition, recommend that children and adolescents aged 6–17 years do 60 minutes or more of moderate-to-vigorous physical activity daily.

[1] "Physical Education," Centers for Disease Control and Prevention (CDC), July 26, 2022. Available online. URL: www.cdc.gov/healthyschools/physicalactivity/physical-education.htm. Accessed March 15, 2024.

BENEFITS OF PHYSICAL ACTIVITY

Regular physical activity can help children and adolescents improve cardiorespiratory fitness, build strong bones and muscles, control weight, reduce symptoms of anxiety and depression, and reduce the risk of developing health conditions such as:

- heart disease
- cancer
- type 2 diabetes
- high blood pressure (HBP)
- osteoporosis
- obesity

CONSEQUENCES OF PHYSICAL INACTIVITY

Physical inactivity can:

- lead to energy imbalance (e.g., expend less energy through physical activity than consumed through diet) and increase the risk of becoming overweight or obese
- increase the risk of factors for cardiovascular disease, including hyperlipidemia (e.g., high cholesterol and triglyceride levels), HBP, obesity, insulin resistance, and glucose intolerance
- increase the risk of developing type 2 diabetes
- increase the risk of developing breast, colon, endometrial, and lung cancers
- lead to low bone density, which, in turn, leads to osteoporosis

PHYSICAL ACTIVITY BEHAVIORS OF YOUNG PEOPLE

- Less than one-quarter (24%) of children aged 6–17 participate in 60 minutes of physical activity daily.
- In 2017, only 26.1 percent of high school students participated in at least 60 minutes per day of physical activity on all seven days of the previous week.
- In 2017, 51.1 percent of high school students participated in muscle-strengthening exercises (e.g., push-ups, sit-ups,

weight lifting) three or more days during the previous week.

- In 2017, 51.7 percent of high school students attended physical education classes in an average week, and only 29.9 percent attended physical education classes daily.

RECOMMENDATIONS FOR PHYSICAL ACTIVITY

- **Aerobic**. For children and adolescents, most of the 60 minutes or more per day should be either moderate- or vigorous-intensity aerobic physical activity and should include vigorous-intensity physical activity at least three days a week.
- **Muscle-strengthening**. As part of their 60 minutes or more of daily physical activity, children and adolescents should include muscle-strengthening physical activity at least three days a week.
- **Bone-strengthening**. Children and adolescents should include bone-strengthening physical activity at least three days a week as part of their 60 minutes or more of daily physical activity.

These guidelines state that children and adolescents be provided opportunities and encouragement to participate in physical activities that are appropriate for their age, enjoyable, and offer variety.

The national recommendation for schools is to have a comprehensive approach to physical education and physical activity. This approach is called "Comprehensive School Physical Activity Programs."

PHYSICAL ACTIVITY AND ACADEMIC ACHIEVEMENT

- Students who are physically active tend to have better grades, school attendance, cognitive performance (e.g., memory), and classroom behaviors (e.g., on-task behavior).

- Higher physical activity and physical fitness levels are associated with improved cognitive performance (e.g., concentration, memory) among students.[2]

[2] "Physical Activity Facts," Centers for Disease Control and Prevention (CDC), July 26, 2022. Available online. URL: www.cdc.gov/healthyschools/physicalactivity/facts.htm. Accessed March 15, 2024.

Chapter 44 | Helping Children Maintain Healthy Habits

Healthy habits are the building blocks of lifelong well-being for children and teens. Healthy eating and physical activity are important for growth and development and to prevent chronic health conditions. They can also help boost students' academic performance. But eating well and being active are only part of the picture. For good mental and physical health, kids also need plenty of sleep and limited screen time. Parents, guardians, and teachers can help children and teens develop healthy habits with these tips.

ENSURE ADEQUATE SLEEP

Children and teens need more sleep than adults, and the amount varies by age. Too little sleep is associated with obesity, partly because inadequate sleep may make us eat more and be less physically active. See the recommended amounts of sleep by age and suggested habits to improve sleep (www.cdc.gov/sleep/features/getting-enough-sleep.html).

REDUCE SCREEN TIME

In young people, too much screen time is associated with poor sleep, weight gain, lower grades in school, and poor mental health. Reducing screen time can help free up time for individual and family activities, improve sleep, and limit cues to eat unhealthy food. Limit the time children and teens watch television, play video games, or use a smartphone or tablet. Instead, encourage children and teens to find fun activities to do with their friends and family members or on their own that involve more activity.

DEVELOP HEALTHY EATING HABITS

The following points are recommended to help children and teens develop healthy eating habits:

- Provide plenty of vegetables, fruits, and whole-grain products.
- Choose lean meats, poultry, fish, lentils, and beans for protein.
- Include low-fat or nonfat milk or dairy products, such as cheese and yogurt.
- Encourage your family to drink water instead of sugary drinks.
- Limit added sugar and saturated fat.

Additionally, you can:

- Encourage kids to eat a healthy breakfast and lunch, whether at home or at school.
- Review school menus with your kids and encourage them to try new foods.
- Model healthy eating at home.

LIMIT SNACKS WITH LOTS OF SALT, ADDED SUGAR, AND SATURATED FAT

Limiting snacks with high amounts of saturated fat, added sugar, and salt can help support healthy eating habits. For everyday snacks, try these easy-to-prepare options:

- one cup of carrots, broccoli, or bell peppers with two tablespoons of hummus
- a medium apple or banana with one tablespoon of peanut butter
- one cup of blueberries or grapes with half a cup of plain, low-fat yogurt
- one-fourth cup of tuna wrapped in a lettuce leaf

HELP CHILDREN AND TEENS STAY ACTIVE

In addition to being fun, regular physical activity has many health benefits, including the following:

- strengthening bones and muscles
- decreasing blood pressure
- reducing the risk of several chronic diseases, including type 2 diabetes and obesity
- reducing the risk of depression
- boosting academic performance by improving attention and memory
- helping regulate body weight and reduce body fat

Children aged three through five years should be active throughout the day. Children and adolescents aged six through 17 should be physically active for at least 60 minutes each day. Include aerobic activity, which is anything that makes their heart beat faster. Also, include bone-strengthening activities such as running or jumping and muscle-strengthening activities such as climbing or push-ups.

To help children and teens get enough physical activity, do the following:

- Make physical activity part of your family's daily routine by walking or playing active games together.
- Encourage children and teens to find fun activities to do alone or with friends and family, such as walking or riding bikes.
- Take young people to places where they can be active, such as public parks or playgrounds, community baseball fields, or community basketball courts.
- Encourage your child to participate in school or community physical activity or sports programs.[1]

[1] "Tips to Support Healthy Routines for Children and Teens," Centers for Disease Control and Prevention (CDC), July 22, 2023. Available online. URL: www.cdc.gov/healthyweight/children/index.html. Accessed March 15, 2024.

Part 7 | Home and Community Safety

Chapter 45 | Childproofing Your Home

Each year, children sustain injuries from hazards in and around the home. The good news is that the risk of injury can be minimized or prevented by following recommended safety practices, using child products that adhere to safety standards, and employing child-safety devices. Most safety devices are readily available and relatively inexpensive. For them to be effective, proper installation and re-engagement after use are essential. It's crucial to follow installation instructions meticulously. Additionally, keep in mind that no device is entirely childproof; determined toddlers have been known to overcome or disable them. Below are safety practices, recommended products meeting safety standards, and child-safety devices designed to reduce injuries to young children. The numbers correspond to those in the images.

- **Use infant sleep products that meet the U.S. Consumer Product Safety Commission (CPSC) mandatory standards (see Figure 45.1 (1)) for your child**. These products include bassinets, cradles, baby cribs, play yards, or bedside sleepers. Place your baby on a firm, flat sleep surface, lying on their back, and alone without any additional items in the sleeping area.
- **Use cordless window coverings (see Figure 45.1 (2)) in homes with young children to help prevent strangulation**. Children can accidentally wrap window covering cords around their necks or pull on cords that are accessible but not clearly visible, leading to entanglement in loops. Cordless options, including affordable choices, are widely available at

major retailers and online. If replacing corded window coverings with cordless ones isn't feasible, contact the Window Covering Safety Council (WCSC) at 800-506-4636 or visit https://windowcoverings.org for a free repair kit. Use tension devices to secure continuous loops and bead chains to the floor or wall. Note that WCSC retrofit kits do not address the risk of dangling pull cords common with many window blinds; trim pull cords to minimize any dangling.

- **Use window guards and safety netting (see Figure 45.1 (3)) to prevent falls from windows, balconies, decks, and landings, as window screens are not sufficient for preventing children from falling out of windows.** Regularly check these safety devices to ensure they are secure, correctly installed, and well-maintained. Limit window openings to four inches or less, including the spacing between window guard bars. If you install window guards, ensure at least one window in each room remains easily accessible for escape during a fire.
- **Use anchors to prevent furniture and appliance tip-overs (see Figure 45.1 (4)).** Furniture, televisions, and ranges can topple over and pose a crushing hazard to young children. Accidents resulting in injuries or fatalities often occur when children climb on or pull themselves up using items like television stands, shelves, bookcases, dressers, desks, chests, and ranges. For enhanced safety, anchor these items to the floor or secure them to a wall. Install antitip brackets for freestanding ranges and stoves to prevent scalding and crushing injuries.
- **Use safety latches and locks (see Figure 45.2 (5)) on cabinets and drawers in kitchens, bathrooms, and other areas to prevent poisonings and other injuries.** These safety devices help restrict access to medicines, laundry detergent, household cleaners, matches, cigarette lighters, knives, and other sharp objects. Even products with child-resistant packaging should be stored

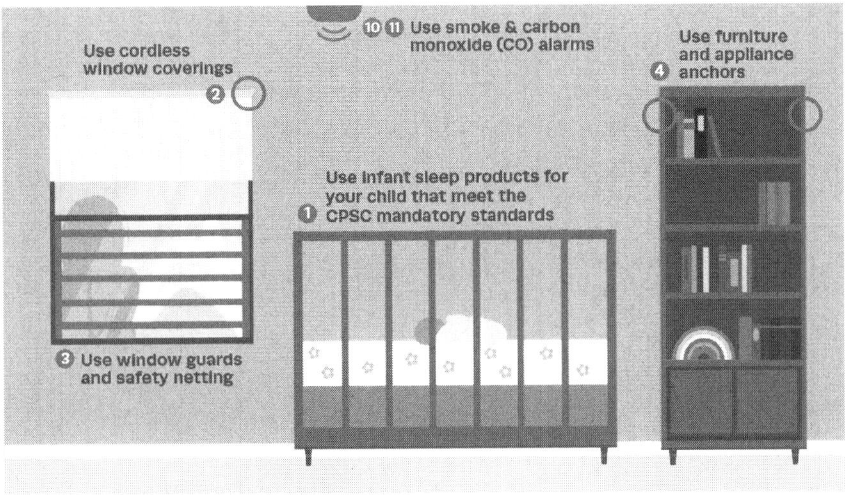

Figure 45.1. Childproofing Bedroom
U.S. Consumer Product Safety Commission (CPSC)

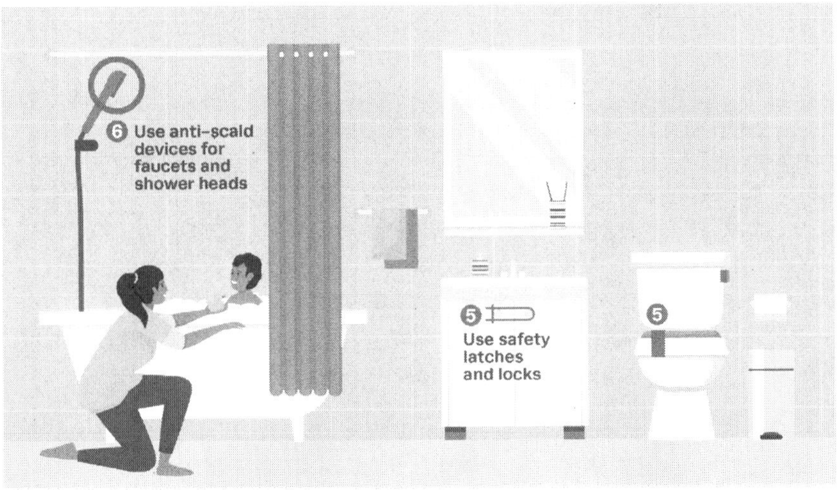

Figure 45.2. Childproofing Bathroom
U.S. Consumer Product Safety Commission (CPSC)

securely and out of reach, as such packaging is not always childproof. If you suspect your child has ingested a poisonous substance, contact the poison control hotline at 800-222-1222. Choose safety latches and locks that are easy for adults to install and use but sturdy enough to withstand children's attempts to open them.

- **Give constant supervision and stay within reach when your baby is bathing.** Children can drown quickly, so it's crucial to maintain constant supervision when they're in or around water. To prevent burns, adjust your water heater to a temperature of 120 °F (48.88 °C) or lower. Additionally, install antiscald devices (see Figure 45.2 (6)) on faucets and showerheads to reduce the risk of scalding or burns.
- **Use multiple layers of protection with pools and spas (see Figure 45.3 (7)).** Most toddler drownings occur in backyard pools, so it's crucial to take preventive measures. Always check the pool first if your child goes missing. The access from the back of your house may need to serve as a barrier to delay your child's access to the pool. Doors leading to the pool should have self-closing, self-locking mechanisms or alarms. Other effective pool barriers include power safety covers, pool alarms, self-closing and self-latching pool gates, isolation and perimeter fences, and pool covers. After each use, ensure that barriers are reestablished to prevent unsupervised access to the pool or spa.
- **Use safety gates (see Figure 45.4 (8)) to help prevent falls down stairs and to keep children from entering rooms and other areas with possible dangers.** Use safety gates that meet current child-safety standards. Pet gates should never be used as child-safety gates. Replace older safety gates that have V shapes large enough to entrap a child's head and neck. Look for safety gates that children cannot dislodge easily but that adults can open and close without difficulty. For the top of stairs, only use gates that screw to the wall.

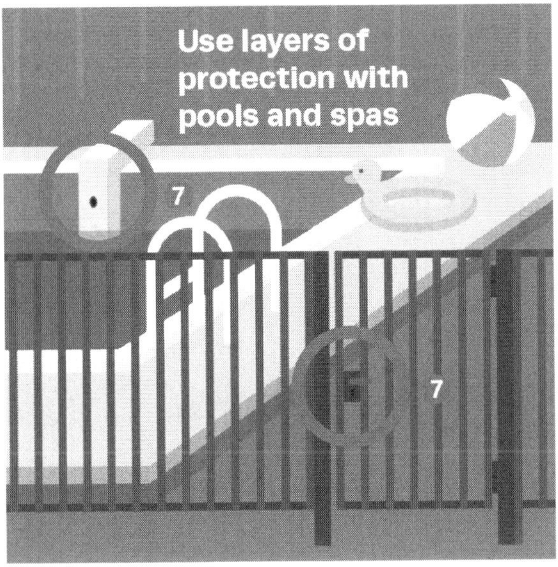

Figure 45.3. Childproofing Pool

U.S. Consumer Product Safety Commission (CPSC)

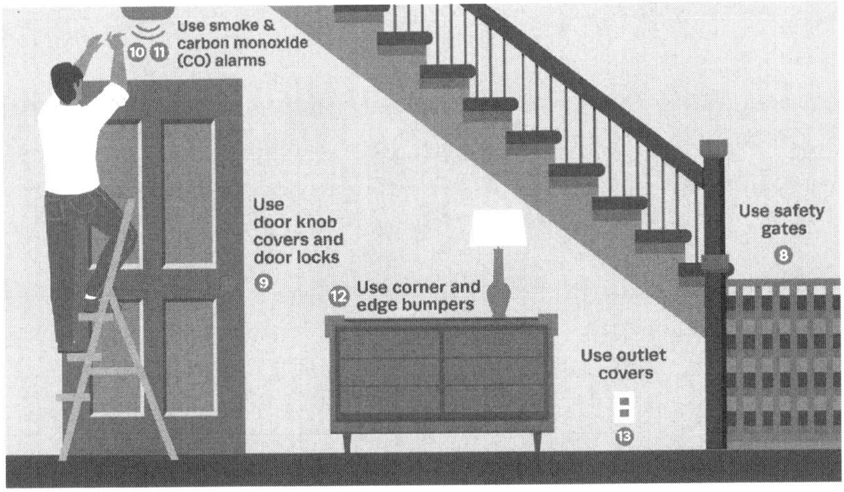

Figure 45.4. Childproofing Hallway

U.S. Consumer Product Safety Commission (CPSC)

- **Use doorknob covers and door locks (see Figure 45.4 (9)) to help prevent children from entering rooms and other areas with possible dangers.** Doorknob covers and door locks can help keep children away from hazardous places. Ensure the doorknob cover is sturdy and allows a door to be opened quickly by an adult in case of emergency.
- **Use smoke alarms (see Figures 45.1 and 45.4 (10)) on every level of your home, inside each bedroom, and outside sleeping areas to alert you to fires.** Smoke alarms are essential safety devices for protection against fire deaths and injuries. Check smoke alarms once a month to make sure they are working. Change batteries at least once a year, or consider using sealed, 10-year batteries for smoke alarms because these do not require yearly battery changes.
- **Use a carbon monoxide (CO) alarm (see Figures 45.1 and 45.4 (11)) to help prevent CO poisoning even when the home does not have fuel-burning appliances.** All consumers should install CO alarms outside of bedrooms near each sleeping area of the home, even if the home does not have any fuel-burning appliances. Test regularly and change batteries at least once a year.
- **Use corner and edge bumpers (see Figure 45.4 (12)) to help prevent injuries from falls against the sharp edges of furniture and fireplaces.** Be sure to look for bumpers that stay securely on furniture or hearth edges.
- **Use outlet covers and outlet plates (see Figure 45.4 (13)) to help prevent electrical shock. Outlet covers and outlet plates can help protect children from electrical shock and possible electrocution.** Ensure outlet protectors cannot be easily removed by children and are large enough so children cannot choke on them. If you are replacing receptacles, use a tamper-resistant type.[1]

---

[1] "Childproofing Your Home—Several Safety Devices to Help Protect Your Children from Home Hazards," U.S. Consumer Product Safety Commission (CPSC), March 22, 2023. Available online. URL: www.cpsc.gov/safety-education/safety-guides/kids-and-babies/Childproofing-Your-Home. Accessed March 13, 2024.

Chapter 46 | Essentials of Safe, Stable, Nurturing Environments

Experiencing significant adversity in childhood, such as being exposed to violence and victimization, has damaging effects on a child's general well-being and lifelong health. The harmful health effects of childhood exposure to serious adversities, such as physical abuse and neglect, witnessing domestic violence, parental substance abuse, and maternal depression, can accumulate over time. On the other hand, social relationships and environments that are secure, supportive, and relatively free of threat can promote healthy child development and encourage adaptive responses to adverse childhood experiences. Developmental, behavioral, and biological research has clearly demonstrated the link between early exposure to stressful events and conditions and impaired neurological, physiological, and psychosocial systems, contributing to a wide array of mental and physical health problems.

DEFINING SAFE, STABLE, NURTURING RELATIONSHIPS AND ENVIRONMENTS

One especially important domain of risk and resiliency involves social interactions and environmental contexts associated with family and caregiving relationships. Children and youth experience much of their world through relationships with parents and caregivers. These relationships are fundamental to the healthy development of physical, emotional, social, behavioral, and intellectual capacities. Conversely, social relationships and environments that are secure, supportive, and relatively free of threat can promote healthy child development and encourage adaptive responses to adverse childhood experiences.

Each of the three dimensions of safe, stable, nurturing relationships represents a significant aspect of the social and physical environments that protect children and promote their optimal healthy development. Each can be thought of as being on a relational and environmental continuum or dichotomy.

"Safety" represents the absence of threat, neglect, and violence and refers to the extent to which children are free from fear and harm within their social and physical environments. Acts of physical abuse, child neglect, harsh or hostile parenting practices, and family drug and alcohol abuse, for example, represent markers of an unsafe family environment.

"Stability" refers to consistency and predictability in the child's environment. Frequent residential moves, household changes, inconsistent childcare, and life events that create volatile or stressful family conditions, such as divorce and job loss, can threaten stability. An unpredictable and chaotic family environment can diminish a child's sense that the world is trustworthy, dependable, and fair and can interfere with a caregiver's ability to parent effectively.

"Nurturing" is characterized by availability, sensitivity, and warmth in responding to a child's needs. Nurturing relationships with caregivers contribute to a child's self-esteem, confidence, social competencies, and emotional development. The nurturing dimension can range from warm and supportive contexts to those characterized by hostility and rejection. Emotional abuse reduces nurturing relationship qualities, whereas supportive interactions, adequate monitoring, social involvement, and caregivers' demonstrations of warmth increase nurturing.

These three dimensions—safe, stable, and nurturing—overlap, but each represents central and distinct aspects of a child's relationships and environments that are critical for healthy development.

IMPLICATIONS FOR PUBLIC HEALTH POLICY

According to a nationally representative study, almost one in four children and adolescents aged 5–15 years in the United States lived in family environments with only modest levels of safety, stability, and nurturance, while about 1 in 15 had consistently low levels across multiple domains. A shortage of safe, stable, nurturing relationships appears to most heavily burden older adolescents and children living in nontraditional family structures. These deficits in the basic foundations of healthy child and adolescent development have crucial implications for the future functioning of these young people.

Relationships and environments that are free of violence and threats are paramount to child and adolescent well-being. Strategies focused on helping families maintain stable and nurturing home environments are important, too, but these results underscore the importance of having a specific focus on reducing exposure to violence and other family conditions that threaten a child's safety—such as harsh parenting and family drug and alcohol problems—as a core component of prevention and intervention efforts to protect children and promote their healthy development.[1]

[1] Office of Juvenile Justice and Delinquency Prevention (OJJDP), "The Prevalence of Safe, Stable, Nurturing Relationships among Children and Adolescents," U.S. Department of Justice (DOJ), September 1, 2017. Available online. URL: https://ojjdp.ojp.gov/sites/g/files/xyckuh176/files/pubs/249197.pdf. Accessed March 13, 2024.

Chapter 47 | Child Abuse and Neglect Prevention

Chapter Contents

Section 47.1 | Understanding and Preventing Adverse Childhood Experiences

WHAT ARE ADVERSE CHILDHOOD EXPERIENCES?

Adverse childhood experiences (ACEs) are potentially traumatic events that occur in childhood (0–17 years). For example, ACEs may take many forms, including:

- experiencing violence, abuse, or neglect
- witnessing violence in the home or community
- having a family member attempt or die by suicide

Also included are aspects of the child's environment that can undermine their sense of safety, stability, and bonding, such as growing up in a household with:

- substance use problems
- mental health problems
- instability due to parental separation or household members being in jail or prison

WHAT ARE THE CONSEQUENCES?

Adverse childhood experiences can have lasting, negative effects on health and well-being in childhood and life opportunities, such as education and job potential, well into adulthood. These experiences can increase the risks of injury, sexually transmitted infections (STIs), maternal and child health problems (including teen pregnancy, pregnancy complications, and fetal death), involvement in sex trafficking, and a wide range of chronic diseases and leading causes of death, such as cancer, diabetes, heart disease, and suicide.

ACEs and associated social determinants of health, such as living in under-resourced or racially segregated neighborhoods, can cause toxic stress (extended or prolonged stress). Toxic stress from ACEs can negatively affect children's brain development, immune systems, and stress-response systems. These changes can affect children's attention, decision-making, and learning.

RISK AND PROTECTIVE FACTORS OF ADVERSE CHILDHOOD EXPERIENCES

The following content explores risk factors (things that increase the likelihood of experiencing ACEs) and protective factors (things that protect people and decrease the possibility of experiencing ACEs). Individual, family, and community factors can affect the likelihood of these experiences, but they may or may not be direct causes of ACEs. Because ACEs include many different types of experiences, including abuse, neglect, household challenges, and other traumatic events that may occur outside the home, such as bullying, teen dating violence (TDV), and witnessing community violence, there are many risk and protective factors that apply to the range of different ACEs.

The following sections list examples of the many common risk and protective factors that are related to multiple ACEs but may not be related to all ACEs. It is also important to note that experiencing some ACEs can increase the risk of experiencing other ACEs. Although some risk and protective factors are at the individual and family level, no child or individual is at fault for the ACEs they experience. The term "caregiver" is used throughout to refer to parents and those who care for children but may not be biological parents.

Risk Factors

INDIVIDUAL AND FAMILY RISK FACTORS

- families experiencing caregiving challenges related to children with special needs (e.g., disabilities, mental health issues, chronic physical illnesses)
- children and youth who do not feel close to their parents/caregivers and feel like they cannot talk to them about their feelings
- youth who start dating early or engaging in sexual activity early
- children and youth with few or no friends or with friends who engage in aggressive or delinquent behavior
- families with caregivers who have a limited understanding of children's needs or development

- families with caregivers who were abused or neglected as children
- families with young caregivers or single parents
- families with low income
- families with adults with low levels of education
- families experiencing high levels of parenting stress or economic stress
- families with caregivers who use spanking and other forms of corporal punishment for discipline
- families with inconsistent discipline and/or low levels of parental monitoring and supervision
- families that are isolated from and not connected to other people (extended family, friends, neighbors)
- families with high conflict and negative communication styles
- families with attitudes accepting of or justifying violence or aggression

COMMUNITY RISK FACTORS

- communities with high rates of violence and crime
- communities with high rates of poverty and limited educational and economic opportunities
- communities with high unemployment rates
- communities with easy access to drugs and alcohol
- communities where neighbors do not know or look out for each other and there is low community involvement among residents
- communities with few community activities for young people
- communities with unstable housing and where residents move frequently
- communities where families frequently experience food insecurity
- communities with high levels of social and environmental disorder

Protective Factors

INDIVIDUAL AND FAMILY PROTECTIVE FACTORS

- families who create safe, stable, and nurturing relationships, meaning children have a consistent family life where they are safe, taken care of, and supported
- children who have positive friendships and peer networks
- children who do well in school
- children who have caring adults outside the family who serve as mentors/role models
- families where caregivers can meet the basic needs of food, shelter, and health services for children
- families where caregivers have college degrees or higher
- families where caregivers have steady employment
- families with strong social support networks and positive relationships with the people around them
- families where caregivers engage in parental monitoring, supervision, and consistent enforcement of rules
- families where caregivers/adults work through conflicts peacefully
- families where caregivers help children work through problems
- families that engage in fun, positive activities together
- families that encourage the importance of school for children

COMMUNITY PROTECTIVE FACTORS

- communities where families have access to economic and financial help
- communities where families have access to medical care and mental health services
- communities with access to safe, stable housing
- communities where families have access to nurturing and safe childcare
- communities where families have access to high-quality preschool
- communities where families have access to safe, engaging after school programs and activities

- communities where adults have work opportunities with family-friendly policies
- communities with strong partnerships between the community and business, health-care, government, and other sectors
- communities where residents feel connected to each other and are involved in the community
- communities where violence is not tolerated or accepted

ACEs do not have a single cause and can take several different forms. Many factors contribute to ACEs, including personal traits and experiences, parents, the family environment, and the community itself. To prevent ACEs and protect children from neglect, abuse, and violence, it is essential to address each of these factors.

HOW TO PREVENT ADVERSE CHILDHOOD EXPERIENCES?

Children growing up with toxic stress may have difficulty forming healthy and stable relationships. They may also have unstable work histories as adults and struggle with finances, jobs, and depression throughout life. These effects can also be passed on to their own children. Some children may face further exposure to toxic stress from historical and ongoing traumas due to systemic racism or the effects of poverty resulting from limited educational and economic opportunities.

HELPING YOUTH AT RISK FOR ADVERSE CHILDHOOD EXPERIENCES

Youth-serving and faith-based organizations, coaches, and caregivers can help prevent and reduce the negative effects of ACEs by creating positive childhood experiences and connecting youth with activities and caring adults that build their sense of safety, confidence, and community. Raising awareness of ACEs in communities and how to prevent these experiences can help children and youth grow up and thrive in a safe, stable environment.[1]

---

[1] National Youth Violence Prevention Resource Center, "Adverse Childhood Experiences (ACEs)," Centers for Disease Control and Prevention (CDC), June 29, 2023. Available online. URL: www.cdc.gov/violenceprevention/aces/fastfact.html. Accessed March 14, 2024.

Section 47.2 | **Preventing Abuse and Neglect**

WHAT ARE CHILD ABUSE AND NEGLECT?

Child abuse and neglect are serious public health problems and adverse childhood experiences (ACEs). They can have long-term effects on health, opportunity, and well-being. This issue includes all types of abuse and neglect of a child under the age of 18 by a parent, caregiver, or another person in a custodial role (such as a religious leader, coach, or teacher) that results in harm, the potential for harm, or threat of harm to a child. There are four common types of abuse and neglect:

- **Physical abuse**. The intentional use of physical force can result in physical injury. Examples include hitting, kicking, shaking, burning, or other shows of force against a child.
- **Sexual abuse**. It involves pressuring or forcing a child to engage in sexual acts. It includes behaviors such as fondling, penetration, and exposing a child to other sexual activities.
- **Emotional abuse**. It refers to behaviors that harm a child's self-worth or emotional well-being. Examples include name-calling, shaming, rejecting, withholding love, and threatening.
- **Neglect**. It is the failure to meet a child's basic physical and emotional needs. These needs include housing, food, clothing, education, access to medical care, and feeling validated and appropriately responded to.

HOW BIG IS THE PROBLEM?

- **Child abuse and neglect are common**. At least one in seven children has experienced child abuse or neglect in the past year in the United States. This is likely an underestimate because many cases are unreported. In 2020, 1,750 children died of abuse and neglect in the United States.
- **Children living in poverty experience more abuse and neglect**. Experiencing poverty can place a lot of stress on

families, which may increase the risk of child abuse and neglect. Rates of child abuse and neglect are five times higher for children in families with low socioeconomic status.

- **Child maltreatment is costly**. In the United States, the total lifetime economic burden associated with child abuse and neglect was about $592 billion in 2018. This economic burden rivals the cost of other high-profile public health problems, such as heart disease and diabetes.

WHAT ARE THE CONSEQUENCES?

Children who are abused and neglected may suffer immediate physical injuries such as cuts, bruises, or broken bones. They may also experience emotional and psychological problems, such as anxiety or posttraumatic stress. Over the long term, children who are abused or neglected are at increased risk for experiencing future violence victimization and perpetration, substance abuse, sexually transmitted infections (STIs), delayed brain development, lower educational attainment, and limited employment opportunities. Chronic abuse may result in toxic stress, which can alter brain development and increase the risk for problems such as posttraumatic stress disorder (PTSD) and difficulties with learning, attention, and memory.

HOW CAN WE PREVENT CHILD ABUSE AND NEGLECT?

Child abuse and neglect are preventable. Certain factors may increase or decrease the risk of perpetrating or experiencing child abuse and neglect. To prevent child abuse and neglect, we must understand and address the factors that put people at risk or protect them from violence. Everyone benefits when children have safe, stable, nurturing relationships and environments. Different types of violence are connected and often share root causes. Child abuse and neglect are linked to other forms of violence through shared risk and protective factors. Addressing and preventing one form of violence may affect the prevention of other forms of violence.

- Strengthen economic support to families:
  - strengthening household financial security
  - family-friendly work policies

- Change social norms to support parents and positive parenting:
  - public engagement and enhancement campaigns
  - legislative approaches to reduce corporal punishment
- Provide quality care and education early in life:
  - preschool enrichment with family engagement
  - improved quality of childcare through licensing and accreditation
- Enhance parenting skills to promote healthy child development:
  - early childhood home visitation
  - parenting skills and family relationship approaches
- Intervene to lessen harms and prevent future risk:
  - enhancing primary care
  - behavioral parents training programs
  - treatment to lessen the harms of abuse and neglect exposure
  - treatment to prevent problem behavior and later involvement in violence[2]

Section 47.3 | **Child Sexual Abuse: Importance of Primary Prevention**

WHAT IS CHILD SEXUAL ABUSE?

Child sexual abuse is a significant public health problem and an adverse childhood experience (ACE). Child sexual abuse refers to the involvement of a child (person less than 18 years old) in sexual activity that violates the laws or social taboos of society and that he/she:

- does not fully comprehend
- does not consent to or is unable to give informed consent to
- is not developmentally prepared for and cannot give consent to

[2] National Youth Violence Prevention Resource Center, "Fast Facts: Preventing Child Abuse & Neglect," Centers for Disease Control and Prevention (CDC), April 6, 2022. Available online. URL: www.cdc.gov/violenceprevention/childabuseandneglect/fastfact.html. Accessed March 14, 2024.

WHAT ARE THE CONSEQUENCES?

Experiencing child sexual abuse can affect how a person thinks, acts, and feels over a lifetime. This can result in short- and long-term physical, mental, and behavioral health consequences.[3]

HOW TO PREVENT

The basics for parents and caretakers in educating their child about sexual abuse are listed below.

Educate Yourself

It is helpful to learn the facts about healthy sexual development as well as child sexual abuse. First, be sure you are comfortable talking about the topic. If you are comfortable using the words, your child will feel that and know they can talk to you. A conversation like this does not need to be a big "talk" but can be something you address gradually. If you are relaxed and easy to talk to, you can be an approachable adult whom your child can ask questions or voice any concerns.

Learn about Healthy Development

It is also helpful to know the typical behaviors for each stage of a child's development. Understand the normal stages of development for preschool, elementary, middle school children, and young teens. Learn the signs of sexual abuse. It will be easier to identify normal behaviors and behaviors that might be of concern. Do not wait until it is too late to learn the signs of sexual abuse.

Talk to Your Child or Teen

Conversations with your child or teen should be open, casual, and ongoing. As your child's understanding of the world grows, conversations can also grow.

[3] National Youth Violence Prevention Resource Center, "Fast Facts: Preventing Child Sexual Abuse," Centers for Disease Control and Prevention (CDC), April 6, 2022. Available online. URL: www.cdc.gov/violenceprevention/childsexualabuse/fastfact.html. Accessed March 14, 2024.

HOW TO TALK TO YOUR CHILD

Discussions about sexuality and sexual abuse can start long before a child reaches puberty. The sooner a parent initiates conversations about healthy sexual development, how the body changes, and sexual abuse, the better. Here are some tips on starting the conversation:

- **Names for body parts**. Properly naming and talking openly about body parts helps children gain respect for their bodies and the bodies of others. These conversations help children avoid feeling ashamed or embarrassed by their bodies and prevent secrecy and silence. Teaching children the names of body parts also gives them the language to ask questions or talk to you about any worries and concerns.
- **Model healthy boundaries**. Teaching your child that it is okay to say no to being touched and to respect when someone tells them no lets them set and respect healthy boundaries. If it is helpful, talk with other adults about boundaries and ask them to respect if a child says no to a hug or other physical affection. This sends a consistent message about respecting each other's boundaries. Be sure to respect a child's boundaries in play and affection.
- **Be sure talks are ongoing**. There is no need to put everything into one big talk about sex. Talking openly about developing bodies, boundaries, and sexuality can be part of ongoing everyday conversations.
- **Be involved in your child's life**. Being engaged in your child's activities, asking about what they are doing, getting to know the parents of your child's friends, and knowing the other adults your child might talk to help you stay connected and involved.
- **Talk about media and technology**. As technology use increases, it is an ever-growing part of children's and teens' lives. Asking questions about technology you do not understand, talking about what your child is doing, and supervising access—especially during the younger

years—will help you monitor what your child sees and hears. Like teaching children to cross the street, it takes time to teach them how to be online safely.

HOW TO TALK TO YOUR TEEN

As a child becomes a teenager, conversations about preventing sexual abuse can become more complicated. Teenagers begin to look for relationships outside the family for friends, security, and advice. They may also feel confused or embarrassed about their developing sexuality, making it more difficult to talk to parents or guardians. As teens go through these stages of exploration, they are also more at risk. Answering questions and being approachable is one way to help keep teens safe.

- **Be realistic and educate yourself.** When teens seek information about sex, their friends may not be reliable sources. Parents can try talking with their teens and letting them know they are available. If a teen is resistant to talking, parents can ask if there is someone else they would feel comfortable with and/or find books or videos with age-appropriate information.
- **Do not put off conversations.** Parents can find small ways to let their teens know they are available to talk. Even if the teen does not want to talk, you are letting them know you are approachable.
- **Explain consent.** It is important for teens to know they have the right to give or refuse consent, regardless of their relationship status. They can say no at any time. It is just as important that they respect the rights of others to say yes or no.

Family and Community Safety

FAMILY SAFETY PLANNING

One way to protect your children is to create a family safety plan. A safety plan gets everyone in the family on the same page and lets you begin important conversations about boundaries, healthy interactions, and how to talk about changing expectations as children grow older. Here are some ideas to get started:

- **Educate everyone in the family**. Make sure every adult knows about healthy sexual development in children and the warning signs of child sexual abuse. Teach children the proper names for body parts so they are aware of their own bodies.
- **Start talking**. Talk with your children and teens and let them know you are open to questions. If you have used the words out loud, they will be more comfortable coming to you with concerns.
- **Set clear family boundaries**. Establish clear family guidelines for personal privacy, respect, safety, healthy communications, and behavior. Talk about these guidelines and model respect for them. Equally important are conversations about what to do when someone ignores or violates a guideline within or outside the family. As a child grows older, boundaries and guidelines may need to change.
- **Get safe adults involved**. Identify people your child can talk to outside the family if there is a concern. Ensure no one in your family is isolated. However, if even a close friend or relative seems too friendly or overly interested, ask more questions. They may not be safe to trust with your child.
- **Know your local resources**. Learn about the agencies in your area and how to contact them. Consider making a list of resources for everyone to have.

SAFETY IN THE COMMUNITY

Organizations working with children and teens focus on creating safe environments for them to grow, explore, learn, and have fun. Part of their commitment is to ensure children and teens are safe while participating in organization-sponsored activities.

- **Check out the organizations your child attends**. To prevent risk, organizations create policies and cultures where child sexual abuse is discussed, addressed, and prevented. Each organization will be different (e.g., summer camp, religious organization, or after-school program) because of the organization's mission, the age of the children or teens they serve, and the activities they offer.

- **Promote safe policies**. If you are a part of an organization working with children or teens, you can help promote policies that support children and keep them safer. The Centers for Disease Control and Prevention (CDC) established six components of effective child sexual abuse prevention:
    - screening and selecting employees and volunteers
    - guidelines on interactions between individuals
    - monitoring behavior
    - ensuring safe environments
    - responding to inappropriate behavior, breaches in policy, and allegations and suspicions of child sexual abuse
    - training about child sexual abuse prevention
- **Encourage organizations to collaborate**. Organizations can also work together to create safer communities for all children and families.

SAFETY IN SCHOOLS

Safety at school is important. Whether at the K-12 or college level, schools offer a unique opportunity to address sexual abuse, sexual assault, and sexual misconduct for students in their care—both in preventing and responding to these issues.

- **Know your state laws**. For schools working with children and teens, adults are mandated to report any suspicion of sexual abuse against a child in their care to law enforcement or child protective services. Each state has different laws on mandatory reporting of sexual abuse against children.
- **Be aware of federal protections**. Federal laws protect students from sexual abuse, sexual assault, and sexual

misconduct, helping to provide safe, supportive learning environments.

- Title IX prohibits sex-based discrimination in all education programs or activities that receive federal financial assistance, including situations of sexual assault and misconduct. It applies to public and private schools, from kindergarten through postsecondary. The Title IX coordinator for a district or school can provide additional information about a school's grievance procedures.
- The Clery Act requires colleges and universities to prepare an annual security report with campus crime statistics and to inform the campus community where they can find information about registered sex offenders. Many colleges and universities have developed protocols and memorandums of understanding with local police to coordinate community responses to any student who reports sexual assault.

- **Know the school's policies**. In addition to the criminal justice system addressing sexual assault, schools have processes to ensure student safety. Schools may classify sexual misconduct as policy violations, often more broadly defined than criminal offenses, which could result in suspension or expulsion. The school administration can provide additional interim measures such as changing a residence on campus, issuing no-contact orders on campus, adjusting class schedules, and restricting access to certain campus events.
- **Talk about prevention**. Prevention is key to school safety. Colleges are required under the Clery Act to provide bystander intervention programs and other prevention strategies. Many K-12 schools offer school-based prevention programs in collaboration with local and national prevention organizations, local rape crisis centers, state and territory coalitions, and child

advocacy centers. These programs and initiatives focus on efforts to prevent child sexual abuse and sexual assault of adults before anyone is harmed.[4]

Section 47.4 | **Abusive Head Trauma**

Abusive head trauma (AHT), which includes shaken baby syndrome, is a preventable and severe form of physical child abuse that results in an injury to the brain of a child. AHT often happens when a parent or caregiver becomes angry or frustrated because of a child's crying. It is caused by violent shaking and/or blunt impact. The resulting injury can cause bleeding around the brain or on the inside back layer of the eyes. Data show the following:

- AHT is a leading cause of physical child abuse deaths in children under five years of age in the United States.
- Babies less than one year of age are at the greatest risk of injury from AHT.
- AHT accounts for about one-third of all child maltreatment deaths.

Crying, including long periods of inconsolable crying, is a normal behavior in infants. Shaking, throwing, or hitting a baby is never the right response to crying.

WHAT ARE THE CONSEQUENCES OF ABUSIVE HEAD TRAUMA?

Nearly all victims of AHT suffer serious, long-term health consequences. Examples include the following:

- vision problems
- developmental delays
- physical disabilities
- hearing loss

[4] The Dru Sjodin National Sex Offender Public Website (NSOPW), "How to Prevent," U.S. Department of Justice (DOJ), August 18, 2023. Available online. URL: www.nsopw.gov/safety-and-education/how-to-prevent#3-0. Accessed March 14, 2024.

At least one of every four babies who experience AHT dies from this form of child abuse.

HOW TO PREVENT ABUSIVE HEAD TRAUMA

Anyone can play a role in preventing AHT. Understanding the dangers of shaking or hitting a baby's head against something, knowing the risk factors and the triggers for abuse, and finding ways to support parents and caregivers in the community are all ways to prevent AHT. The Centers for Disease Control and Prevention (CDC) has developed a technical package, *Preventing Child Abuse and Neglect: A Technical Package for Policy, Norm, and Programmatic Activities* (www.cdc.gov/violenceprevention/pdf/CAN-Prevention-Technical-Package.pdf), that identifies a number of strategies to help states and communities prioritize prevention activities based on the best available evidence.

If you are a parent or caregiver, do the following:

- Understand that infant crying is worse in the first few months of life but will improve as the child grows.
- Try calming a crying baby by rocking gently, offering a pacifier, singing or talking softly, walking with a stroller, or driving in the car.
- If the baby does not stop crying, check for signs of illness and call the doctor if you think the child is sick.
- If you are getting upset, focus on calming yourself down. Put the baby in a safe place and walk away to calm down, checking on the baby every 5–10 minutes.
- Call a friend, relative, neighbor, or parent helpline for support.
- Never leave your baby with a person who is easily irritated, has a temper, or has a history of violence.[5]

---

[5] National Youth Violence Prevention Resource Center, "Preventing Abusive Head Trauma," Centers for Disease Control and Prevention (CDC), April 6, 2022. Available online. URL: www.cdc.gov/violenceprevention/childabuse-andneglect/Abusive-Head-Trauma.html. Accessed March 14, 2024.

Chapter 48 | Child Safety and Injury Prevention

Chapter Contents

MOTOR VEHICLE CRASHES: A LEADING CAUSE OF DEATH FOR CHILDREN

In 2021, 711 child passengers aged 12 and younger were killed in motor vehicle crashes in the United States, and in 2020, more than 63,000 were injured. Of the children who were killed in a crash, 36 percent were not buckled up. Parents and caregivers can make a lifesaving difference by ensuring that their children are properly buckled on every trip.

RISK FACTORS FOR CHILD PASSENGERS

Age

Restraint use (such as car seat, booster seat, or seat belt use) varies by age.

- Restraint use typically decreases as children get older.
    - In a study from 2021, where researchers observed children riding in cars, they found the following data:
        - Less than 1 percent of children under the age of one were not buckled up.
        - Six percent of children one to three years old were not buckled up.
        - Eleven percent of children four to seven years old were not buckled up.
        - Thirteen percent of children 8–12 years old were not buckled up.
    - Being unrestrained in a vehicle increases the risk of being killed in a crash. In a study from 2023 using fatal crash data, researchers found the following:
        - Thirty percent of zero- to three-year-olds killed in crashes were not buckled up.
        - Thirty-six percent[§] of 8- to 12-year-olds killed in crashes were not buckled up.
- Also, among children who are buckled up in child restraints, many graduate too soon to the next stage of

child passenger safety. An example is when children stop using a booster seat before the seat belt fits them correctly. Age-appropriate restraint use typically decreases as children get older.

§Restraint status was known for 209 of the 242 child passenger vehicle occupants aged 8–12 who were killed in crashes in 2021. Among the 209 child passengers (aged 8–12) for which restraint status was known, 76 (36%) were unrestrained. Restraint status was known for 206 of the 223 child passenger vehicle occupants aged zero to three who were killed in crashes in 2021. Among the 206 child passengers (aged 0–3) for whom restraint status was known, 61 (30%) were unrestrained.

Rural versus Urban Location

Children in rural areas are typically at higher risk of being killed in a crash. The following are the facts according to combined data from 2015 to 2019:

- Child passenger death rates were highest in the most rural counties (4.5 per 100,000 population) and lowest in the most urban counties (0.9).
- Death rates among children who were not using age-appropriate restraints were highest in the most rural counties (2.9 per 100,000 population) and lowest in the most urban counties (0.5).

Studies also indicate that children in rural areas are more likely to be incorrectly restrained than children in urban areas.

- A multistate study using data from car seat check events found that child restraint misuse was more common in rural locations (91%) than in urban locations (83%). Similar to racial and ethnic disparities, there are likely several factors for these differences.

Alcohol-Impaired Driving

Alcohol-impaired driving is a major threat to all road users, including child passengers.

- In 2021, 25 percent of deaths among child passengers (aged 14 and younger) involved an alcohol-impaired driver.

- Among all child passengers (aged 14 and younger) who were killed in crashes, a higher proportion of those riding with alcohol-impaired drivers were unrestrained (43%)¶ compared with children riding with drivers who had no alcohol in their system (38%).
- Other studies* have also found an association between driver alcohol use and child passengers being unrestrained. For example, one study among children under two years old who were killed in crashes found that the odds of the child being unrestrained were 2.2 times higher when the driver had been drinking alcohol than when the driver had not been drinking.

¶These percentages are based on child passenger vehicle occupants for which restraint status was known.
**The Quinlan et al. study assessed drivers with a blood alcohol content (BAC) ≥0.08 g/dL. The Huang et al. study assessed drivers who tested positive for alcohol. About 22 percent of these drivers had a BAC lower than ≥0.08 g/dL.*

Driver Seat Belt Use

Restraint use among children is associated with their driver's seat belt use.

- In 2021, 69 percent[††] of child passengers aged 14 and younger killed in crashes who rode with unbuckled drivers were also not buckled up, compared with 26 percent of children riding with buckled drivers.
- Researchers who observed adults and children riding in cars in 2021 found that 95 percent of children aged seven and younger who were driven by a buckled driver were restrained, compared with 77 percent of children driven by an unbuckled driver.
- Many other studies assessing different child age groups or specific geographic locations have also found strong associations between unrestrained drivers and unrestrained child passengers.

††These percentages are based on child passenger vehicle occupant and driver dyads for which restraint status was known.

Car Seat and Booster Seat Misuse

Car seats and booster seats are often used incorrectly, which can make them less effective.

- Researchers who observed children riding in cars in 2011 estimated that 46 percent of car seats and booster seats are used incorrectly in a way that could reduce their effectiveness. Car seat misuse estimates are even higher at 59 percent when booster seats are excluded. The most common errors were:
  - incorrect recline angle for rear-facing car seats
  - loose installation for all car seats
  - loose harness for all car seats
  - harness behind the child's arms, legs, or back in forward-facing car seats
  - improper lap belt position for booster seats
  - improper shoulder belt position for booster seats
- Some smaller studies indicate that misuse could be 85 percent or more in some areas.[1]

KNOW THE STAGES

Ensure children are properly buckled in a car seat, booster seat, or seat belt—whichever is appropriate for their age, weight, and height.

- Use a rear-facing car seat from birth until ages two to four.
  - Infants and toddlers should be buckled in a rear-facing car seat with a harness in the back seat until they reach the maximum weight or height limit of their car seat. This offers the best possible protection.
  - Check the car seat manual and labels on the car seat for weight and height limits.
  - Never place a rear-facing car seat in the front seat. Front passenger airbags can injure or kill young children in a crash.

---

[1] National Center for Injury Prevention and Control (NCIPC), "Keep Child Passengers Safe on the Road," Centers for Disease Control and Prevention (CDC), October 14, 2022. Available online. URL: www.cdc.gov/injury/features/child-passenger-safety/index.html. Accessed March 15, 2024.

- After outgrowing their rear-facing car seat, use a forward-facing car seat until at least the age of five.
  - When children outgrow their rear-facing car seat, they should be buckled in a forward-facing car seat with a harness and a top tether in the back seat.
  - Children should stay in their forward-facing car seat until they reach the maximum weight or height limit of this seat.
  - Check the car seat manual and labels on the car seat for weight and height limits.
- After outgrowing their forward-facing car seat, use a booster seat until the seat belt fits properly.
  - When children outgrow their forward-facing car seat, they should be buckled in a belt-positioning booster seat with a seat belt in the back seat until the seat belt fits properly without a booster seat.
  - A seat belt fits properly when the lap belt is across the upper thighs (not the stomach), and the shoulder belt is across the center of the shoulder and chest (not across the neck or face, and not off the shoulder). This usually occurs when children are between 9 and 12 years old.
- When the seat belt fits properly without a booster seat, use a seat belt on every trip.
  - Children no longer need to use a booster seat when the seat belt fits them properly. A seat belt fits properly when the lap belt is across the upper thighs (not the stomach), and the shoulder belt is across the center of the shoulder and chest (not across the neck or face and not off the shoulder).
  - Proper seat belt fit usually occurs when children are between 9 and 12 years old.
  - Seat belt fit can vary by vehicle, so check seat belt fit in all vehicles where the child will ride to ensure the child no longer needs to use a booster seat. Sometimes a child might need a booster seat in one vehicle but not in a different vehicle.

- Keep children properly buckled in the back seat through age 12 for the best possible protection.[2]

Section 48.2 | **Pedestrian and Bicycle Safety**

EVERYONE IS A PEDESTRIAN

Everyone has different preferences when it comes to transportation, but at one time or another, everyone is a pedestrian. When drivers maintain safe speeds and practice other safe driving behaviors, safer walking environments are created for you, your loved ones, and others in your community.

KEEPING YOUR KIDS SAFE WHILE THEY WALK

- **Elementary school children are very active and impulsive.** Although they are learning and growing, school-age children 10 and younger still need guidance and supervision when playing and walking near traffic. For more information, visit the Prevent Pedestrian Crashes: Parents and Caregivers of Elementary School Children website (www.nhtsa.gov/sites/nhtsa.gov/files/811027.pdf).
- **Strengthen your traffic safety knowledge by teaching and reinforcing your children's pedestrian safety habits.** For more information, visit the "Five tips to keep your children safe on their way to and from school" website (www.nhtsa.gov/school-bus-safety/keeping-children-safe).
- **The colorful pamphlet will help you teach young children safety tips for crossing the street and things to remember when walking.** For more information, visit the A Kid's Guide to Safe Walking website (www.nhtsa.gov/sites/nhtsa.gov/files/811026.pdf).

[2] "Child Passenger Safety: Get the Facts," Centers for Disease Control and Prevention (CDC), September 11, 2023. Available online. URL: www.cdc.gov/transportationsafety/child_passenger_safety/cps-factsheet.html. Accessed March 15, 2024.

- **Remind your preteens and teens that walking around traffic requires the same critical thinking skills as riding a bike or driving a car: stop, look left-right-left, be safe, and be seen.** For more information, visit the Tips for Preteens and Teens: Prevent Pedestrian Crashes website (www.nhtsa.gov/sites/nhtsa.gov/files/11146b-preventpedestriancrashes.pdf).[3]

Understand that the road is a shared space, and bicyclists should follow the same rules and responsibilities as drivers:

- Ride in a straight line, single file, in the same direction as traffic.
- Obey all traffic signs and signals.
- Stop and look left-right-left for traffic before entering a street.
- Use bike lanes whenever available.

Bikers should always wear a helmet that fits level on the head and low on the forehead, one or two finger widths above the eyebrows. Also, adjust the slider on both side straps to form a V shape under and slightly in front of the ears, and lock the slider if possible. Before heading out on the road for the first time, or if it has been a while since your last bike ride, practice in a safe area. In some areas, traffic gardens are available. Communities and schools have worked with designers to turn playgrounds and lots into miniature street networks, allowing children to learn to navigate and use streets in a comfortable space free of cars. The goal of traffic gardens is to teach children about road safety so they become adults who truly understand how streets work—and how to be safe on them.

Maybe it is time we rethink the phrase, "It's like riding a bike." It is often used to describe a task that is easy to accomplish if you learned it once. But what happens if you never learned the correct

[3] "Pedestrian Safety," National Highway Traffic Safety Administration (NHTSA), December 16, 2016. Available online. URL: www.nhtsa.gov/road-safety/pedestrian-safety. Accessed March 18, 2024.

way to ride a bike? Well, it is never too late to relearn. Here are some more tips:

- Check your bike.
  - Tires should be properly inflated.
  - Brakes should be checked before you get on your bike.
- Be visible.
  - Wear bright colors, reflective materials at night and in low-light conditions.
  - Make sure your reflector is visible, and consider adding a light to your bicycle.[4]

BICYCLING IS FUN, HEALTHY, AND A GREAT FAMILY ACTIVITY

A bicycle is not a toy; it is a vehicle! Some bike crashes can cause serious injuries, and most are related to the behavior of the bicyclist or the motorist. There are several things you can do to prevent a crash and protect your brain if a crash occurs.

RULES OF THE ROAD—BICYCLING ON THE ROAD

In all states, bicycles on the roadway are considered vehicles, and bicyclists are drivers with the same rights and responsibilities as motorists to follow the rules of the road. When riding, always do the following:

- **Go with the traffic flow**. Ride on the right in the same direction as other vehicles. Go with the flow—not against it.
- **Obey all traffic laws**. A bicycle is a vehicle, and you are the driver. When you ride in the street, obey all traffic signs, signals, and lane markings.
- **Yield to traffic**. Most drivers on a smaller road must yield (wait) for traffic on a major or larger road. If there is no stop sign or traffic signal, and you are coming from a smaller roadway (out of a driveway, from a sidewalk, a bike path, etc.), you must slow down and

[4] "Learn to Bike Safely," National Highway Traffic Safety Administration (NHTSA), May 14, 2020. Available online. URL: www.nhtsa.gov/learn-bike-safely. Accessed April 10, 2024.

look to see if the way is clear before proceeding. Yield to pedestrians in a crosswalk.

- **Be predictable**. Ride in a straight line, not in and out of cars. Signal your moves to others.
- **Stay alert at all times**. Use your eyes and ears. Watch out for potholes, cracks, wet leaves, storm grates, railroad tracks, or anything that could make you lose control of your bike. Listen for traffic and avoid dangerous situations; do not use personal electronics when you ride.
- **Look before turning**. When turning left or right, always look behind you for a break in traffic and signal before making the turn. Watch for left- or right-turning traffic.
- **Watch for parked cars**. Ride far enough out from the curb to avoid the unexpected from parked cars (such as doors opening or cars pulling out).

TIPS FOR SAFE RIDING

Before riding, make sure you, your family, and the bicycles are ready to ride. Be a "role model" for other adults and children. Remember to do the following:

- **Wear a bicycle helmet**. Everyone—at every age—should wear bicycle helmets.
- **Adjust your bicycle to fit**. Stand over your bicycle. There should be one to two inches between the rider and the top tube (bar) if using a road bike and three to four inches if using a mountain bike. The seat should be level front to back, and the height should be adjusted to allow a slight bend at the knee when the leg is fully extended. The handlebar height should be level with the seat.
- **Check your equipment**. Before riding, inflate the tires properly and check that the brakes work.
- **See and be seen**. Whether it's daytime, dawn, dusk, bad weather, or night, make yourself visible to others. Wear neon, fluorescent, or other bright colors when riding to

be most easily seen. Wear something that reflects light, such as reflective tape or markings, or flashing lights. Remember, just because you can see a driver does not mean the driver can see you.
- **Control the bicycle.** Ride with two hands on the handlebars, except when signaling a turn. Place books and other items in a bicycle carrier or backpack.
- **Watch for and avoid road hazards.** Look for hazards such as potholes, broken glass, gravel, puddles, leaves, and dogs. All these hazards can cause a crash.
- **Use verbal and nonverbal communication.** This includes eye contact with drivers, turn signals, pointing to road hazards for bicyclists behind you, and stating "passing on your left" or "on your left."
- **Avoid riding at night.** It is hard for road users to see bicyclists at dusk, dawn, and nighttime. Use reflectors on the front and rear of your bicycle. White lights and red rear reflectors or lights are required by law in all states.

WHERE TO RIDE SAFELY

- Use bike lanes or bike paths, if available.
  - While bicycles are allowed on many roads, riders may feel safer being separated from traffic. A lane or path is a safer choice than riding on a sidewalk.
  - Riding on sidewalks puts you in a place where cars do not look for or expect to see moving traffic.
  - Sidewalk riding puts you at risk for crashes at driveways and intersections.
- Children younger than 10 years old cannot consistently make the decisions necessary to safely ride unsupervised in the street. Therefore, they are safer riding away from traffic.
- The following are the instructions for anyone riding on a sidewalk:
  - Check the law in your state or jurisdiction to ensure sidewalk riding is allowed.
  - Watch for vehicles coming out of or turning into driveways.

- Stop at corners of sidewalks and streets to look for cars and to make sure the drivers see you before crossing.
- Enter a street at a corner and not between parked cars. Alert pedestrians that you are nearby, saying, "passing on your left," or use a bell or horn.[5]

Section 48.3 | **Drowning Prevention**

DROWNING IS A LEADING CAUSE OF DEATH FOR CHILDREN

Keeping children safe in and around water allows everyone to enjoy summer water activities. Drowning is the leading cause of death for children aged one to four years and the second leading cause of unintentional injury death for children aged 5–14 years. Drowning can happen in seconds and is often silent. It can occur in any body of water, including pools, lakes, bathtubs, and water-filled buckets. However, drowning is preventable.

CONSIDERATIONS FOR WATER SAFETY

Swimming lessons can reduce the risk of drowning. Consider enrolling children in swimming lessons and consider lessons for yourself to improve your swimming skills and comfort in the water. It is never too late to learn to swim, and the benefits increase as we age.

Keep in mind that children who have had swimming lessons still need close and constant supervision when in or around water, even when a lifeguard is present. An adult should always be within arm's length of a child who is in or near water. When supervising children, a responsible adult should avoid distracting activities such as reading, using the phone, and consuming alcohol or drugs because drowning happens quickly and quietly.

Even nonfatal drowning can result in long-term health problems and costly hospital stays. Drowning injuries can cause brain damage and other serious outcomes, including long-term disability. For

[5] "Bicycle Safety Tips," National Highway Traffic Safety Administration (NHTSA), January 2013. Available online. URL: www.nhtsa.gov/sites/nhtsa.gov/files/811557.pdf. Accessed April 23, 2024.

every child under the age of 18 who dies from drowning, another seven receive emergency department care for nonfatal drowning. Nearly 40 percent of drownings treated in emergency departments require a hospital stay or transfer for further care. This is four times higher than the number of other unintentional injuries that require follow-up care.

POOLS AND NATURAL WATER

Home swimming pools need a four-sided fence at least four feet high that fully encloses the pool and separates it from the house. The fence should have a self-closing and self-latching gate. All toys that might attract a child should be removed from the pool when no one is using it.

Floaties, armbands, or water wings do not prevent children from drowning and can easily slip off, especially when kids jump into the water. Water wings can produce a false sense of safety for parents and children and can inhibit a child's ability to learn to swim. A life jacket approved by the U.S. Coast Guard is more protective.

About 40 percent of drowning deaths among children aged 5–14 occur in natural water. More than half of fatal and nonfatal drownings among people 15 years and older occur in natural or open waters such as lakes, rivers, or oceans. Wearing properly fitted life jackets can be beneficial for many activities in and around natural water, not just boating. When in or around open or natural water—whether in a boat or in the water—children and adults are best protected by wearing life jackets approved by the U.S. Coast Guard that are well-fitted to their size and fully fastened when boating. Over 80 percent of people who drowned while boating in 2021 were not wearing a life jacket.

Drowning is preventable. Follow these key prevention steps:

- Properly fence home swimming pools.
- Learn how to swim and teach children how to swim.
- Supervise children closely and constantly when they are in or near water.
- Wear a properly fitted life jacket.[6]

[6] National Center for Injury Prevention and Control (NCIPC), "Summer Swim Safety," Centers for Disease Control and Prevention (CDC), June 12, 2023. Available online. URL: www.cdc.gov/injury/features/drowning/index.html. Accessed April 9, 2024.

LEARN HOW TO KEEP CHILDREN SAFER AROUND POOLS AND SPAS

Supervise Children: Always Watch Children in or near Water, Never Leave Them Unattended

Always watch children when they are in or near water and never leave them unattended. Designate an official water watcher, an adult tasked with supervising children in the water. That should be their only task; they should not read, text, or play games on their phone. Have a phone close by at all times in case you need to call for help, and if a child is missing, check the pool first.

Even if a lifeguard is present, parents and caregivers should still be designated water watchers. When any lifeguard chair is empty, the remaining lifeguards may not be able to see the entire pool, and when lifeguards are seated in low chairs, their view can be blocked by patrons in the pool.

Learn to Swim: Teach Children How to Swim

Swimming is not only fun; it is also a lifesaving skill. Enroll children in swimming lessons; many free or reduced-cost options are available from your local Young Men's Christian Association (YMCA), USA Swimming chapter, or Parks and Recreation Department.

Know Your Drains: Teach Children to Stay Away from Drains

Do not play or swim near drains or suction outlets, especially in spas and shallow pools. Never enter a pool or spa with a loose, broken, or missing drain cover. Children's hair, limbs, jewelry, or bathing suits can get stuck in a drain or suction opening. When using a spa, be sure to locate the emergency vacuum shutoff before getting in the water.

Install Safety Devices: Install Barriers, Covers, and Alarms

Proper fences, barriers, alarms, and covers can be lifesaving devices. A fence of at least four feet in height should surround the pool or spa on all sides and should not be climbable for children. The water should only be accessible through a self-closing, self-latching gate. Teach children never to climb over the gate or fence. Install a door alarm from the house to the pool area, and keep pool and spa covers in working order.

Get Certified: Know How to Perform Cardiopulmonary Resuscitation on Children and Adults

Often, bystanders are the first to aid a drowning victim, so learning cardiopulmonary resuscitation (CPR) can help save a life. Once you are CPR certified, make sure to keep your certification current. CPR classes are available through many hospitals, community centers, or by contacting the American Red Cross.

Take the Pledge: Take the Pool Safely Pledge!

Before heading to the pool or spa with your family, remember to take the Pool Safely Pledge. This online call to action is a reminder to stay safer around the water.[7]

Section 48.4 | Poisoning and Drug Overdose

Unintentional pediatric poisoning deaths of children under the age of five increased by 66 percent to 98 in 2021. This increase was largely linked to narcotics and psychodysleptics. Deaths in this category nearly doubled in one year, from 33 in 2021 to 59 in 2022. This National Poison Prevention Week (March 17–23, 2024) marks 62 years since the first national observation. There are growing risks associated with these substances, with pediatric poisoning deaths in the United States rising steadily since 2019 from a low of 17 deaths in 2018, the lowest since the Consumer Product Safety Commission (CPSC) was created in 1972. Additionally, there were an estimated 68,600 emergency department–treated injuries in children under the age of five in 2022, a nearly 10 percent increase from the estimated 62,600 injuries in 2021. Nearly seven out of 10 poisonings occurred in the home. The CPSC encourages family members and caregivers to identify hazards in the home that could be a poisoning danger and keep them out of a child's sight and reach.

[7] "Safety Tips," U.S. Consumer Product Safety Commission (CPSC), May 6, 2012. Available online. URL: www.poolsafely.gov/parents/safety-tips. Accessed April 9, 2024.

SAFETY TIPS FOR PARENTS AND CAREGIVERS

- Laundry packets:
    - Store laundry packets in their original containers and out of a child's sight and reach.
    - Do not let children handle laundry detergent packets.
- Button cell or coin batteries:
    - Keep products with accessible batteries away from children if the battery compartments do not have a screw closure or if the compartment is damaged.
    - Check your home's toys to ensure battery compartments are secured.
    - Do not allow children to play with or be in contact with button cell or coin batteries.[8]

More than 90 percent of the time, poisonings happen in people's homes. The majority of these poisonings occur in the kitchen, bathroom, and bedroom. That is why it is important to follow simple steps to prevent poisonings at home. Teach your family to never touch or put anything in their mouths unless they know what it is. Below are additional tips on how to keep poisonous items safe in your home.

- Medicines:
    - Keep all medicines, as well as potentially poisonous substances, in locked cabinets or out of the reach of children.
    - Keep medicines in their original containers, properly labeled, and store them appropriately.
    - Never share prescription medicines. If you are taking more than one drug at a time, check with your health-care provider or pharmacist, or call the toll-free Poison Help line (1-800-222-1222), which connects you to your local poison center, to find out more about possible drug interactions.

[8] "Poison Prevention," U.S. Consumer Product Safety Commission (CPSC), October 3, 2022. Available online. URL: www.cpsc.gov/Safety-Education/Safety-Education-Centers/Poison-Prevention-Information-Center. Accessed April 10, 2024.

- Carbon monoxide (CO):
  - Have a working CO detector in your home. The best places for a CO detector are near bedrooms and close to furnaces.
- Household products:
  - Household cleaners and disinfectants can make you sick when not used properly. Always follow the instructions on the product label to ensure safe and effective use.
  - Bleach is especially toxic and should not be mixed with anything other than water.
  - Do not use food containers (such as cups or bottles) to store household cleaners and other chemicals or products.
  - Do not use bleach on food products.
  - Avoid using household cleaners and disinfectants on hands or skin improperly.
- Chemicals:
  - Keep antifreeze and all chemicals and household products in their original containers.
  - Never mix household or chemical products together. Doing so can create a dangerous gas.
- Back to school and art supplies:
  - Some art products are mixtures of chemicals. They can be dangerous if not used correctly. Make sure children use art products safely by reading and following directions.
  - Do not eat or drink while using art products.
  - Wash skin after contact with art products.
  - Clean equipment. Wipe tables, desks, and counters.
  - Keep art products in their original containers.
- Food:
  - Wash fruits and vegetables with running water.
  - Do not wash meat, poultry, or eggs.
  - Never use commercial cleaning products on food or food packaging.
  - Wash your hands and work surfaces before, during, and after preparing food.
  - Wash hands and counters before preparing all food.

    - Store food at the proper temperatures. Refrigerated foods should not be left out at temperatures above 40 °F (5 °C).
    - Use clean utensils for cooking and serving.
- Animals and insects:
    - Know what poisonous snakes live in your area and wear proper attire (boots, etc.) when hiking outdoors.
    - Check the label on any insect repellent. Be aware that most contain N-diethyl-meta-toluamide (DEET), which can be poisonous in large quantities.
- Plants, mushrooms, and berries:
    - Be sure that everyone in your family can identify poisonous mushrooms and plants.
    - Call your local poison center to learn about common poisonous plants in your area.[9]

Section 48.5 | Fire Safety and Burn Prevention

The relative risk of children dying in a fire is now lower than that of the general population. This reduced risk may be attributed, in part, to an increase in public fire education and prevention efforts by fire departments and other fire safety organizations.

MAKE A FIRE ESCAPE PLAN

It is important to have a plan when there are children in your home. Children sometimes need help getting out of the house. They may not know how to escape or what to do unless an adult shows them.

[9] "Prevention Tips," Health Resources and Services Administration (HRSA), October 6, 2010. Available online. URL: https://poisonhelp.hrsa.gov/what-you-can-do/prevention-tips. Accessed April 10, 2024.

- **Have a plan for young children who cannot get outside alone**. You must wake babies and young children and help them get out. In your plan, discuss who will help each child get out safely.
- **It is important to find two ways out of every room in your home in case the first exit is blocked or dangerous to use.**
- **Choose a meeting place outside your home**. Children should know what to do when they hear a smoke alarm, and no adult is around. Help them practice going to the outside meeting place. Teach them to never go back inside a building that is on fire.

KEEP CHILDREN SAFE FROM FIRE AND BURNS

Some children are curious about fire. The following are simple steps you can take to keep you and the people you love safer from fire and burns:

- **Space heaters and stovetops can cause terrible burns**. Keep children at least three feet away from stoves, heaters, or anything that gets hot.
- **Keep smoking materials locked up in a high place**. Never leave cigarette lighters or matches where children can reach them.
- **Never play with lighters or matches when you are with your children**. Children may try to do the same things they see you do.[10]

Teach children the following things:

- Only adults should use matches and lighters.
- Even small fires can spread very quickly.
- Fire is a tool, not a toy, and must only be used by adults.
- Make your home safer by:
    - inspecting it for fire hazards
    - keeping lighters and matches away from children
    - supervising children

[10] "Fire Safety for Children," U.S. Fire Administration (FA), April 1, 2023. Available online. URL: www.usfa.fema.gov/prevention/home-fires/at-risk-audiences/children. Accessed March 18, 2024.

- having working smoke alarms on every level and inside and outside all sleeping areas
- planning and practicing your home fire escape plan[11]

MESSAGES TO SHARE WITH KIDS

- **Fires burn fast and hot; smoke can make a room dark.**
- **You should know two ways out of every room and two ways out of your house.**
- **Before you open a door, feel it.** If it is hot, use your other exit.
- **Stay low and get to your exit if you smell or see smoke or if your smoke alarm sounds.**
- **Stay outside.** Do not go back inside for anything.
- **Never touch matches, lighters, or candles.** If you find matches or lighters, tell an adult.
- **If you get burned, put the burn under cool water for three to five minutes.** Tell an adult right away about your burn.[12]

Section 48.6 | Fall Prevention

Falls are the leading cause of nonfatal injuries for all children aged 0–19. Every day, approximately 8,000 children are treated in U.S. emergency rooms for fall-related injuries. This adds up to almost 2.8 million children each year. However, injuries from falls can be prevented, and you can play a key role in protecting the children you love.

To keep kids safe on a playground, ensure they use playground equipment that is properly designed and maintained and has a safe, soft landing surface below. This can help reduce the likelihood of injury if your little one trips and falls while playing.

[11] "Youth Firesetting," U.S. Fire Administration (FA), May 24, 2023. Available online. URL: www.usfa.fema.gov/prevention/arson/prevent-youth-firesetting. Accessed April 10, 2024.
[12] See footnote [10].

Also, use home safety devices, such as guards on windows above ground level, stair gates, and guard rails. Falls can happen at home as well as at the playground, so these safety devices can help keep a busy, active child from taking a dangerous tumble.

When your child is quickly growing and developing, they may go from not being mobile one day to suddenly rolling over on their own and crawling soon after. Be aware of your child's level of mobility and anticipate their actions. Just because your toddler has not tried to crawl down the stairs yet does not mean they will not try tomorrow.

Simple precautions can help prevent injury. Make sure your child wears protective gear when playing active sports, such as wrist guards, knee and elbow pads, and a helmet when in-line skating. This gear can reduce the likelihood of sports-related injuries and help keep your child in the game. Close supervision of children in your care is a critical step to prevent injury from falls, whether you are at home or out to play. It is important to supervise young children at all times around fall hazards, such as stairs and playground equipment.

When it comes to a child you love, you naturally want to protect them from harm. It is within your power to help them live to their full potential without experiencing the pain and suffering that injuries can cause.[13]

Although injury death rates have declined in the past two decades for children aged 1–14, unintentional injuries remain the leading cause of death for children aged one to four and aged five to 14. Nonfatal injuries continue to be significant causes of child morbidity, disability, and reduced quality of life. The economic cost (medical expenses and productivity losses) of injuries among children under the age of 15 in 2019 was $396 billion. In 2020, there were 4,272 fatal injuries and nearly 3 million emergency department (ED) visits for nonfatal injuries among children aged 1–14. The leading causes of injury differ for children and adolescents.

---

[13] "Protect the Ones You Love from Falls," Centers for Disease Control and Prevention (CDC), December 10, 2016. Available online. URL: www2c.cdc.gov/podcasts/media/pdf/ProtecttheOnesYouLove-Falls.pdf. Accessed March 18, 2024.

- Among children aged one to four and aged 5–14, falls were the leading cause of injury-related ED visits in 2019–2020.
- For children aged 5–14, being struck (see Figure 48.1) by or against an object or person was the second leading cause of injury-related ED visits in 2019–2020. For children aged one to four, there was no significant difference between being struck by or against an object or person and natural or environmental factors.
- In 2019–2020, there were 54 ED visits for falls per 1,000 children aged one to four and 28 ED visits for falls per 1,000 children aged 5–14. Falls accounted for 39 percent of initial injury-related ED visits for children aged one to four and 29 percent of initial injury-related ED visits for children aged 5–14.
- The rates of injury-related ED visits resulting from being struck by or against an object or person were 19 visits per 1,000 for children aged one to four and aged 5–14.
- Injury-related ED visits for injuries caused by natural or environmental factors, including insect and animal bites, were 12 visits per 1,000 for children aged one to four and 6 visits per 1,000 for children aged 5–14.

Note: *Visits are the initial visit to the ED for the injury. "Struck" denotes being struck by or against an object or person, "natural or environmental" denotes injuries caused by natural or environmental factors such as insect or animal bites, and "cut or pierced" denotes injuries caused by cutting or piercing from instruments or objects.*

DEATH RATES AMONG CHILDREN AGED 1–14 BY CAUSE OF DEATH AND AGE GROUP, 2021

- From 2011 to 2021, the all-cause death rate among children aged one to four declined from 26.3 deaths per 100,000 to 25.0 deaths per 100,000. The injury-related death rate among children aged one to four decreased from 11.4 deaths per 100,000 in 2011 to 9.5 deaths per 100,000 in 2019 but did not change significantly through 2021 at 11.2 deaths per 100,000.

- The all-cause death rate among children aged 5–14 increased from 13.2 deaths per 100,000 in 2011 to 14.3 deaths per 100,000 in 2021. The injury-related death rate increased from 5.5 deaths per 100,000 in 2011 to 6.0 deaths per 100,000 in 2019 but did not change significantly through 2021 at 7.0 deaths per 100,000.
- In 2021, unintentional injuries (accidents) were the leading cause of death for children aged one to four (8.5 deaths per 100,000) and aged 5–14 (4.2 deaths per 100,000). The second leading cause of death was birth defects among children aged one to four (2.7 deaths per 100,000) and cancer among children aged 5–14 (1.9 deaths per 100,000).
- Among both younger and older children, males have higher death rates than females. In 2021, males aged one to four had a death rate of 27.0 per 100,000 compared with 22.9 deaths per 100,000 for females. Among children aged 5–14, males had a death rate of 16.4 deaths per 100,000 compared with 12.2 per 100,000 for females.[14]

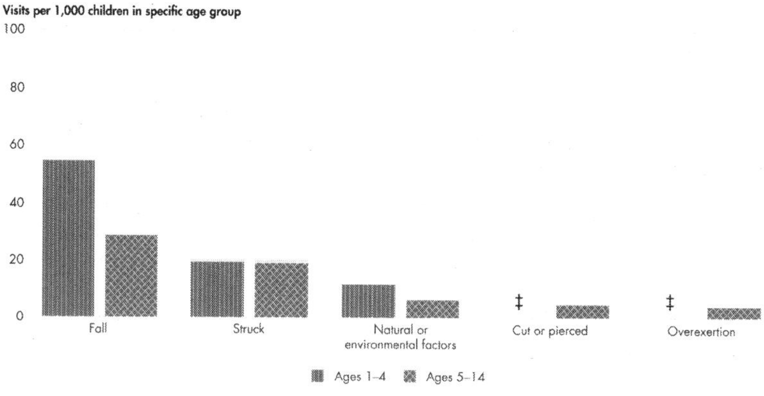

Figure 48.1. Emergency Department Visit Rates for Children Ages 1–4 and 5–14 by Leading Causes of Injury, 2019–2020

Federal Interagency Forum on Child and Family Statistics
‡ Reporting standards not met; the estimate is considered unreliable.

[14] "Child Injury and Mortality," Federal Interagency Forum on Child and Family Statistics, July 27, 2017. Available online. URL: www.childstats.gov/americaschildren/phys7.asp. Accessed March 18, 2024.

Section 48.7 | **Secondhand Smoke Prevention**

SECONDHAND SMOKE THREATENS OUR CHILDREN

Secondhand smoke comes from lit cigarettes and cigars and from the smoke breathed out by smokers. When children breathe secondhand smoke, it is as if they are smoking, too. Secondhand smoke contains thousands of chemicals, many of which are poisons that stay in the body. What do these poisons do? The U.S. Surgeon General asked scientists to investigate. They found that secondhand smoke harms everyone, especially children. They also learned that:

- an estimated 58 million nonsmoking Americans, including 14 million children aged 3–11 years, are exposed to secondhand smoke
- they breathe it at home, day care, and in cars
- children are almost twice as likely as nonsmoking adults to be exposed to secondhand smoke

Here are just a few of the chemicals and poisons in tobacco smoke (see Figure 48.2).

HOW DOES SECONDHAND SMOKE HURT OUR CHILDREN?

- Tobacco smoke harms babies, even before they are born. It harms children, too, because their lungs and bodies are still growing.
- Babies who breathe secondhand smoke are more likely to die unexpectedly from sudden infant death syndrome (SIDS), also called "crib death."
- Babies and children who breathe secondhand smoke are sick more often with bronchitis, pneumonia, and ear infections.
- For children with asthma, breathing secondhand smoke can trigger an attack. The attack can be severe enough to send a child to the hospital. Sometimes an asthma attack is so severe that a child dies.

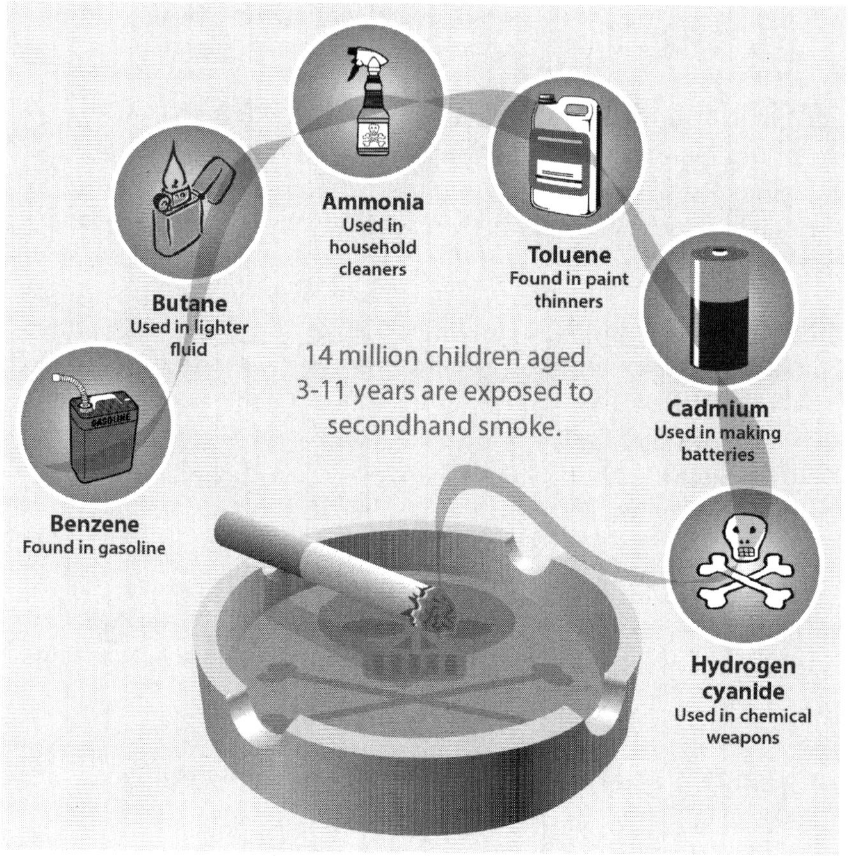

Figure 48.2. Chemicals and Poisons in Tobacco Smoke

Centers for Disease Control and Prevention (CDC)

CHILDREN CANNOT HIDE FROM SECONDHAND SMOKE AT HOME

Smoking in another room, such as a bathroom or bedroom, pollutes all the air in your home. In an apartment, smoke in one room can go through the whole building (see Figure 48.3).

- Smoking outside in a hall or stairwell does not protect children inside. Smoke goes under doors, windows, and through cracks.
- To protect the children inside, homes and apartment buildings must be smoke-free.

No amount of secondhand smoke is safe. Even when you cannot smell it, cigarette smoke can still harm your child.

- Opening a window or using a fan does not protect children.
- Air purifiers and air fresheners do not remove smoke's poisons.
- Smoke from one cigarette can stay in a room for hours. Do not smoke at home, even when children are not there.

Allowing people to smoke in only one room does not protect children. Smoke from halls and stairs gets inside, too.

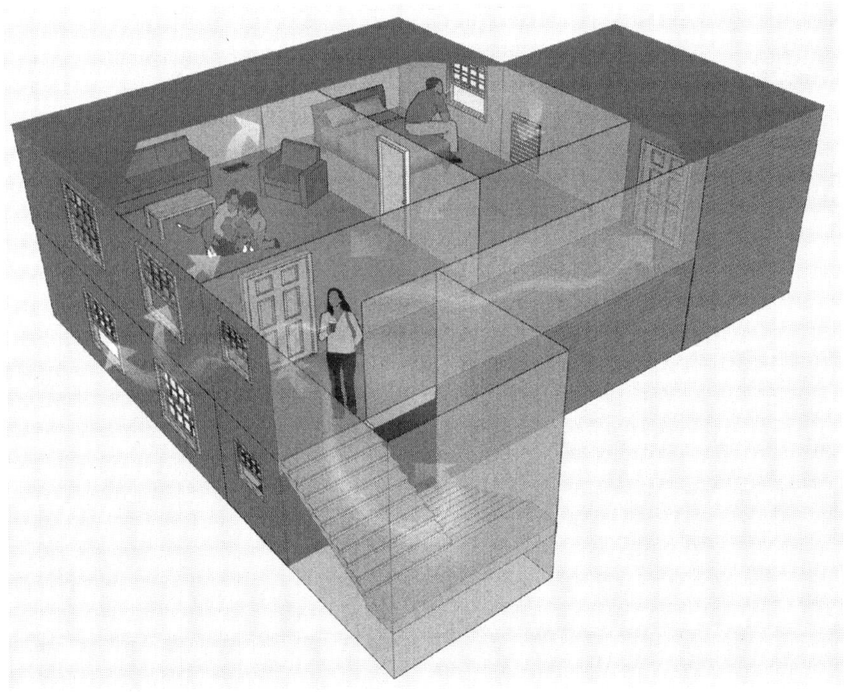

Figure 48.3. Secondhand Smoke at Home
Centers for Disease Control and Prevention (CDC)

PROTECTING CHILDREN FROM SECONDHAND SMOKE EVERYWHERE

- **At home**. If you take care of children in your home, do not allow anyone to smoke there. Do not let babysitters or family and friends smoke around your children.
- **In daycare**. Make sure smoking is not allowed in your child's day care.
- **At school**. Make sure your child's school is smoke-free inside and out. All school events should be "No Smoking."
- **In public**. Choose restaurants and businesses that are smoke-free. "No Smoking" sections in restaurants do not protect children from secondhand smoke.
- **In your car**. Do not allow anyone to smoke if children are riding in your car. Rolling down a window does not protect them.

SIMPLE STEPS TO PROTECT YOUR CHILDREN FROM SECONDHAND SMOKE

Children respect and learn from your actions and words. As caregivers, we teach our children by the choices we make.

- Ask people not to smoke around your children.
- Support family and friends who also want to stop smoking.
- Decide to have a smoke-free home and car, and ask family and friends to respect your decision.
- Get rid of all ashtrays in your home.
- Teach your children to stay away from secondhand smoke. Encourage your teens not to smoke.
- Make the decision to quit smoking. Get help from your doctor, family, and friends. Call this free quit-line: 800-QUIT-NOW (1-800-784-8669).[15].

[15] "How We Can Protect Our Children from Secondhand Smoke, a Parents Guide," Centers for Disease Control and Prevention (CDC), January 1, 2019. Available online. URL: www.cdc.gov/tobacco/basic_information/secondhand_smoke/protect_children/pdfs/general-population-p.pdf. Accessed March 18, 2024.

Chapter 49 | Internet and Screen Time Safety for Children

Chapter Contents

POTENTIAL RISK OF HARM FROM CONTENT EXPOSURE

Extreme, inappropriate, and harmful content continues to be easily and widely accessible by children and adolescents. This content can be spread through direct pushes, unwanted exchanges, and algorithmic designs. In certain tragic cases, childhood deaths have been linked to suicide- and self-harm-related content and risk-taking challenges on social media platforms. This content may be especially risky for children and adolescents already experiencing mental health difficulties.

Despite social media providing a sense of community for some, a systematic review of more than two dozen studies found that some social media platforms show live depictions of self-harm acts such as partial asphyxiation, leading to seizures, and cutting, leading to significant bleeding. These studies found that discussing or showing this content can normalize such behaviors, including through the formation of suicide pacts and posting of self-harm models for others to follow.

Social media may also perpetuate body dissatisfaction, disordered eating behaviors, social comparison, and low self-esteem, especially among adolescent girls. A synthesis of 20 studies demonstrated a significant relationship between social media use and body image concerns and eating disorders, with social comparison as a potential contributing factor. Social comparison driven by social media is associated with body dissatisfaction, disordered eating, and depressive symptoms. When asked about the effect of social media on their body image, nearly half (46%) of adolescents aged 13–17 said social media makes them feel worse, 40 percent said it makes them feel neither better nor worse, and only 14 percent said it makes them feel better.

Additionally, roughly two-thirds (64%) of adolescents are often or sometimes exposed to hate-based content. Among adolescent girls of color, one-third or more report exposure to racist content or language on social media platforms at least monthly. In a review of 36 studies, a consistent relationship was found between cyberbullying via social media and depression among children and adolescents, with adolescent females and sexual minority youth more likely to report experiencing incidents of cyberbullying. Nearly 75 percent of adolescents say social media sites are only doing a fair-to-poor job of addressing online harassment and cyberbullying.

Social media platforms can also be sites for predatory behaviors and interactions with malicious actors who target children and adolescents, such as adults seeking to sexually exploit children, financially extort them through the threat or actual distribution of intimate images, or sell illicitly manufactured fentanyl. Adolescent girls and transgender youth are disproportionately affected by online harassment and abuse, which is associated with negative emotional effects such as feeling sad, anxious, or worried. Nearly six in ten adolescent girls say they have been contacted by a stranger on certain social media platforms in ways that make them feel uncomfortable.

POTENTIAL RISK OF HARM FROM EXCESSIVE AND PROBLEMATIC USE

Excessive and problematic use of social media can harm children and adolescents by disrupting important healthy behaviors. Social media platforms are often designed to maximize user engagement, which has the potential to encourage excessive use and behavioral dysregulation. Features such as push notifications, autoplay, infinite scroll, quantifying and displaying popularity (i.e., likes), and algorithms that leverage user data to serve content recommendations are examples of these features that maximize engagement. According to one model, nearly a third (31%) of social media use may be attributable to self-control challenges magnified by habit formation.

Further, some researchers believe that social media exposure can overstimulate the reward center in the brain and, when the stimulation becomes excessive, can trigger pathways comparable to addiction. Small studies have shown that people with frequent and problematic social media use can experience changes in brain structure similar to changes seen in individuals with substance use or gambling addictions. In a nationally representative survey of girls aged 11–15, one-third or more say they feel addicted to a social media platform. Over half of teenagers report that it would be hard to give up social media. Nearly three in four teenagers believe that technology companies manipulate users to spend more time on their devices. In addition, according to a survey of eighth and tenth graders, the average time spent on social media is three and a half hours per day; one in four spends more than five hours per day, and one in seven spends more than seven hours per day on social media.

Excessive and problematic social media use, such as compulsive or uncontrollable use, has been linked to sleep problems, attention problems, and feelings of exclusion among adolescents. Sleep is essential for the healthy development of adolescents. A systematic review of 42 studies on the effects of excessive social media use found a consistent relationship between social media use and poor sleep quality, reduced sleep duration, sleep difficulties, and depression among youth. Poor sleep has been linked to altered neurological development in adolescent brains, depressive symptoms, and suicidal thoughts and behaviors. On a typical weekday, nearly one in three adolescents reports using screen media until midnight or later. While screen media use encompasses various digital activities, social media applications are the most commonly used by adolescents.[1]

Children of first-time mothers and those in home-based childcare log the most screen time. Children's average daily time spent watching television or using a computer or mobile device increased from 53 minutes at the age of 12 months to more than 150 minutes at three years, according to an analysis by researchers at the National Institutes of Health (NIH), the University at Albany, and the New York University Langone Medical Center. By the age of eight, children were more likely to log the highest amount of screen time if they had been in home-based childcare or were born to first-time mothers. The study appears in *JAMA Pediatrics*.

[1] "High Amounts of Screen Time Begin as Early as Infancy, NIH Study Suggests," National Institutes of Health (NIH), November 25, 2019. Available online. URL: www.nih.gov/news-events/news-releases/high-amounts-screen-time-begin-early-infancy-nih-study-suggests. Accessed March 18, 2024.

"Our results indicate that screen habits begin early," said Edwina Yeung, Ph.D., the study's senior author and an investigator in the Epidemiology Branch of the NIH's *Eunice Kennedy Shriver* National Institute of Child Health and Human Development (NICHD). "This finding suggests that interventions to reduce screen time could have a better chance of success if introduced early."

The American Academy of Pediatrics (AAP) recommends avoiding digital media exposure for children under 18 months of age, introducing children 18–24 months of age to screen media slowly, and limiting screen time to an hour a day for children from two to five years of age. In a study, researchers found that 87 percent of the children had screen time exceeding these recommendations. However, while screen time increased throughout toddlerhood, by the age of seven and eight, screen time fell to under one and a half hours per day. The researchers believe this decrease relates to time consumed by school-related activities.[2]

CHILDREN AND SCREEN TIME

Screen time used to mean sitting around and watching TV. For kids, too much time in front of the TV is linked to obesity and trouble in school. But screen time now includes smartphones, tablets, and other handheld devices, which are everywhere.

These new screens pose new challenges for parents, says Dr. Jenny Radesky, a pediatrician at the University of Michigan. "There is so much content available now on something a child can carry from room to room," she explains. Almost all this new technology was designed for adults, not children, Radesky says. For example, a study by her team analyzed ads on YouTube channels marketed to kids. They found that more than half featured age-inappropriate ads, such as those for violent video games. Parents may find it hard to know how much time their kids really spend on handheld devices. Another study from Radesky's team found that

[2] "Social Media and Youth Mental Health," U.S. Department of Health and Human Services (HHS), May 20, 2023. Available online. URL: www.hhs.gov/sites/default/files/sg-youth-mental-health-social-media-advisory.pdf. Accessed March 18, 2024.

young children who had their own tablets used them almost two hours a day. However, only about a third of their parents accurately guessed that amount.

Researchers are exploring how this type of media use affects kids' developing brains. They are interested in whether the use of phones and tablets alters the brain's executive functioning, Radesky explains, including the ability to focus on important tasks, resist distractions, and use self-control.

"Devices like tablets give you lots of stuff that is really exciting, all at once, with no waiting," Radesky says. Researchers want to know if that gets in the way of kids doing harder tasks that help them build life skills. Studies have already shown that too much media use can affect other aspects of kids' health, including mental health and physical activity.

"And sleep is a major one," adds Radesky. "A lot of studies have shown that the more kids use media, especially around bedtime, the worse their sleep is." But some uses of handheld devices can have benefits. Kids can use video chat to talk with relatives who live far away. Some educational apps and programs designed especially for children can help them in school.

So how can parents find a balance? "There are ways to set some limits about how much time they can spend on devices," Radesky says. You can set timers. Some apps let you stop content from continuing to play automatically.

SETTING SCREEN TIME BOUNDARIES

- Set a good example. Be a role model and limit your own screen time.
- Create a house rule that limits screen time and enforce it.
- Do not allow screens during meals or homework.
- Give your kids alternatives to screen time. Suggest playing outside, finding a new hobby, or learning a sport.
- Do other activities together, such as family board games, puzzles, or going for a walk.
- Do not put a TV or computer in your child's bedroom or let them go to bed with a portable device.

It can be hard for parents to track what their children are doing on portable screens. However, adults can model thinking critically about what they see when watching TV or other media with their kids. You can talk about what you like and do not like about a show or ad. You can point out when and why you think something is false or misleading. This can help kids learn these skills and use them on their own.[3]

Section 49.2 | **Benefits and Risks of Online Gaming**

A study of nearly 2,000 children found that those who reported playing video games for three hours per day or more performed better on cognitive skills tests involving impulse control and working memory compared to children who had never played video games. Published in JAMA Network Open, this study analyzed data from the ongoing Adolescent Brain Cognitive Development (ABCD) study, supported by the National Institute on Drug Abuse (NIDA).

"Numerous studies have linked video gaming to behavior and mental health problems," said NIDA director Dr. Nora Volkow. "This study suggests there may also be cognitive benefits associated with this popular pastime, which are worthy of further investigation."

Scientists at the University of Vermont, Burlington, analyzed data obtained when children entered the ABCD study at ages 9 and 10 years. The research team examined survey, cognitive, and brain imaging data from nearly 2,000 participants from within the larger study cohort.

The three-hour threshold was selected as it exceeds the American Academy of Pediatrics (AAP) screen-time guidelines, which recommend that video gaming time be limited to one to two hours

[3] *NIH News in Health*, "Delving into Devices—Children and Screen Time," National Institutes of Health (NIH), February 2, 2022. Available online. URL: https://newsinhealth.nih.gov/2022/02/delving-into-devices. Accessed March 18, 2024.

per day for older children. Investigators found that the children who reported playing video games for three or more hours daily were faster and more accurate on cognitive tasks than those who never played. In the gamer group, functional magnetic resonance imaging (MRI) brain imaging analyses found higher brain activity in regions of the brain associated with attention and memory. This group also had more brain activity in frontal brain regions associated with more cognitively demanding tasks and less brain activity in brain regions related to vision.

While prior studies have reported associations between video gaming and increases in depression, violence, and aggressive behavior, this study did not find that to be the case. There were reports of higher mental health and behavioral issues in this cohort, but the authors could not confirm whether this trend reflected a true association or chance. They note this will be an important measure to continue to track and understand as these children mature.[4]

BENEFITS OF ONLINE GAMING

Playing video games can positively affect a player's cognitive, emotional, and social skills. It can help children and teens enhance their problem-solving and strategizing skills. Multiplayer team games may help youth learn how to cooperate with others. Youth who play video games may also improve their motor skills and creativity. Video games provide a space for players to work out their emotions, boost their mood, and ease anxiety. Additionally, gaming can be a place to make new friends and socialize.

RISKS OF ONLINE GAMING

While gaming has the potential for positive benefits, it is also a place where cyberbullying can happen. If someone is not performing well in a game, other players may curse or make negative remarks that can turn into bullying or even exclude the person from playing together.

[4] "Do Video Games Improve Cognitive Performance?" National Institutes of Health (NIH), November 11, 2022. Available online. URL: https://nihrecord.nih.gov/2022/11/11/do-video-games-improve-cognitive-performance. Accessed March 18, 2024.

The anonymity of players and the use of avatars allow users to create alter egos or fictional versions of themselves, which is part of the fun of gaming. However, it also allows users to harass, bully, and sometimes gang up on other players. When players are anonymous, it can be difficult to hold them accountable when they bully others and use the game as a tool of harassment. Some players may use the game as a means to harass others or to get their personal information, such as usernames and passwords. They can even make others' personal information available online through a tactic called doxing. "doxing." can compromise not just a child's information but their parents' information as well, making them targets of bullying and harassment.

Gamers often use online gaming communities and social media to connect with other players, learn tips and tricks, share strategies, create teams or guilds, and connect while they play or watch others play. These types of online communities are also places where cybercriminals may seek to cause harm, for instance, by posting links that appear to be game-related but are actually computer viruses or malware (software designed to disrupt, damage, or gain access to a computer), or where predators may seek access to children.

PREVENT CYBERBULLYING FOR GAMERS

Gaming can be a fun, safe, and positive environment for all. Parents can help prevent cyberbullying of their children who play video games by:

- playing the game with your child or observing the game to understand how it works and what a child is exposed to in the game
- checking in periodically with your child about who is online, playing the game with them
- knowing which gaming communities, social media, and apps your child uses while gaming and their security risks which you can research online
- helping your child set the privacy and security settings for their games and apps

- teaching children about safe digital behavior, including not clicking on links from strangers; not downloading bots (software for automated tasks) or clicking on links in gaming forums; not sharing personal information such as emails, phone numbers, addresses, and passwords; not participating in bullying behavior of other players; and what to do if they observe or experience cyberbullying
- establishing rules about how much time a child can spend playing video games
- keeping an open line of communication about your child's digital life

There are things that gamers can do if they are experiencing cyberbullying or see it happen to others while gaming:

- Tell the player who is bullying to stop.
- Block the player who is bullying from the game and unfriend them on social media and in gaming communities.
- Report the player who is bullying to the game group, team, platform, community, or developers.
- Take a break from playing the game.
- Tell a parent or trusted adult and get some support.[5]

[5] StopBullying.gov, "Cyberbullying and Online Gaming," U.S. Department of Health and Human Services (HHS), December 11, 2023. Available online. URL: www.stopbullying.gov/cyberbullying/cyberbullying-online-gaming. Accessed March 18, 2024.

Section 49.3 | Keeping Children Safe Online

WHAT UNIQUE RISKS ARE ASSOCIATED WITH CHILDREN?

When a child uses your computer, normal safeguards and security practices may not be sufficient. Children present additional challenges due to their natural characteristics: innocence, curiosity, desire for independence, and fear of punishment. You need to consider these characteristics when determining how to protect your data and the child.

You may think that because the child is only playing a game, researching a term paper, or typing a homework assignment, they cannot cause any harm. But what if, when saving their paper, the child deletes a necessary program file? Or what if they unintentionally visit a malicious web page that infects your computer with a virus? These are just two possible scenarios. Mistakes happen, but children may not realize what they have done or may not tell you what happened because they are afraid of getting punished.

Online predators present another significant threat, particularly to children. Because the nature of the internet is so anonymous, it is easy for people to misrepresent themselves and manipulate or trick other users (see Avoiding Social Engineering and Phishing Attacks for some examples). Adults often fall victim to these ploys, and children, who are usually much more open and trusting, are even easier targets. Another growing problem is cyberbullying. These threats are even greater if a child has access to email or instant messaging programs, visits chat rooms, or uses social networking sites.

WHAT CAN YOU DO?

- **Be involved.** Consider activities you can work on together, whether it is playing a game, researching a topic you had been talking about (e.g., family vacation spots, a particular hobby, or a historical figure), or putting together a family newsletter. This will allow you to supervise your child's online activities while teaching them good computer habits.
- **Keep your computer in an open area.** If your computer is in a high-traffic area, you will be able to easily monitor

the computer activity. Not only does this accessibility deter children from doing something they know they are not allowed to do, it also gives you the opportunity to intervene if you notice a behavior that could have negative consequences.

- **Set rules and warn about dangers**. Make sure your child knows the boundaries of what they are allowed to do on the computer. These boundaries should be appropriate for the child's age, knowledge, and maturity and may include rules about how long they are allowed to be on the computer, what sites they are allowed to visit, what software programs they can use, and what tasks or activities they are allowed to do. You should also talk to children about the dangers of the internet so that they recognize suspicious behavior or activity. Discuss the risks of sharing certain types of information (e.g., that they are home alone) and the benefits of only communicating and sharing information with people they know. The goal is not to scare them but to make them more aware. Make sure to include the topic of cyberbullying in these discussions.
- **Monitor computer activity**. Be aware of what your child is doing on the computer, including which websites they are visiting. If they are using email, instant messaging, or chat rooms, try to get a sense of who they are corresponding with and whether they actually know them.
- **Keep lines of communication open**. Let your child know that they can approach you with any questions or concerns about behaviors or problems they may have encountered on the computer.
- **Consider partitioning your computer into separate accounts**. Most operating systems give you the option of creating a different user account for each user. If you are worried that your child may accidentally access, modify, or delete your files, you can give them a separate account and decrease the amount of access and number of

privileges they have. If you do not have separate accounts, you need to be especially careful about your security settings. In addition to limiting functionality within your browser, avoid letting your browser remember passwords and other personal information. Also, it is always important to keep your virus definitions up to date.

- **Consider implementing parental controls**. You may be able to set some parental controls within your browser. For example, internet browsers allow you to restrict or allow certain websites to be viewed on your computer, and you can protect these settings with a password. There are other resources you can use to control and monitor your child's online activity. Some ISPs offer services designed to protect children online. Contact your ISP to see if any of these services are available. There are also special software programs you can install on your computer. Different programs offer various features and capabilities, so you can find one that best suits your needs.[6]

[6] Cybersecurity and Infrastructure Security Agency (CISA), "Keeping Children Safe Online," U.S. Department of Homeland Security (DHS), January 23, 2023. Available online. URL: www.cisa.gov/news-events/news/keeping-children-safe-online. Accessed June 29, 2024.

Chapter 50 | **Outdoor Play and Safety**

Chapter Contents

Section 50.1 | Supporting Outdoor Play and Exploration for Infants and Toddlers

BENEFITS OF OUTDOOR PLAY IN EARLY CARE AND EDUCATION SETTINGS

Healthy Bodies

Outdoor play is a great way to get children moving and staying physically active, which protects their health in childhood and throughout life. Children learn through free play and need opportunities to take risks, test their limits, and learn new skills. Being physically active by playing outdoors and in nature can help children develop strong bodies and meet important developmental milestones for movement and physical development. Time spent in bright sunlight can also reduce nearsightedness.

Healthy Minds

Moving and staying active are important for having a healthy brain. Playing and exploring the outdoors can give children new experiences. Being outdoors often enables children to try different games and practice skills that help them meet milestones in learning, language, and emotions. Studies show that time spent playing outside can help children by improving their grades, attention spans, and behavior.

WAYS TO KEEP CHILDREN SAFE AND HEALTHY WHILE PLAYING OUTSIDE

Playing outside comes with many benefits, but it also comes with possible risks from exposure to sun, heat, and bugs and from health and safety hazards associated with playgrounds and water play.

Protect Children from Sun and Heat

Sunburns can happen even on cloudy or cool days. To protect their skin, keep children in the shade and encourage them to wear wide-brimmed hats, sunglasses, and clothes that cover their arms and legs. Sunscreen is not recommended for babies who are six months old or younger. Keep younger babies who cannot use sunscreen out of direct sunlight by finding shade and dressing them in sun-protective clothing.

Protect Children from Bug Bites

Outdoor activities can increase the risk of bug bites. Bugs, including mosquitoes, ticks, fleas, and flies, can spread germs. Using an insect repellent registered by the Environmental Protection Agency (EPA) can help protect children from bug bites:

- Find the right insect repellent by using the EPA's search tool.
- Always follow label instructions.
- Apply the insect repellent to your hands first and only use enough to cover the child's exposed skin.
- Do not apply the insect repellent to children's hands, eyes, or mouth or to cuts or irritated skin.
- Wash your hands immediately after.
- Apply insect repellent after applying sunscreen.

Protect Children from Injuries on the Playground

Playgrounds are great places for children to play and explore risks and limits, but they can also put children at risk for injuries. On the playground, using certain types of equipment, such as monkey bars, climbing equipment, and swings, is more likely to lead to concussions and other brain injuries.

For a safe and fun playground experience, seek out playgrounds with:

- equipment that is right for the child's age
- soft material below equipment, such as wood chips, sand, or mulch
- guardrails to help prevent falls

Look out for things in the play area that can trip the children, such as tree stumps or rocks. If outdoor play includes riding tricycles or bicycles or using rollerblades, skateboards, or similar wheeled equipment, be sure that children use well-fitting helmets. While playing outdoors, children may encounter stray or wild animals. Keep children away from snakes, rodents, and other animal hazards.

Protect Children from Drowning

Drowning can happen quickly and quietly anywhere there is water. Adults play a key role in protecting children from drowning and other recreational water-related injuries by closely and constantly supervising them:

- Avoid distracting activities such as reading or using a phone while supervising children in or near water.
- Take extra precautions to supervise children who have medical conditions or who might be affected by side effects of medications.[1]

Section 50.2 | Playing by the Rules: Playground Safety Precautions

The U.S. Consumer Product Safety Commission (CPSC) has long recognized the potential hazards associated with playground equipment, with over 200,000 estimated emergency room–treated injuries annually. A study of playground equipment–related incidents indicated that falls are the most common hazard pattern (44 percent of injuries), followed by equipment-related hazards such as breakage, tip-over, design, and assembly (23%). Other hazard patterns involved entrapment and colliding with other children or stationary equipment. Playground-related deaths involved entanglement of ropes, leashes, or clothing; falls; and effects from equipment tip-over or structural failure.

[1] "Outdoor Play and Safety for Children in ECE," Centers for Disease Control and Prevention (CDC), May 3, 2023. Available online. URL: www.cdc.gov/earlycare/resources/outdoor-play-and-safety.html. Accessed March 15, 2024.

IMPORTANCE OF SUPERVISION

Parents and playground supervisors should be aware that not all playground equipment is appropriate for all children who may use the playground. Supervisors should look for posted signs indicating the appropriate age of the users and direct children to equipment appropriate for their age (see Table 50.1). Toddlers and preschool-age children require more attentive supervision than older children.[2]

Table 50.1. Examples of Age-Appropriate Equipment

Toddler: Ages 6–23 Months	**Preschool: Ages 2–5 Years**	**Grade School: Ages 5–12 Years**
• climbing equipment under 32" high • ramps • single file step ladders • slides • spiral slides less than 360° • spring rockers • stairways • swings with full bucket seats	• certain climbers • horizontal ladders less than or equal to 60" high for ages 4 and 5 • merry-go-rounds • ramps • rung ladders • single file step ladders • slides • spiral slides up to 360° • spring rockers • stairways • swings—belt, full bucket seats (2–4 years), and rotating tire	• arch climbers • chain or cable walks • free-standing climbing events with flexible parts • fulcrum seesaws • ladders—horizontal, rung, and step • overhead rings • merry-go-rounds • ramps • ring treks • slides • spiral slides more than one 360° turn • stairways • swings—belt and rotating tire • track rides • vertical sliding poles

IS YOUR PUBLIC PLAYGROUND A SAFE PLACE TO PLAY?

Each year, more than 200,000 children go to U.S. hospital emergency rooms with injuries associated with playground equipment. Most injuries occur when a child falls from the equipment onto

[2] "Public Playground Safety Handbook," U.S. Consumer Product Safety Commission (CPSC), December 29, 2015. Available online. URL: www.cpsc.gov/s3fs-public/325.pdf. Accessed April 16, 2024.

the ground. Use this simple checklist to help make sure your local community or school playground is a safe place to play:

Public Playground Safety Checklist

- Make sure surfaces around playground equipment have at least 12 inches of wood chips, mulch, sand, or pea gravel or are mats made of safety-tested rubber or rubber-like materials.
- Check that protective surfacing extends at least six feet in all directions from play equipment. For swings, ensure surfacing extends, in back and front, twice the height of the suspending bar.
- Make sure play structures more than 30 inches high are spaced at least nine feet apart.
- Check for dangerous hardware, such as open "S" hooks or protruding bolt ends.
- Ensure spaces that could trap children, such as openings in guardrails or between ladder rungs, measure less than 3.5 inches or more than 9 inches.
- Check for sharp points or edges on equipment.
- Look out for tripping hazards, such as exposed concrete footings, tree stumps, and rocks.
- Make sure elevated surfaces, such as platforms and ramps, have guardrails to prevent falls.
- Check playgrounds regularly to ensure equipment and surfacing are in good condition.
- Carefully supervise children on playgrounds to make sure they are safe.[3]

---

[3] "Public Playground Safety Checklist," U.S. Consumer Product Safety Commission (CPSC), September 28, 2016. Available online. URL: www.cpsc.gov/safety-education/safety-guides/playgrounds/public-playground-safety-checklist. Accessed March 18, 2024.

Section 50.3 | Sun Safety

Spending time outside is a great way to be physically active, reduce stress, and get vitamin D. By protecting your skin from the sun, you can work and play outside without raising your skin cancer risk. Most skin cancers are caused by too much exposure to ultraviolet (UV) light. UV rays are invisible radiation that comes from the sun, tanning beds, and sunlamps. They can damage skin cells. Protection from UV rays is important all year, not just during the summer. UV rays can reach you on cloudy and cool days, reflecting off surfaces such as water, cement, sand, and snow. In the continental United States, UV rays tend to be strongest from 10 a.m. to 4 p.m. daylight saving time (9 a.m. to 3 p.m. standard time). The UV Index forecasts the strength of UV rays each day. If the UV Index is three or higher in your area, protect your skin from too much exposure to the sun.

HOW TO PROTECT YOUR SKIN FROM THE SUN

Shade

You can reduce your risk of sun damage and skin cancer by staying in the shade under an umbrella, tree, or other shelter. Your best bet to protect your skin is to use sunscreen or wear protective clothing when you are outside—even when you are in the shade.

Clothing

When possible, wear long-sleeved shirts and long pants and skirts to provide protection from UV rays. If wearing this type of clothing is not practical, try to wear a T-shirt or a beach cover-up. Clothes made from tightly woven fabric offer the best protection. A wet T-shirt offers much less UV protection than a dry one, and darker colors may offer more protection than lighter colors. Some clothing is certified under international standards as offering UV protection.

Hat

For the most protection, wear a hat with a brim all the way around that shades your face, ears, and the back of your neck. A tightly woven fabric, such as canvas, protects your skin from UV rays. Avoid straw hats with holes that let sunlight through. A darker hat may offer more UV protection. If you wear a baseball cap, you should also protect your ears and the back of your neck by wearing clothing that covers those areas, using sunscreen, or staying in the shade.

Sunglasses

Sunglasses protect your eyes from UV rays and reduce the risk of cataracts. They also protect the tender skin around your eyes from sun exposure. The best protection comes from sunglasses that block both Ultraviolet A (UVA) and Ultraviolet B (UVB) rays. Regardless of cost, most sunglasses sold in the United States meet this standard. Wrap-around sunglasses work best because they block UV rays from sneaking in from the side.

Sunscreen

Put on broad-spectrum sunscreen that filters out both UVA and UVB rays and has a sun protection factor (SPF) of 15 or higher before you go outside. Do not forget to apply a thick layer on all exposed skin. Get help for hard-to-reach places such as your back. Remember, sunscreen works best when combined with other options.

Sunscreen is not recommended for babies who are six months old or younger. The U.S. Food and Drug Administration (FDA) recommends keeping infants out of the sun during midday and using protective clothing if they have to be in the sun.

- **SPF**. Sunscreens are assigned an SPF, which is a number that rates how well they filter out UV rays. Higher numbers indicate more protection. You should

use a broad-spectrum sunscreen with an SPF of 15 or higher.
- **Reapplication**. Sunscreen wears off. Reapply it if you stay in the sun for more than two hours, after swimming, sweating, or toweling off.
- **Expiration date**. Check the sunscreen's expiration date. Sunscreen without an expiration date has a shelf life of no more than three years. Its shelf life is shorter if it has been exposed to high temperatures.

SUN SAFETY TIPS FOR SCHOOLS

Recess and other outdoor activities during the day can put students at risk if their skin is not protected from too much sun exposure. Teachers and school administrators can take steps to protect students from getting skin cancer later in life.

Increase Shade

- Provide shade structures or trees.
- Move outdoor activities to shaded areas.
- Plan for shade when developing or renovating school buildings, playgrounds, or athletic fields.

Promote Sun-Safe Behaviors

- Encourage students to wear hats, sunglasses, and sunscreen outdoors.
- Try to avoid scheduling outdoor activities when the sun is strongest.
- Provide outdoor activity breaks, so students can reapply sunscreen and get water.[4]

[4] "Sun Safety," Centers for Disease Control and Prevention (CDC), April 18, 2023. Available online. URL: www.cdc.gov/cancer/skin/basic_info/sun-safety.htm. Accessed March 18, 2024.

Chapter 51 | Child Protection in Disasters and Emergencies

Disasters can be especially stressful for children and teens. Young people are less likely to understand the events affecting them, have less control and decision-making opportunities than adults, and often have less experience coping with highly stressful situations. Children and teens are more likely to experience trauma due to a disaster, as they are more likely to be severely injured, have little to no knowledge of safety precautions, and understand less about the situation.

As a parent or guardian, there are steps you can take to ensure your child is better equipped to respond to disasters and cope with common reactions.

DISASTER PLANNING FOR FAMILIES

You and your family can take several steps before a disaster occurs to ensure your child's safety and resilience in case of an emergency event. No matter your child's age, try to include them in planning for emergencies by encouraging their participation in the following steps:

- **Create emergency kits for your family**. Discuss what you may need during an emergency and ensure there are enough supplies for all household members, including pets.

- **Develop an emergency evacuation and reunification plan for events where your home may not be safe, or family members are separated.** Decide on an alternative meeting location that is recognizable for all household members.
- **Discuss safety drills that your child may experience in school.** Encourage them to find strategies they learned during safety drills that could be incorporated into your household emergency plans.

COMMON REACTIONS IN YOUNG PEOPLE

Disasters can be just as frightening and stressful for children and teens as they are for adults. Just like adults, young people can experience reactions as they attempt to cope with anxiety, frustration, and fear. These reactions can occur for a few weeks to a month after the event and should be monitored.

The following reactions are common for children and teens of all ages:

- experiencing issues sleeping, having nightmares, or not wanting to sleep alone
- expressing extreme concern for the well-being of others or fear that the disaster is not over
- expressing fear of being separated from parent or caregiver
- feeling detached, isolated, or vulnerable
- engaging in violent, aggressive, or dangerous activities or play
- losing interest in activities they previously enjoyed
- being unable to complete tasks they completed before, such as talking, walking, reading, or writing
- complaining of headaches, stomachaches, or muscle aches often
- going through abrupt and radical changes in attitude and shifts in relationships with family and friends
- repeatedly wanting to talk about and play out the event or avoiding all talk of the event

HELPING YOUR CHILD COPE

While reactions to disasters are common, children and teens may be unable to cope with their own feelings, thoughts, and behaviors. Parents and caregivers can help their children process and identify their emotions and reactions through the following strategies:

- **Encourage your child to express their thoughts, feelings, and concerns**. Encourage drawing or coloring as an emotional outlet for children who cannot express themselves verbally and discuss their work with them.
- **Create and follow routines throughout the day**. This makes your child know what to expect.
- **Let your child make choices about small things throughout the day**. This helps them feel in control. This can include choices over what they eat, wear, or play.
- **Avoid extended separations from your child**. For brief separations, help your child express their feelings and explain where you are going and when you will return. If you must be separated for an extended amount of time, have your child stay with familiar people in a familiar environment.
- **Engage in positive activities together where you give your child undivided attention**. Try to include family members and friends to encourage interpersonal relationships.
- **Help your child process nervousness, stress, or frustration through activities such as stretching, running sports, and deep breathing exercises.**
- **Provide age-appropriate, consistent explanations in response to questions or concerns from your child**. Remain matter-of-fact with your responses and avoid voicing your own fears or concerns.
- **Limit your child's access to dangerous and high-risk activities.**
- **Limit your child's access to media coverage of the event and monitor their use of television, radio,**

Internet, and social media. If possible, steer your child toward positive media coverage of the event.
- **Set an example by taking care of yourself, making time for stress management activities, and discussing your own emotions and reactions with a loved one or health-care professional.**

To best support your child after a disaster, it is not recommended to keep them isolated from family and friends for long periods of time, force them to discuss the event before they feel ready, or force them to engage in activities they do not want to.

Supporting your child throughout this period can be frustrating and upsetting, but it is important to know these reactions will often go away on their own and will not seriously affect your child's development and well-being.

WHEN TO SEEK PROFESSIONAL SUPPORT

While behavioral and emotional reactions after a disaster are common, you may consider talking to a health-care professional if your child's reactions continue for more than two to four weeks after the disaster, worsen over time, or affect their usual routines.[1]

[1] "Children and Disasters," Substance Abuse and Mental Health Services Administration (SAMHSA), March 5, 2024. Available online. URL: www.samhsa.gov/dtac/disaster-survivors/children-and-disaster. Accessed March 15, 2024.

Chapter 52 | Safety for Children with Disabilities

Preventing injuries and harm is not very different for children with disabilities compared to children without disabilities. However, finding the right information and learning about the kinds of risks children might face at different ages can be challenging for parents of children with disabilities. Each child is different, and the general recommendations available to keep children safe should be tailored to fit your child's skills and abilities.

There are steps that parents and caregivers can take to keep children with disabilities safe. To keep all children safe, parents and caregivers need to:

- know and learn about what health concerns or special conditions are unique for their child
- plan ways to protect their child and share the plan with others
- remember that their child's needs for protection will change over time

WHAT CAN PARENTS AND CAREGIVERS DO?

Parents or caregivers can talk to their child's doctor or health-care professional about how to keep them safe. Your child's teacher or childcare provider might also have good ideas. Once you have ideas about keeping your child safe, make a safety plan, explain it to your child, and share it with other adults who might be able to help if needed. Here are some things to think about when making a safety plan for your child:

Moving Around and Handling Things

Does your child have challenges with moving around and handling things around them? Sometimes children are faced with unsafe situations, especially in new places. Children who have limited ability to move, see, hear, or make decisions and children who do not feel or understand pain might not realize that something is unsafe or might have trouble getting away. Take a look around the place where your child will be to make sure every area your child can reach is safe. Check your child's clothing and toys—are they suitable for their abilities, not just age and size?

For example, clothing and toys meant for older children might have strings that are not safe for a child who cannot easily untangle themselves, or toys might have small parts that are not safe for children who are still mouthing toys.

Safety Equipment

Do you have the right kind of safety equipment? Safety equipment is often developed based on age and size rather than ability. For example, a major cause of child death is motor vehicle crashes. Keeping your child safe in the car is important. When choosing the right car seat, you might need to consider whether your child has difficulties sitting up or sitting still in the seat, in addition to their age, height, and weight. If you have a child with disabilities, talk to your health-care professional about the best type of car seat or booster seat and the proper seat position for your child. You can also ask a certified child passenger safety technician who is trained in special needs.

The following are other examples of special safety equipment:

- Life jackets may need to be specially fitted for your child.
- Smoke alarms that signal with a light and vibration may be better in a home where there is a child who cannot hear.

- Handrails and safety bars can be put into homes to help a child who has difficulty moving around or a child who is at a greater risk of falling.

Speak to your health-care professional about the right equipment for your child and have this equipment ready and available before you may need it.

Talking and Understanding

Does your child have problems with talking or understanding? Children who have problems communicating might have limited ability to learn about safety and danger. For example, children who cannot hear might miss spoken instructions. Children who have trouble understanding or remembering might not learn about safety as easily as other children. Children who have a hard time communicating might not be able to ask questions about safety. Adults might think that children with disabilities are aware of dangers when they actually are not.

Parents and caregivers may need to find different ways to teach their children about safety, such as:

- showing them what to do
- using pretend play to rehearse
- practicing on a regular basis

Parents and caregivers may need to find different ways to let their children communicate that they are in danger. For example, you might teach your child to use a whistle, bell, or alarm to alert others to danger. Inform adults who take care of your child about these communication methods. It is also useful to contact your local fire department and explain any special circumstances you have so that they do not have to rely on the child or others to explain their special needs in case of an emergency.

Making Decisions

Does your child have problems with making decisions? Children might have limited ability to make decisions either because of developmental delays or limits in their thinking skills or in their ability to stop themselves from doing things that they want but should not do. For example, children with attention deficit hyperactivity disorder (ADHD) or fetal alcohol spectrum disorders (FASDs) might be very impulsive and fail to think about the results of their actions. People often put more dangerous things higher up so that little children cannot reach them. Your older child might be able to reach something that they are not ready to handle safely. Check your child's environment, particularly in new places.

Some children might also have problems distinguishing when situations and people are safe or dangerous. They might not know what to do. Parents and caregivers can give children specific instructions on how to behave in certain situations that might become dangerous.

Moving and Exploring

Does your child have enough chances to move and explore? Children with disabilities often need extra protection. But, just like all children, they also need to move and explore to develop healthy bodies and minds. Some parents of children with special needs worry about their children needing extra protection. It is not possible to protect children from every bump and bruise. Exploring can help children learn what is safe and what might be difficult or dangerous. Being fit and healthy can help children stay safe, and an active lifestyle is important for long-term health.

Children with disabilities might find it hard to take part in sports and active play. For example, equipment may need to be adjusted, coaches may need extra information and support to help a child with a disability, or a communication problem may make it more difficult for some children to play as part of a team.

Talk to your child's teachers, potential coaches, care providers, or health professional about ways to find the right balance between safety and activity.[1]

[1] National Center on Birth Defects and Developmental Disabilities (NCBDDD), "Keeping Children with Disabilities Safe," Centers for Disease Control and Prevention (CDC), September 17, 2019. Available online. URL: www.cdc.gov/ncbddd/disabilityandsafety/child-safety.html. Accessed March 15, 2024.

Part 8 | Additional Help and Information

Chapter 53 | **Glossary of Terms Related to Infant, Toddler, and Child Health**

abusive head trauma (AHT): A term used to describe the constellation of signs and symptoms resulting from violent shaking or shaking and impacting of the head of an infant or small child.

acquired immunodeficiency syndrome (AIDS): A disease of the immune system due to advanced stage of infection with human immunodeficiency virus (HIV). HIV destroys the CD4T lymphocytes, leaving the body vulnerable to life-threatening infections.

adverse childhood experiences (ACEs): Stressful or traumatic events, including abuse and neglect. ACEs are strongly related to the development and prevalence of a wide range of health problems throughout a person's lifespan, including those associated with substance misuse.

allergy: A condition in which the body has an exaggerated response to a substance (e.g., food or drug). Also known as "hypersensitivity."

anticholinergics: A type of medicine relaxes the muscle bands that tighten around the airways. This action opens the airways, letting more air out of the lungs to improve breathing. Anticholinergics also help clear mucus from the lungs.

Apgar score: A scoring system for assessing a newborn's health right after birth. The Apgar score measures five key areas of health: skin color, heart rate, reflexes, muscle tone, and breathing rate.

arthritis: A disease that causes inflammation and pain in the joints.

This glossary contains terms excerpted from documents produced by several sources deemed reliable.

asthma: A chronic medical condition where the bronchial tubes (in the lungs) become easily irritated. This leads to constriction of the airways resulting in wheezing, coughing, difficulty breathing, and production of thick mucus.

autism: A chronic developmental disorder usually diagnosed between 18 and 30 months of age.

bacteria: Bacteria are small single-celled organisms. Bacteria are found almost everywhere on Earth and are vital to the planet's ecosystems. The human body is full of bacteria and in fact is estimated to contain more bacterial cells than human cells. Most bacteria in the body are harmless, and some are even helpful. A relatively small number of species cause disease.

behavior problem: Behavior of the child in the school and/or community that adversely affects socialization, learning, growth, and moral development.

birth weight: The first weight of the fetus or neonate obtained after birth; for live births, birth weight can be measured within the first hour of life before postnatal weight loss has occurred; actual weight is recorded to the degree of accuracy by which it is measured.

bonding: The process of developing lasting emotional ties with one's immediate caregivers; seen as the first and primary developmental achievement of a human being and central to a person's ability to relate to others throughout life.

bronchitis: Inflammation of the main air passages to the lungs. It causes cough, shortness of breath, and chest tightness.

caregiver: One who provides for the physical, emotional, and social needs of a dependent person. The term most often applies to parents or parent surrogates, child care and nursery workers, health-care specialists, and relatives caring for children.

carrier: A person who has a mutated (changed) copy of a gene. This change may cause a disease in that person or in his or her children.

cerebral palsy (CP): A group of neurological disorders that appear in infancy or early childhood and permanently affect body movement, muscle coordination, and balance. CP affects the part of the brain that controls muscle movements.

chickenpox: A disease caused by the varicella-zoster virus (VZV), which results in a blister-like rash, itching, tiredness, and fever.

child abuse and neglect: Defined by the Child Abuse Prevention and Treatment Act (CAPTA) as any recent act or failure to act on the part of a parent or caregiver that results in death, serious physical or emotional harm, sexual abuse, or exploitation, or an act or failure to act that presents an imminent risk of serious harm.

child protective services (CPS): The social services agency designated (in most states) to receive reports, conduct investigations and assessments, and provide intervention and treatment services to children and families in which child maltreatment has occurred.

chromosome: Part of a cell that contains genetic information. Except for sperm and eggs, all human cells contain 46 chromosomes.

cleft lip: A partial or complete fissure of the upper lip; it can be either unilateral or bilateral and can be associated with a cleft of the gum.

cleft palate: A fissure of the palate, resulting from a complete or partial lack of fusion of the palatal shelves (secondary palate), that can affect the hard or soft palate, or both.

constipation: Infrequent or hard stools or difficulty passing stools.

cystic fibrosis (CF): A common hereditary disease in which exocrine (secretory) glands produce abnormally thick mucus. This mucus can cause problems in digestion, breathing, and body cooling.

developmental disability: A diverse group of severe chronic conditions caused by mental and/or physical impairments. People with developmental disabilities may have problems with major life activities such as language, mobility, learning, and independent living.

diabetes: A chronic health condition where the body is unable to produce insulin and properly break down sugar (glucose) in the blood.

diagnostic test: A test used to confirm or rule out the presence of a medical condition.

diarrhea: Passing frequent and loose stools that can be watery.

domestic violence: A pattern of assaultive and/or coercive behaviors, including physical, sexual, and psychological attacks, as well as economic coercion, that adults or adolescents use against their intimate partners. Intimate partners include spouses, sexual partners, parents, children, siblings, extended family members, and dating relationships.

echocardiogram: An ultrasound picture of the heart.

electrocardiogram (ECG or EKG): A test that records the electrical activity of the heart.

emotional maltreatment: A type of maltreatment that refers to acts or omissions, other than physical abuse or sexual abuse, that caused, or could have caused, conduct, cognitive, affective, or other mental disorders. Includes emotional neglect, psychological abuse, mental injury, and so on. Frequently occurs as verbal abuse or excessive demands on a child's performance and may cause the child to have a negative self-image and disturbed behavior.

encephalopathy: A general term describing brain dysfunction.

epilepsy: A group of disorders marked by problems in the normal functioning of the brain. These problems can produce seizures, unusual body movements, a loss of consciousness or changes in consciousness, as well as mental problems or problems with the senses.

fetal alcohol spectrum disorders (FASDs): A group of conditions that can occur in a person whose mother drank alcohol during pregnancy. These effects can include physical problems and problems with behavior and learning. Often, a person with an FASD has a mix of these problems.

fever: The body temperature is raised above normal and is usually a sign of infection or illness.

folic acid: The synthetic form of vitamin B used in fortified foods and supplements; folic acid is more bioavailable than the natural form—folate—found in foods.

***Haemophilus influenzae* type b (Hib):** A type of bacteria that can cause many different kinds of infections. These infections range from mild, such as ear infections, to serious, like bloodstream infections.

health-care provider: Any person, such as a primary care physician, nurse, or therapist, who provides health-care services for you or your baby.

hepatitis: Disease of the liver causing inflammation. Symptoms include an enlarged liver, fever, nausea, vomiting, abdominal pain, and dark urine.

immune system: The complex system in the body responsible for fighting disease. Its primary function is to identify foreign substances in the body (bacteria, viruses, fungi, or parasites) and develop a defense against them.

incubation period: The time from contact with infectious agents (bacteria or viruses) to onset of disease.

Individuals with Disabilities Education Act (IDEA): A law ensuring services to children with disabilities throughout the nation. The IDEA governs how states and public agencies provide early intervention, special education, and related services to eligible infants, toddlers, children, and youth with disabilities.

inflammatory bowel disease (IBD): A general term for any disease characterized by inflammation of the bowel. Examples include colitis and Crohn disease.

influenza (flu): A highly contagious viral infection characterized by sudden onset of fever, severe aches and pains, and inflammation of the mucous membrane.

intervention: An action intended to modify an outcome; a set of techniques and therapies practiced in counseling.

jaundice: A yellowing of the skin and the whites of the eyes, caused by too much bilirubin in the blood. While not a disease, jaundice can signal a liver or gallbladder problem. Newborns can develop jaundice, which is only temporary and goes away.

learning disability: A disorder in basic psychological processes involved in understanding or using language, spoken or written, that may manifest itself in an imperfect ability to listen, think, speak, read, write, spell, or use mathematical calculations. The term includes conditions such as perceptual disability, brain injury, minimal brain dysfunction, dyslexia, and developmental aphasia.

magnetic resonance imaging (MRI): A procedure in which radio waves and a powerful magnet linked to a computer are used to create detailed pictures of areas inside the body. These pictures can show the difference between normal and diseased tissue.

maltreatment: An act or failure to act by a parent, caretaker, or other person as defined under state law which results in physical abuse, neglect, medical neglect, sexual abuse, emotional abuse, or an act or failure to act which presents an imminent risk of serious harm to a child.

neural tube defect (NTD): A failure of the neural tube to close correctly.

newborn screening (NBS): The process of checking babies to identify those who might have certain serious health conditions that can benefit from early treatment or intervention.

otitis media (OM): A viral or bacterial infection that leads to inflammation of the middle ear. This condition usually occurs along with an upper respiratory infection.

pathogens: Organisms (e.g., bacteria, viruses, parasites, and fungi) that cause disease in human beings.

phenylketonuria (PKU): A condition in which babies cannot process a specific amino acid. It can cause serious health problems, including brain damage, if not treated early in life.

physical abuse: Any abuse that results in physical injury to a child. This may include burning, hitting, punching, shaking, kicking, beating, or otherwise harming a child. Although an injury resulting from physical abuse is not accidental, the parent or caregiver may not have intended to hurt the child. The injury may have resulted from severe discipline, including injurious spanking, or physical punishment that is inappropriate to the child's age or condition. The injury may be the result of a single episode or of repeated episodes and can range in severity from minor marks and bruising to death.

pneumonia: Inflammation of the lungs characterized by fever, chills, muscle stiffness, chest pain, cough, shortness of breath, rapid heart rate, and difficulty breathing.

posttraumatic stress disorder (PTSD): A mental health disorder that some people develop after experiencing or witnessing a life-threatening or other traumatic event. PTSD is characterized by pervasive feelings of distress after the event. PTSD is diagnosed if the duration of symptoms is longer than a few months or if symptoms are significantly disrupting daily life.

protective factor: Strengths and resources that appear to mediate or serve as a buffer against risk factors that contribute to maltreatment. These factors may strengthen the parent-child relationships, ability to cope with stress, and capacity to provide for children. Protective factors include nurturing and attachment, knowledge of parenting and of child and youth development, parental resilience, social connections, and concrete supports for parents.

Reye syndrome: Encephalopathy (general brain disorder) in children following an acute illness such as influenza or chickenpox. This condition may result in coma or death.

risk: A risk assessment is a measure of the likelihood that a child will be maltreated in the future, frequently through the use of checklists, matrices, scales, and other methods of measurement.

risk factor: Behaviors and conditions present in the child, parent, or family that will likely contribute to child maltreatment occurring in the future. Major risk factors include substance abuse, domestic/family violence, and mental health problems.

rubella: Also called "German measles." Rubella virus causes rash, mild fever, and arthritis. If a woman gets rubella while she is pregnant, she could have a miscarriage, or her baby could be born with serious birth defects.

safety plan: A casework document developed when it is determined that a child is in imminent or potential risk of serious harm. In the safety plan, the caseworker targets the factors that are causing or contributing to the risk of imminent serious harm to the child and identifies, along with the family, the interventions that will control the safety factors and assure the child's protection.

seizure: Sudden, uncontrolled body movements and changes in behavior that occur because of abnormal electrical activity in the brain.

sexual abuse: According to the Child Abuse Prevention and Treatment Act (CAPTA), sexual abuse is defined as the employment, use, persuasion, inducement, enticement, or coercion of any child to engage in, or assist any other person to engage in, any sexually explicit conduct or simulation of such conduct for the purpose of producing a visual depiction of such conduct; or the rape, and in cases of caretaker or interfamilial relationships, statutory rape, molestation, prostitution, or other form of sexual exploitation of children, or incest with children.

sudden infant death syndrome (SIDS): A term describing the sudden and unexpected death of a baby less than one year old in which the cause was not obvious before investigation. These deaths often happen during sleep or in the baby's sleep area.

Tourette syndrome (TS): A brain-based disorder that starts in childhood in which a person makes involuntary movements and sounds (called "tics").

tumor: An abnormal mass of tissue that results when cells divide more than they should or do not die when they should. Tumors may be benign (not cancer) or malignant (cancer). Also called "neoplasm."

ultrasound: A procedure in which high-energy sound waves are bounced off internal tissues or organs and make echoes. The echo patterns are shown on the screen of an ultrasound machine, forming a picture of body tissues called a "sonogram." Also called "ultrasonography."

vaccine: A product made from very small amounts of weak or dead germs that can cause diseases—for example, viruses, bacteria, or toxins. It prepares your body to fight the disease faster and more effectively so that you will not get sick. Vaccines are administered through needle injections, by mouth, and by aerosol.

virus: A tiny organism that multiplies within cells and causes diseases such as chickenpox, measles, mumps, rubella, pertussis, and hepatitis. Viruses are not affected by antibiotics, the drugs used to kill bacteria.

vitamin: A nutrient that the body needs in small amounts to function and maintain health. Examples are vitamins A, C, and E.

voice: Sound produced by air passing out through the larynx and upper respiratory tract.

well-being: The result of meeting a child's educational, emotional, and physical and mental health needs. Well-being is achieved when families have the capacity to provide for the needs of their children or when families are receiving the support and services needed to adequately meet the needs of their children.

wheezing: Breathing with difficulty, with a whistling noise. Wheezing is a symptom of asthma.

whooping cough (pertussis): Bacterial infectious disease marked by a convulsive spasmodic cough, sometimes followed by a crowing intake of breath.

x-ray: A type of high-energy radiation. In low doses, x-rays are used to diagnose diseases by making pictures of the inside of the body.

Chapter 54 | **Directory of Organizations Providing Information for Parents and Caregivers**

GOVERNMENT ORGANIZATIONS

Agency for Healthcare Research and Quality (AHRQ)
5600 Fishers Ln., 7th Fl.
Rockville, MD 20857
Phone: 301-427-1364
Website: www.ahrq.gov

Centers for Disease Control and Prevention (CDC)
1600 Clifton Rd.
Atlanta, GA 30329-4027
Toll-Free TTY: 888-232-6348
Website: www.cdc.gov

Child Welfare Information Gateway
330 C St., S.W.
Washington, DC 20201
Toll-Free: 800-394-3366
Website: www.childwelfare.gov
Email: info@childwelfare.gov

ChildCare.gov
330 C St., S.W.
4th Fl., Mary E. Switzer Bldg.
Washington, DC 20201
Toll-Free: 800-422-4453
Phone: 202-690-6782
Website: https://childcare.gov
Email: ChildCare.gov@acf.hhs.gov

Clinical Center (CC)
10 Center Dr.
Bethesda, MD 20892
Toll-Free: 800-411-1222
Phone: 301-496-2563
Toll-Free TTY: 866-411-1010
Website: https://clinicalcenter.nih.gov

Resources in this chapter were compiled from several sources deemed reliable; all contact information was verified and updated in July 2024.

Early Childhood Learning and Knowledge Center (ECLKC)
Toll-Free: 866-763-6481
Website: eclkc.ohs.acf.hhs.gov
Email: HeadStart@eclkc.info

***Eunice Kennedy Shriver* National Institute of Child Health and Human Development (NICHD)**
P.O. Box 3006
Rockville, MD 20847
Toll-Free: 800-370-2943
Phone: 301-496-5133
Fax: 866-760-5947
Website: www.nichd.nih.gov
Email: NICHDInformationResourceCenter@mail.nih.gov

Food and Nutrition Service (FNS)
1320 Braddock Pl.
Braddock Metro Center II
Alexandria, VA 22314
Toll-Free: 800-221-5689
Phone: 703-305-2062
Website: www.fns.usda.gov

Health Resources and Services Administration (HRSA)
5600 Fishers Ln.
Rockville, MD 20857
Toll-Free: 877-464-4772
Phone: 301-443-3376
Toll-Free TTY: 877-897-9910
Website: www.hrsa.gov

National Cancer Institute (NCI)
9609 Medical Center Dr.
Rockville, MD 20850
Toll-Free: 800-4-CANCER (800-422-6237)
Website: www.cancer.gov
Email: NCIinfo@nih.gov

National Heart, Lung, and Blood Institute (NHLBI)
P.O. Box 30105
Bethesda, MD 20824
Toll-Free: 877-645-2448
Website: www.nhlbi.nih.gov
Email: nhlbiinfo@nhlbi.nih.gov

National Institute of Allergy and Infectious Diseases (NIAID)
5601 Fishers Ln.
MSC 9806
Bethesda, MD 20892-9806
Toll-Free: 866-284-4107
Phone: 301-496-5717
Toll-Free TDD: 800-877-8339
Fax: 301-402-3573
Website: www.niaid.nih.gov
Email: ocpostoffice@niaid.nih.gov

National Institute of Arthritis and Musculoskeletal and Skin Diseases (NIAMS)
1 AMS Cir.
Bethesda,
MD 20892-3675
Toll-Free: 877-22-NIAMS (877-226-4267)
Phone: 301-495-4484
Fax: 301-718-6366
Website: www.niams.nih.gov
Email: NIAMSinfo@mail.nih.gov

National Institute of Dental and Craniofacial Research (NIDCR)
Toll-Free: 866-232-4528
Website: www.nidcr.nih.gov
Email: nidcrinfo@mail.nih.gov

National Institute of Diabetes and Digestive and Kidney Diseases (NIDDK)
9000 Rockville Pike
Bethesda, MD 20892
Toll-Free: 800-860-8747
Website: www.niddk.nih.gov
Email: healthinfo@niddk.nih.gov

National Institute of Environmental Health Sciences (NIEHS)
P.O. Box 12233 MD. K3-16
Research Triangle Park, NC 27709
Phone: 919-541-3345
Fax: 919-541-4395
Website: www.niehs.nih.gov
Email: webcenter@niehs.nih.gov

National Institute of Neurological Disorders and Stroke (NINDS)
P.O. Box 5801
Bethesda, MD 20824
Toll-Free: 800-352-9424
Website: www.ninds.nih.gov

NIH News in Health
9000 Rockville Pike
Bldg. 31, Rm. 5B52
Bethesda, MD 20892
Phone: 301-451-8224
Website: newsinhealth.nih.gov
Email: nihnewsinhealth@od.nih.gov

Office of Disease Prevention and Health Promotion (ODPHP)
1101 Wootton Pkwy, Ste. 420
Rockville, MD 20852
Website: https://health.gov

Office of Justice Programs (OJP)
810 7th St., N.W.
Washington, DC 20531
Phone: 202-514-2000
Website: www.ojp.gov
Email: askojp@ncjrs.gov

Office on Women's Health (OWH)
1101 Wootton Pkwy.
Rockville, MD 20852
Toll-Free: 800-994-9662
Phone: 202-690-7650
Fax: 202-205-2631
Website: www.womenshealth.gov
Email: womenshealth@hhs.gov

U.S. Department of Education (ED)
400 Maryland Ave., S.W.
Washington, DC 20202
Toll-Free: 800-USA-LEARN
(800-872-5327)
Phone: 202-401-2000
Website: www2.ed.gov

U.S. Department of Justice (DOJ)
950 Pennsylvania Ave., N.W.
Washington, DC 20530
Phone: 202-514-2000
Toll-Free TTY: 800-877-8339
Website: www.justice.gov

PRIVATE ORGANIZATIONS

Action for Healthy Kids®
600 W. Van Buren St., Ste. 720
Chicago, IL 60607
Toll-Free: 800-416-5136
Website: www.actionforhealthykids.org
Email: contactus@actionforhealthykids.org

American Academy of Child and Adolescent Psychiatry (AACAP)
3615 Wisconsin Ave., N.W.
Washington, DC 20016-3007
Phone: 202-966-7300
Fax: 202-464-0131
Website: www.aacap.org
Email: communications@aacap.org

American Academy of Pediatrics (AAP)
345 Park Blvd.
Itasca, IL 60143
Toll-Free: 800-433-9016
Phone: 630-626-6000
Fax: 847-434-8000
Website: www.aap.org
Email: mcc@aap.org

American Association for the Study of Liver Diseases (AASLD)
1001 N. Fairfax St.
4th Fl. Alexandria, VA 22314
Phone: 703-299-9766
Fax: 703-299-9622
Website: www.aasld.org
Email: aasld@aasld.org

American Childhood Cancer Organization (ACCO)
P.O. Box 498
Kensington, MD 20895-0498
Toll-Free: 855-858-2226
Website: www.acco.org
Email: staff@acco.org

American Diabetes Association® (ADA)
2451 Crystal Dr., Ste. 900
Arlington, VA 22202
Toll-Free: 800-DIABETES (800-342-2383)
Website: www.diabetes.org
Email: askada@diabetes.org

American Heart Association (AHA)
7272 Greenville Ave.
Dallas, TX 75231
Toll-Free: 800-AHA-USA-1 (800-242-8721)
Phone: 214-570-5943
Website: www.heart.org

Birth Defect Research for Children, Inc.
976 Lake Baldwin Ln., Ste. 104
Orlando, FL 32814
Phone: 407-895-0802
Website: www.birthdefects.org
Email: staff@birthdefects.org

Child Find of America, Inc.
P.O. Box 277
New Paltz, NY 12561
Toll-Free: 800-I-AM-LOST
(800-426-5678)
Phone: 845-883-6060
Website: childfindofamerica.org
Email: information@
childfindofamerica.org

Childhelp
6730 N. Scottsdale Rd., Ste. 150
Scottsdale, AZ 85253
Toll-Free: 800-4-A-CHILD
(800-422-4453)
Phone: 480-922-8212
Website: www.childhelp.org
Email: info@childhelp.org

Children's Hospice International (CHI)
1800 Diagonal Rd., Ste. 600
Alexandria, VA 22314
Phone: 703-684-0330
Website: www.chionline.org
Email: Info@CHIonline.org

ChildSafe®
3730 IH-10 E.
San Antonio, TX 78220-4225
Phone: 210-675-9000
Fax: 726-200-9199
Website: www.childsafe-sa.org

Cystic Fibrosis Foundation (CF Foundation)
4550 Montgomery Ave., Ste. 1100 N.
Bethesda, MD 20814
Toll-Free: 800-FIGHT-CF
(800-344-4823)
Phone: 301-951-4422
Website: www.cff.org
Email: info@cff.org

Federation for Children with Special Needs (FCSN)
529 Main St. Ste. 1M3
Boston, MA 02129
Toll-Free: 800-331-0688
Phone: 617-236-7210
Fax: 617-241-0330
Website: fcsn.org
Email: info@fcsn.org

National Association for Children's Behavioral Health (NACBH)
201 E. Main St., Ste. 810
Lexington, KY 40507
Phone: 859-402-9768
Website: www.nacbh.org
Email: info@nacbh.org

National Center on Health, Physical Activity and Disability (NCHPAD)
3810 Ridgeway Dr.
Birmingham, AL 35209
Toll-Free: 866-866-8896
Fax: 205-975-0043
Website: www.nchpad.org
Email: nchpad@uab.edu

National Center on Shaken Baby Syndrome (NCSBS)
1433 N. 1075 W., Ste. 110
Farmington, UT 84025
Phone: 801-447-9360
Fax: 801-447-9364
Website: www.dontshake.org
Email: mail@dontshake.org

The National Children's Cancer Society (NCCS)
2900 Frank Scott Pkwy.
W. Ste. 928
Belleville, IL 62223
Toll-Free: 800-532-6459
Phone: 314-241-1600
Fax: 314-241-1996
Website: www.thenccs.org
Email: communications@thenccs.org

National Council on Child Abuse and Family Violence (NCCAFV)
P.O. Box 5222
Arlington, VA 22205
Phone: 202-429-6695
Website: www.nccafv.org
Email: nccafv@aol.com

Planned Parenthood Federation of America (PPFA)
123 William St.
New York, NY 10038
Toll-Free: 800-230-7526
Phone: 212-541-7800
Fax: 212-868-4677
Website: www.plannedparenthood.org
Email: dmca@ppfa.org

Prevent Child Abuse America® (PCAA)
33 N. Dearborn St., Ste. 2300
Chicago, IL 60602
Phone: 312-663-3520
Website: preventchildabuse.org
Email: info@preventchildabuse.org

Spina Bifida Association of America (SBAA)
1600 Wilson Blvd.
Ste. 800
Arlington, VA 22209
Toll-Free: 800-621-3141
Website: www.spinabifidaassociation.org
Email: sbaa@sbaa.org

St. Jude Children's Research Hospital
262 Danny Thomas Pl.
Memphis, TN 38105
Toll-Free: 866-278-5833
TTY: 901-595-1040
Website: www.stjude.org

INDEX

INDEX

Page numbers followed by "n" refer to citation information; by "t" indicate tables; and by "f" indicate figures.

A

Index

B

Index

C

Index

Index

E

G

I

Index

M

P

S

T